BE PREPARED FOR SUCCESS

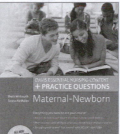

Psychiatric Mental Health

Fundamentals

Maternal-Newborn

Fluid, Electrolyte and Acid-Base Imbalances
CONTENT REVIEW PLUS PRACTICE QUESTIONS
Allison Hale | Mary Jo Hovey

Pediatric Nursing
CONTENT REVIEW PLUS PRACTICE QUESTIONS
Margot R. De Sevo

Don't have time to read your textbook?
Try the Essential Nursing Content + Practice Questions series

Content Review | Case Studies | NCLEX®-Prep

"The most essential facts you will ever need from a trusted series."
—Amazon student reviewer

SAVE 20%
+ FREE SHIPPING

Use Promo Code:
REVIEW20

Order today online at
www.FADavis.com

Pediatric **Success**

NCLEX®-Style Q&A Review

THIRD EDITION

Beth Richardson, PhD, RN, CPNP, FAANP
Associate Professor Emeritus
Indiana University School of Nursing
Indianapolis, Indiana
Pediatric Nurse Practitioner
HealthNet
Indianapolis, Indiana

 F.A. Davis Company • Philadelphia

F. A. Davis Company
1915 Arch Street
Philadelphia, PA 19103
www.fadavis.com

Printed in the United States of America

Last digit indicates print number: 10 9 8 7 6 5 4 3 2 1

Acquisitions Editor: Jacalyn Sharp
Senior Content Project Manager: Julia L. Curcio
Electronic Project Editor: Sandra A. Glennie
Illustration and Design Manager: Carolyn O'Brien

As new scientific information becomes available through basic and clinical research, recommended treatments and drug therapies undergo changes. The author(s) and publisher have done everything possible to make this book accurate, up to date, and in accord with accepted standards at the time of publication. The author(s), editors, and publisher are not responsible for errors or omissions or for consequences from application of the book, and make no warranty, expressed or implied, in regard to the contents of the book. Any practice described in this book should be applied by the reader in accordance with professional standards of care used in regard to the unique circumstances that may apply in each situation. The reader is advised always to check product information (package inserts) for changes and new information regarding dose and contraindications before administering any drug. Caution is especially urged when using new or infrequently ordered drugs.

I thank my children, Jason, Sarah, and Walker; my grandchildren, Caroline, Darren, Sadie, and Sam; and my friends, especially David, for all their love and support.

To students, graduates, and colleagues: thank you for all you do in caring for children and their families.

Contributors to Previous Editions

Susan P. Wade, MSN, RN, CPN, CCRN
Clinical Assistant Professor
Indiana University
Purdue University
Fort Wayne, Indiana

Sherrilyn Coffman, DNS, RN, CPN
Professor and Assistant Dean
Nevada State College
Henderson, Nevada

Dawn Marie Daniels, DNS, RN, PHCNS-BC
Clinical Nurse Specialist
Riley Hospital for Children
Indianapolis, Indiana

Mary Jo Eoff, RN, MSN, CPNP
Clinical Instructor
Indiana University
Indianapolis, Indiana

Joyce Foresman-Capuzzi, BSN, RN, CEN, CPN, CCRN, CTRN, CPEN, SANE-A, EMT-P
Clinical Nurse Educator/Emergency
Department
Lankenau Hospital
Wynnewood, Pennsylvania

Paige Johnson, RN, MSN, MPH, CRNP
Pediatric Nurse Practitioner
Children's Mercy Hospital, Department of
Hematology/Oncology
Kansas City, Missouri

Dominique Leveque, MSN, RN, CPNP, FNP-C
Workplace Health Services
Clarian Health Partners
Indianapolis, Indiana

Christina Bittles McCarthy, MSN, RN, CPNP
Pediatric Nurse Practitioner
Indiana University, Department of
Orthopedic Surgery
Indianapolis, Indiana

Patricia A. Normandin, RN, MSN, CEN, CPN, CPEN, DNP(c)
Pediatric Nursing Instructor
University of Massachusetts, Lowell
Lowell, Massachusetts

Julie A. Poore, RN, MSN
Visiting Lecturer
Indiana University
Indianapolis, Indiana

Susan P. Wade, MSN, RN, CPN, CCRN
Clinical Assistant Professor
Indiana University
Purdue University
Fort Wayne, Indiana

Cele Walter, BSN, RN, CPN, NCSN
High School Nurse
Paul VI High School
Haddonfield, New Jersey

Candace F. Zickler, RN, MSN, CPNP
Supervisor, Health Services
Metropolitan School District of Perry
Township
Indianapolis, Indiana

Reviewers for Previous Editions

Jacoline Sommer Albert, ADN, RN, BScN, DI
Senior Instructor
The Aga Khan University
Karachi, Pakistan

Monique Alston-Davis, MSN, Ed, CPN
Assistant Professor
Montgomery College
Silver Spring, Maryland

Cathryn J. Baack, PhD, RN, CPNP
Assistant Professor
MedCentral College of Nursing
Mansfield, Ohio

Joyce Beard, MSN, PHCNS-BC, NCSN, RN
Assistant Clinical Professor
University of North Carolina, Pembroke
Pembroke, North Carolina

Vicky H. Becherer, MSN, RN
Assistant Teaching Professor
University of Missouri, St. Louis
St. Louis, Missouri

Stacee Bertolla, RN, MSN, CPNP
Instructor
University of South Alabama
Mobile, Alabama

María del Rosario C. Biddenback, RN, MSN, FNP-C
Professor
Napa Valley College
Napa, California

Kathleen Borge, MS, RNC
Faculty Chair, Women and Children's Health
Samaritan Hospital
Troy, New York

Pam Bowden, RN, MS, PNP
Faculty
North Hennepin Community College
Brooklyn Park, Minnesota

Twila J. Brown, PhD, RN
Assistant Professor
Southeast Missouri State University
Cape Girardeau, Missouri

Katherine Bydalek, MSN, FNP-BC, PhD
Assistant Professor
University of South Alabama
Mobile, Alabama

Dena Christianson, MSN, PNP
Adjunct Faculty
Nova Southeastern University
Fort Lauderdale, Florida

Karen Clancy, MS, RN, CNP
Clinical Instructor
Ohio State University
Neonatal Nurse Practitioner
Columbus Children's Hospital
Columbus, Ohio

Myra L. Clark, MS, FNP-C
Assistant Professor
North Georgia College and State University
Dahlonega, Georgia

Lori Clay, MSN, RN
Assistant Professor
Arkansas State University
Jonesboro, Arkansas

Sallie Coke, PhD, APRN, CPNP, CFNP
Associate Professor
Georgia College and State University
Milledgeville, Georgia

Georgina Colalillo, MS, RN, CNE
Associate Professor, Nursing Department
Queensborough Community College
Bayside, New York

Judith Drumm, DNS, RN, CPN
Professor/Nursing
Palm Beach Atlantic University
West Palm Beach, Florida

Elizabeth Fiske, PhD, RN, NNP-BC, PCNS, BC
Associate Professor
Carson-Newman University
Jefferson City, Tennessee

Jennifer Bell Frank, MSN, APRN, BC
Instructor
Jacksonville State University
Jacksonville, Alabama

Marianne Fraser, MSN, RN, BC
Assistant Professor
University of Utah
Salt Lake City, Utah

Susan Golden, MSN, RN
Nursing Faculty
Eastern New Mexico University, Roswell
Roswell, New Mexico

Heather Janiszewski Goodin, PhD, RN, AHN-BC
Professor
Capital University
Columbus, Ohio

Kathy L. Ham, RN, EdD
Assistant Professor
Southeast Missouri State University
Cape Girardeau, Missouri

Brenda J. Walters Holloway, APRN, FNP, DNSc
Clinical Assistant Professor
University of South Alabama
Spanish Fort, Alabama

Teresa L. Howell, DNP, RN, CNE
Associate Professor of Nursing
Morehead State University
Morehead, Kentucky

Mary C. Kishman, PhD, RN
Associate Professor
College of Mount St. Joseph
Cincinnati, Ohio

Katherine R. Kniest, RN, MSN, CNE
Professor
William Rainey Harper College
Palatine, Illinois

Robyn Leo, MSN
Associate Professor
Worcester State College
Worcester, Massachusetts

Barbara J. MacDougall, MSN, ARNP
Nova Southeastern University
Ft. Lauderdale, Florida

Sheila Matye, MSN, RN, CNE
Associate Clinical Professor
Montana State University, College of Nursing
Great Falls, Montana

Kathleen T. Mohn, RN, MSEd, CLNC
Instructor
College of Southern Nevada
Las Vegas, Nevada

Jennifer Morton, MS, MPH, RN
Assistant Professor
University of New England
Portland, Maine

Irene Owens, MSN, APRN
Instructor
Lake Sumter Community College
Leesburg, Florida

Brenda Pavill, RN, FNP, PhD, IBCLC
Professor
Misericordia University
Dallas, Pennsylvania

Delia Pittman, PhD
Nursing Professor
MidAmerica Nazarene University
Olathe, Kansas

Janine T. Reale, MS, RN, CNE
Instructor, Nursing Faculty
Rivier University
Nashua, New Hampshire

Deborah A. Roberts, RN, BSN, MSN, EdD
Instructor
Sonoma State University, Department of Nursing
Sonoma, California

Rebecca L. Shabo, RN, PNP-BC, PhD
Associate Professor
Kennesaw State University
Kennesaw, Georgia

Cynthia A. Shartle, RN, MSN, APRN, BC-FNP
ADN Faculty
South Texas College
McAllen, Texas

Patsy M. Spratling, RN, MSN
Nursing Instructor
Holmes Community College
Ridgeland, Mississippi

Linda Strong, MSN, RN, CPNP, CNE
Assistant Professor, Pediatric Nursing
Cuyahoga Community College
Cleveland, Ohio

Bev Valkenier, BScN, RN, MSN
Lecturer
University of British Columbia
Vancouver, British Columbia, Canada

Linda Walters, RN, MSN, PhD (a.b.d.)
Nursing Instructor
Indiana State University
Terre Haute, Indiana

Elizabeth M. Wertz, RN, BSN, MPM, EMT-P, PHRN, FACMPE
Chief Executive Officer
Pediatric Alliance, PC
Carnegie, Pennylvania

Sarah Whitaker, DNS, RN
Nursing Program Director
Dona Ana Community College
Las Cruces, New Mexico

Barbara White, RN, MSN, CCRN
Nursing Instructor
Southwestern Michigan College
Dowagiac, Michigan

Contents

Fundamentals of Critical Thinking Related to Test Taking: The RACE Model

1

Pediatric Success: NCLEX®-Style Q&A Review is designed to help you, the student, complete your nursing program as well as succeed on the NCLEX-RN® examination.

This book applies critical-thinking skills primarily to multiple choice questions and to some alternate test items. It provides practice test questions and test-taking hints to help you analyze each item and choose the correct response.

Another book in the Success series, *Fundamentals Success* by Nugent and Vitale, explains critical thinking and the RACE Model, which are used in each book in the series. This information will help you answer questions on tests in your nursing courses and on the NCLEX-RN® examination. The key to successful studying is knowing the material that will be covered on the examinations. Course notes should be studied every night and corresponding readings done before class. This will help you learn the material and retain it longer. Once you know the material, it is important for you to be able to answer primarily multiple choice questions correctly. The RACE Model will help you succeed with answering questions.

HOW TO USE THIS REVIEW BOOK

The book contains 14 chapters, a final comprehensive examination, and practice questions online. Test-taking hints are included with each question.

This chapter, Chapter 1, provides guidelines for course test preparation and includes an example of how to use the RACE Model.

Chapter 2 focuses on pharmacology and has been included because of the expressed need of students for extra testing in this area. In the NCLEX-RN® test plan (www. ncsbn.org), pharmacology and management of care have a large number of test items. This chapter includes questions centered on what the student nurse caring for children of all ages needs to know about administering medications, drug actions, dosages, expected effects, adverse effects, and teaching families. Chapter 3 covers growth and development of children from infancy through adolescence. Chapter 4 covers material on issues related to pediatric health. Chapters 5 through 13 follow pediatric health problems through each of the body systems. Each chapter contains practice questions, answers, and rationales for the correct answer, including test-taking hints, keywords, and abbreviations.

Chapter 14, "Leadership and Management," relates to pediatric nursing. Graduates need to have a working knowledge of issues in these areas. Chapter 15 is a final 100-question comprehensive examination. There are also questions available online that you can access free for 30 days. Questions in this book are written primarily at the application and analysis level and are either multiple choice, with four response choices, or alternate item format. Nursing faculty members write tests in these formats to familiarize students with the NCLEX-RN® examination style.

Test Preparation

One of the most important strategies for you is to study your course materials thoroughly and know the assigned concepts for each examination in your class. It is best to study daily so that you really learn the material. Don't wait and try to learn it all at once. The more time you spend studying the topic, the better you will retain the material.

After you feel confident that you know the material, choose the chapter(s) in this book that correspond(s) with the assigned test material in your nursing course. Answer the practice questions to determine your level of knowledge about the topic. Carefully review the questions you miss, making sure you read and understand the rationale for choosing the wrong distracter and why the correct response is indeed correct. The rationales provide a great deal of information about the correct and incorrect options, which helps you understand the content more completely. The test-taking hints are strategies to help you logically determine the correct response. If you still feel uncomfortable with the content area, review that chapter in your textbook for better understanding. This method of preparing for an examination will help you identify your strengths and areas to focus on as you continue to study.

You may want to start with Chapter 2, "Pharmacology," because you will be administering medications to children throughout your pediatric nursing course. This chapter will help you focus on teaching strategies for families of children receiving medications, differences in delivering drugs to children, and calculating dosages.

RACE Model

The RACE Model is a critical-thinking strategy to be used when answering multiple choice questions. The RACE Model helps you analyze the question stem and determine the correct response. For more detailed information about the RACE Model, see *Test Success: Test-Taking Techniques for Beginning Nursing Students* by Nugent and Vitale.

The RACE Model comprises:

R - Recognize the keywords in the stem.

A - Ask what the question is asking the nurse to do.

C - Critically analyze each option in relation to the information in the stem.

E - Eliminate as many options as possible to narrow your choice to the correct response.

Some students believe they know the material but have difficulty choosing the correct response when answering multiple choice questions. Using the RACE Model will greatly increase your chances of choosing the correct response. To use it effectively during timed tests, you need to practice. Using the RACE Model as you prepare yourself with the chapter tests will help you. Following is a sample question:

1. A 6-month-old is being seen in the clinic for a well-child checkup. The parents want to know about starting solid foods. How should the nurse counsel them?
   1. "Since you started rice cereal from a spoon 2 months ago, you can add a new strained vegetable each week."
   2. "Introduce some mashed fruits first. After the infant is eating that well, start vegetables and rice cereal."
   3. "Infants do best eating solids if you spoon-feed a new strained vegetable every other day to see what their preferences are."
   4. "Add rice cereal to each bottle. Next you can add fruits and vegetables fed by spoon."

Using the RACE Model:

R - The client in the stem is the parent.

A - The parents want to know how to add solid foods to their infant's diet.

C - Infants start rice cereal between 4 and 6 months. This is fed to the infant by spoon unless there is an indication to place it in the bottle. That is not stated in the stem of this question. Either strained fruits or vegetables are added to the infant's diet at about 6 months of age. The infant stays on that choice for several days to determine whether the infant is allergic.

E - Now you can eliminate choices 2, 3, and 4 because they do not contain choices that you know are correct. The remaining choice is 1, the correct response.

Pharmacology

KEYWORDS

The following words include English vocabulary, nursing/medical terminology, concepts, principles, or information relevant to content specifically addressed in the chapter or associated with topics presented in it. English dictionaries, your nursing textbooks, and medical dictionaries such as *Taber's Cyclopedic Medical Dictionary* are resources that can be used to expand your knowledge and understanding of these words and related information.

Acetaminophen (Tylenol)
Albuterol (Proventil)
Amoxicillin (Amoxil)
Amoxicillin/clavulanate potassium (Augmentin)
Amphotericin B
Anticholinergic
Baclofen
Diphenhydramine (Benadryl)
Benzoyl peroxide
Carbamazepine (Tegretol)
Chlorhexidine (Hibiclens)
Ciprofloxacin (Cipro)
Collagenase (Santyl)
Cyclophosphamide (Cytoxan)
Dexamethasone (Decadron)
Diclofenac (Voltaren)
Digoxin (Lanoxin)
Diltiazem (Cardizem)
Erythromycin
Filgrastim (Neupogen)
Gamma globulin
Gentamicin (Garamycin)
Growth hormone
Ibuprofen (Advil, Motrin)
Ifosfamide (Ifex)

Indomethacin (Indocin)
Intradermal
Isotretinoin (Accutane)
Levothyroxine (Synthroid)
Lindane (Kwell, G-Well)
Mesna (Mesnex)
Metoclopramide (Reglan)
Morphine sulfate (Duramorph)
Nasal decongestant
NPH insulin
Oxybutynin (Ditropan)
Pancreatic enzymes
Penicillin
Phenytoin (Dilantin)
Prednisone
Prostaglandin E
Pyrantel pamoate (Antiminth)
Ribavirin (Virazole)
Rifampin (Rifadin)
Salicylic acid
Sympathomimetic
Terbinafine (Lamisil)
Trimethoprim/sulfamethoxazole (Septra, Bactrim)
Vancomycin
Vastus lateralis

ABBREVIATIONS

Cerebral palsy (CP)
grain (gr)
gram (g)

milligram (mg)
pound (lb)

CONVERSIONS

1 fl ounce = 30 mL (fluid volume)   1 kg = 2.2 lb
1 g = 15 gr   1 L = 1000 mL
1 g = 1000 mg   1 lb = 454 g
1 gr = 60 mg (or 65 mg for Tylenol or   1 lb = 16 ounces
  aspirin)   1 mg = 1000 mcg
1 in = 2.54 cm   1 ounce = 28 g (weight)

QUESTIONS

1. A child is to receive phenytoin (Dilantin) 100 mg IV for seizure prophylaxis. Which intervention is appropriate when administering this drug?
   1. Mix it in dextrose 5% in water and give over 1 hour.
   2. Administer no faster than 2 mg/kg/min.
   3. Do not use an inline filter.
   4. Monitor temperature prior to and after administration.

2. The parent of a child who is being discharged from the clinic wants to know if there is a difference between Advil and ibuprofen, saying, "I can buy ibuprofen over the counter at a cheaper price than Advil." What is the nurse's best response?
   1. "Advil and ibuprofen are two different drugs with similar effects."
   2. "There is no difference between the two medications, so you should use whichever one is cheaper."
   3. "Similarities exist between the drugs, but you need to consult the health-care provider about the specific order."
   4. "Ibuprofen is usually cheaper, so you should use it."

3. What time would the nurse most likely see signs and symptoms of hypoglycemia after administering NPH insulin at 0730?
   1. 0930 to 1030.
   2. 1130 to 1430.
   3. 1130 to 1930.
   4. 1530 to 1930.

4. Morphine sulfate (Duramorph) 2 mg IV q2h prn for pain is ordered for a 12-year-old who has had abdominal surgery. Which is the most appropriate nursing action?
   1. Administer the morphine sulfate (Duramorph) using a syringe pump over 1 hour.
   2. Encourage the child to use incentive spirometer every hour during the day and when awake at night.
   3. Ask the health-care provider to change the medication to meperidine (Demerol).
   4. Administer the morphine sulfate (Duramorph) with Benadryl (diphenhydramine) to prevent itching.

5. The parent of a child who is being treated for *Haemophilus influenzae* meningitis tells the nurse that the family is being treated prophylactically with rifampin (Rifadin). Which should the nurse include in teaching about this medication?
   1. "The drug will change the color of the urine to orange-red, and it will cause staining."
   2. "Adverse effects of the drug may cause urinary retention."
   3. "The drug is given to treat meningitis."
   4. "You will need to continue taking the drug for 7 days."

6. A 2-year-old child has been prescribed amoxicillin (Amoxil) bid for treatment of pharyngitis. Which statement indicates that the parent knows how to give the medication?
   1. "If I miss giving my child a dose at breakfast, I will double up on the dose at night."
   2. "I will give the medication at breakfast and dinner."
   3. "I know that amoxicillin (Amoxil) is a pill, but sometimes my child will not take it."
   4. "I will continue giving the amoxicillin (Amoxil) for 10 days even after my child is better."

7. A nurse is caring for a child who is receiving amphotericin B IV daily for a fungal infection. Prior to starting the therapy, which should the nurse review?
   1. Aspartate aminotransferase and alanine aminotransferase serum levels.
   2. Serum amphotericin level.
   3. Serum protein and sodium levels.
   4. Blood urea, nitrogen, and creatinine levels.

8. Which toxicity is specific to gentamicin (Garamycin)?
   1. Hepatatoxicity.
   2. Ototoxicity.
   3. Myocardial toxicity.
   4. Neurotoxicity.

9. A nurse is administrating vancomycin intravenously and sets the pump to infuse the medication over 90 minutes. Which adverse reaction is the nurse trying to prevent?
   1. Vomiting.
   2. Headache.
   3. Flushing of the face, neck, and chest.
   4. Hypertension.

10. The parents of an 8-year-old come to the clinic and ask the nurse if their child should receive growth hormone to boost short stature. Which is the nurse's best response?
    1. "Growth hormone only works if the child has short bones."
    2. "Can your child remember to take the pills every day?"
    3. "Test results are required before growth hormone can be started in children."
    4. "How tall do you think your child should be?"

11. A child has been receiving prednisone for the past 3 weeks, and the parent wants to stop the medication. What is the nurse's best response?
    1. "There is no problem in stopping the medication since the child's symptoms are gone."
    2. "It is dangerous for steroids to be stopped suddenly."
    3. "Your child may develop severe psychological symptoms when prednisone is stopped suddenly."
    4. "Stopping the prednisone will require blood work."

12. A child who has been diagnosed with hypothyroidism is started on levothyroxine (Synthroid). Which should be included in the nurse's teaching plan?
    1. The child will have more energy the next day after starting the medication.
    2. Optimal effectiveness of the medication may not occur for several weeks.
    3. The medication should be taken once a day at any time.
    4. The medication should be taken with milk.

13. Which should the nurse include in the discharge teaching plan for a child beginning growth hormone therapy?
    1. The child is expected to grow 3 to 5 inches during the first year of treatment.
    2. The parents must measure the child's weight and height weekly.
    3. The child will need to continue the therapy until he or she is 21 years old.
    4. There are no side effects from taking growth hormones.

14. The onset of Humalog insulin is:
    1. 10 to 15 minutes.
    2. 30 minutes to 1 hour.
    3. 1 to 2 hours.
    4. 2 to 4 hours.

15. Which should the nurse include in the teaching plan for a child started on metoclopramide (Reglan)?
    1. The drug increases gastrointestinal motility.
    2. The drug decreases tone in the lower esophageal sphincter.
    3. The drug prevents diarrhea.
    4. The drug induces the release of acetylcholine.

16. The nurse will monitor a child on high-dose prednisone for:
    1. Diabetes.
    2. Deep vein thrombosis.
    3. Nephrotoxicity.
    4. Hepatotoxicity.

17. A nurse is administering cyclophosphamide (Cytoxan) to a child with leukemia. Which action by the nurse would be appropriate?
    1. Monitoring serum potassium levels.
    2. Checking for hematuria.
    3. Obtaining daily weights.
    4. Obtaining neurological checks every 4 hours.

18. A nurse is giving ifosfamide (Ifex) as chemotherapy for a child who has leukemia. Mixed in with the ifosfamide (Ifex) is mesna (Mesnex). Mesna is given for which reason?
    1. As combination chemotherapy.
    2. As an antiarrhythmic.
    3. To prevent hemorrhagic cystitis.
    4. To increase absorption of the chemotherapy.

19. Which should a nurse anticipate be prescribed in chelation therapy for a child receiving frequent blood transfusions?
    1. Dalteparin sodium (Fragmin).
    2. Deferoxamine (Desferal).
    3. Diclofenac (Voltaren).
    4. Diltiazem (Cardizem).

20. Why is filgrastim (Neupogen) given to a child who has received chemotherapy?
    1. Reduce fatigue level.
    2. Prevent infection.
    3. Reduce nausea and vomiting.
    4. Increase mobilization of stem cells.

21. A child comes to the clinic for diphtheria, pertussis, and tetanus (DTaP) and inactivated poliovirus vaccines. The child does not appear ill but has a temperature of 101°F (38.3°C). The nurse should take which action?
    1. Withhold the vaccines and reschedule when the child is afebrile.
    2. Administer acetaminophen (Tylenol) and give the vaccines.
    3. Give the vaccines and instruct the parent to give acetaminophen (Tylenol) every 4 hours as needed.
    4. Have the health-care provider order an antibiotic and give the vaccine.

22. Which of the following would the nurse instruct the parent about treating a pediculosis infestation?
    1. Apply spinosad (Natroba) to the scalp, leave it in place for 4 minutes, and then add water.
    2. Apply chlorhexidine (Hibiclens) to the scalp with sterile gloves and leave on overnight.
    3. Apply terbinafine (Lamisil) as a thin layer to the scalp twice a day for 5 days.
    4. Apply collagenase (Santyl) to the scalp with cotton applicator, leave in place overnight, then shampoo.

23. Amoxicillin (Amoxil) 250 mg PO twice a day is prescribed to treat strep throat in a child who weighs 42 lb. The desired dose is 50 mg/kg/day. The nurse determines that:
    1. The prescribed dose is too low.
    2. The prescribed dose is too high.
    3. The prescribed dose is safe.
    4. Not enough information is given to determine the safe dose.

24. A child with a heart defect is placed on a maintenance dose of digoxin (Lanoxin) elixir. The dose is 0.07 mg/kg/day, and the child's weight is 16 lb. The medication is to be given two times a day. The nurse prepares how much digoxin (Lanoxin) for the morning dose?
    1. 0.25 mg.
    2. 0.37 mg.
    3. 0.5 mg.
    4. 2.5 mg.

25. Ciprofloxacin (Cipro) 300 mg daily is ordered for a child with a urinary tract infection. The medication comes 250 mg/5 mL. How much of the medication will the nurse prepare to give to the child?
    1. 1.2 mL.
    2. 3 mL.
    3. 6 mL.
    4. 12 mL.

26. A nurse is caring for a child with congenital heart disease who is being treated with digoxin (Lanoxin). Which is included in the family's discharge teaching?
    1. Make sure the medication is taken with food.
    2. Repeat the dose if the child vomits.
    3. Take the child's pulse prior to administration.
    4. Weigh the child daily.

27. Which medication is the most effective treatment for acne?
    1. Salicylic acid.
    2. Benzoyl peroxide.
    3. Fluconazole (Diflucan).
    4. Clotrimazole (Lotrimin).

28. Which would the nurse include when teaching an adolescent female beginning isotretinoin (Accutane) therapy?
    1. Apply a thin layer to the affected skin twice a day.
    2. Use Dove Sensitive Skin soap for added benefit.
    3. A pregnancy test will be done prior to starting treatment.
    4. Keep lips moistened to prevent inflammation.

29. Which medication is used for the treatment of spasticity in cerebral palsy (CP)?
    1. Dexamethasone (Decadron).
    2. Baclofen (Lioresal)
    3. Diclofenac (Voltaren).
    4. Carbamazepine (Tegretol).

30. Which assessment should be a priority to monitor in a child receiving a narcotic for pain relief?
    1. Respirations.
    2. Bowel sounds.
    3. Blood pressure.
    4. Oxygen saturation.

31. Which is the correct method to instill eardrops in a 5-year-old?
    1. Pull the pinna of the ear downward and back for instillation.
    2. Place cotton tightly in the ear after instillation.
    3. Have the child remain upright after instillation.
    4. Pull the pinna of the ear upward and back for instillation.

32. A health-care provider has ordered amoxicillin (Amoxil) 500 mg IVPB q8h for a child with tonsillitis. Which action by the nurse is appropriate?
    1. Question the order because the route is incorrect.
    2. Give the medication as ordered.
    3. Call the health-care provider because the dosing frequency is incorrect.
    4. Call the health-care provider and question the dose of the drug.

33. Which should the nurse do first for a child diagnosed with conjunctivitis and ordered to have eye ointment applied three times a day?
    1. Remove any discharge from the affected eye.
    2. Ensure the ointment is at room temperature.
    3. Hold the tip of the eye ointment tube parallel to the eye.
    4. Wash hands with soap and water.

34. Which instruction about nose drops should be included in the teaching plan for the parents of a child with nasopharyngitis?
    1. "Do not use the drops for any other family member."
    2. "Administer the drops as often as necessary until the nasal congestion subsides."
    3. "Insert the dropper tip as far back as possible in the nasal passage."
    4. "You can save the drops for the next time your child has the same symptoms."

35. Trimethoprim/sulfamethoxazole (Septra, Bactrim) should be given with:
    1. Breakfast and dinner.
    2. A snack.
    3. Glass of water.
    4. Glass of juice.

36. An IV infusion of gamma globulin 2 g/kg over 12 hours has been ordered for a 22-lb child. Which dose is correct?
    1. 11 g.
    2. 20 g.
    3. 22 g.
    4. 44 g.

37. Lindane (Kwell) shampoo is used only once because it can cause:
    1. Hypertension.
    2. Seizures.
    3. Elevated liver functions.
    4. Alopecia.

38. Which is essential for the nurse to teach the parent regarding administration of albendazole (Albenza)?
    1. Fever and rash are common adverse effects.
    2. The medication kills the eggs in about 48 hours.
    3. The drug should be given with a meal.
    4. The dose should be repeated in 2 weeks.

39. A 6-month-old is prescribed 2.5% hydrocortisone for topical treatment of eczema. The nurse instructs the parent not to use the cream for more than a week. What is the primary reason for this instruction?
   1. Adverse effects, such as skin atrophy and fragility, can occur with long-term treatment.
   2. If after a week there is no improvement, then a stronger dose is required.
   3. The drug loses its efficacy after prolonged use.
   4. If no improvement is seen after a week, an antibiotic should be prescribed.

40. A 15-kg child is started on cephalexin (Keflex) for treatment of cellulitis. The dose is 40 mg/kg/day, given twice a day. The nurse has a bottle of Keflex that indicates there are 250 mg/5 mL. How many milliliters must the nurse draw up for each dose?
   1. 2.5 mL.
   2. 6 mL.
   3. 12 mL.
   4. 20 mL.

41. A child with hives is prescribed diphenhydramine (Benadryl) 5 mg/kg per day in divided doses every 6 hours. The child weighs 40 lb. How many milligrams should the nurse give for each dose?
   1. 4.5 mg.
   2. 11.45 mg.
   3. 22.73 mg.
   4. 50 mg.

42. When is the best time to give furosemide (Lasix)?
   1. 8:00 a.m.
   2. 12 noon.
   3. 6:00 p.m.
   4. Bedtime.

43. Which assessment finding should the nurse observe following administration of albuterol (Proventil)?
   1. Decrease in wheezing.
   2. Decrease in respiratory rate from 34 to 22.
   3. Decrease in blood pressure.
   4. Decrease in heart rate.

44. A child in the emergency room is being treated with albuterol (Proventil) aerosol treatments for an acute asthma attack. She requires treatments every 2 hours. Which adverse effect of the medication would the nurse expect?
   1. Lethargy and bradycardia.
   2. Decreased blood pressure and dizziness.
   3. Nervousness and tachycardia.
   4. Increased blood pressure and fatigue.

45. A child with cystic fibrosis (CF) is placed on an oral antibiotic to be given four times a day for 14 days. Which of the following schedules is the most appropriate?
   1. 8 a.m., 12 p.m., 4 p.m., 8 p.m.
   2. 7 a.m., 1 p.m., 7 p.m., 12 midnight.
   3. 9 a.m., 1 p.m., 5 p.m., 9 p.m.
   4. 10 a.m., 2 p.m., 6 p.m., 10 p.m.

46. Which is the best area for the tuberculin skin test to be placed?
   1. Upper thigh.
   2. Scapular area.
   3. Back.
   4. Ventral forearm.

47. A hospitalized child is to receive 75 mg of acetaminophen (Tylenol) for fever of 101°F (38.3°C). If the acetaminophen (Tylenol) is 160 mg per 5 mL, how much will the nurse administer?
1. 0.4 mL.
2. 1.5 mL.
3. 2.3 mL.
4. 3 mL.

48. Which is a toxic reaction in a child taking digoxin (Lanoxin)?
1. Weight gain.
2. Tachycardia.
3. Nausea and vomiting.
4. Seizures.

49. A 10-month-old with heart failure weighs 10 kg. Digoxin (Lanoxin) is prescribed as 10 mcg/kg/day to be given every 12 hours. How much is given for each dose?
1. 10 mcg.
2. 50 mcg.
3. 100 mcg.
4. 500 mcg.

50. Why is indomethacin (Indocin) given to a preterm neonate?
1. Encourage ductal closure.
2. Prevent hypertension.
3. Promote release of surfactant.
4. Protect the immature liver.

51. Which drug is most important in treating an infant with transposition of the great vessels?
1. Digoxin (Lanoxin).
2. Antibiotics.
3. Prostaglandin E.
4. Diuretics.

52. Penicillin is given to a 2-year-old prior to dental work. The child weighs 44 lb. The order is for 25 mg/kg to be given 2 hours before the procedure. The penicillin comes in 250 mg/5 mL. How much of the medication will the nurse administer?
1. 2.5 mL.
2. 5 mL.
3. 10 mL.
4. 15 mL.

53. Which is the most common adverse reaction to erythromycin?
1. Weight gain.
2. Constipation.
3. Mouth sores.
4. Nausea and vomiting.

54. A child who weighs 20 kg is to receive 8 g of gamma globulin over 12 hours for the treatment of idiopathic thrombocytopenia purpura. The concentration is 8 g in 300 mL of normal saline. How many milliliters per hour will the child receive?
1. 12 mL/hr.
2. 25 mL/hr.
3. 50 mL/hr.
4. 40 mL/hr.

55. The treatment for a child with sinus bradycardia is atropine 0.02 mg/kg/dose. How much should the nurse give a child who weighs 20 kg?
1. 0.02 mg.
2. 0.04 mg.
3. 0.2 mg.
4. 0.4 mg.

56. The effect of atropine is:
    1. Anticholinergic.
    2. As a beta-adrenergic agonist.
    3. As a bronchodilator.
    4. Sympathomimetic.

57. A common adverse reaction to atropine is:
    1. Diarrhea.
    2. Increased urine output.
    3. No tears when crying.
    4. Lethargy.

58. Which should the nurse include in teaching parents about administering pancreatic enzymes to their child?
    1. The enzymes may be chewed or swallowed.
    2. The capsules may be opened and sprinkled over acidic food.
    3. Give the same amount of the medicine with meals and snacks.
    4. Store the enzymes in the refrigerator.

59. Common side effects of oxybutynin (Ditropan) are:
    1. Increase in heart rate and blood pressure.
    2. Sodium retention and edema.
    3. Constipation and dry mouth.
    4. Insomnia and hyperactivity.

60. Ribavirin (Virazole) is prescribed for a hospitalized child with respiratory syncytial virus (RSV). The nurse prepares to administer the medication by which route?
    1. Oral.
    2. Subcutaneous.
    3. Intramuscular.
    4. Nebulizer.

61. A child has an infusion of dextrose 5% via a line with a volume control chamber on the pump. The nurse knows this system is used for administration of intravenous solutions for which reason?
    1. Prevent accidental fluid overload.
    2. Reduce the potential for bacterial infection.
    3. Make administering of intravenous fluids easier.
    4. Is less costly.

ANSWERS AND RATIONALES

The correct answer number and rationale for why it is the correct answer are given in **boldface blue type.** Rationales for why the other possible answer options are incorrect also are given, but they are not in boldface type.

1. 1. Mix intravenous doses in normal saline as mixtures precipitate with dextrose 5% in water.
   2. **Phenytoin (Dilantin) should be given slowly (1–2 mg/kg/min) via pump. Rapid infusion may cause hypotension, arrhythmias, and circulatory collapse.**
   3. An inline filter is recommended.
   4. Continuous monitoring of electrocardiogram, blood pressure, and respiratory status is essential because of potential side effects.

   TEST-TAKING HINT: The test taker must know both the side effects of the drug and how to administer it safely.

2. 1. This does not answer the parent's question.
   2. This is not a true statement because Advil is enteric coated, and not all ibuprofens are enteric coated.
   3. **This response answers the question and tells the parent the physician is the only one who can change a name brand to a generic drug.**
   4. The nurse should not make that judgment. The physician should be consulted.

   TEST-TAKING HINT: The nurse needs to answer the parent's question and be aware that a physician chooses name brand or generic.

3. 1. Peak time for regular insulin is 2 to 3 hours.
   2. Peak time for Semilente insulin is 4 to 7 hours.
   3. **Peak time for NPH insulin is 4 to 12 hours.**
   4. Peak time for Lente insulin is 8 to 12 hours.

   TEST-TAKING HINT: NPH insulin works in an intermediate range; select an appropriate period of time.

4. 1. Giving morphine sulfate (Duramorph) over 1 hour takes too long to relieve the pain. It can be given by slow IV push.
   2. **Because morphine sulfate (Duramorph) can depress respirations and the child has just had abdominal surgery, deep breathing should be encouraged.**
   3. Meperidine (Demerol) is not used in children because of the risk of induced seizures.

4. One of the side effects of morphine sulfate (Duramorph) is itching, and diphenhydramine (Benadryl) is a good medication to give as needed in case of itching. It should not be given together with the morphine sulfate (Duramorph).

   TEST-TAKING HINT: The test taker must be aware of the major side effects of morphine (Duramorph) and the age of the client who is receiving the morphine (Duramorph).

5. 1. **Rifampin (Rifadin) causes an orange-red discoloration of body fluids, including urine. Knowledge of this can decrease anxiety when such discoloration occurs.**
   2. Urinary retention is not a side effect. Rifampin (Rifadin) is metabolized in the liver and should be used with caution in clients with elevated liver enzymes.
   3. The drug is ordered prophylactically to guard against developing meningitis.
   4. The drug is given for 2 days as prophylactic treatment.

   TEST-TAKING HINT: Associate the "R" in rifampin (Rifadin) with the red in orange-red body fluids.

6. 1. Missed doses should be given as soon as possible and not doubled with the next dose.
   2. Doses of antibiotics should be taken at regular intervals over 24 hours without interrupting sleep to maintain maximum blood levels.
   3. Attempting to have the child take it whole could cause the child to aspirate.
   4. **A full course of the antibiotic must be taken to decrease the risk of resistance to the antibiotic or recurrence of the infection.**

   TEST-TAKING HINT: The test taker must know specific information about antibiotic therapy.

7. 1. Liver damage is not associated with amphotericin therapy.
   2. Serum levels of the drug are not done.
   3. The drug should not cause a change in sodium or protein levels.
   4. **The drug tends to be nephrotoxic. Elevation of blood urea, nitrogen, and creatinine levels indicates renal damage. If these levels are elevated, the health-care provider must be notified to determine if the drug must be withheld for the day.**

12

TEST-TAKING HINT: This drug is nephrotoxic. Some nurses refer to the drug as "amphoterrible."

8. 1. Hepatic and neurological toxicities are more common in fluoroquinolones.
   2. **Nephrotoxicity and ototoxicity are the most significant adverse effects.**
   3. Myocardial toxicity is not a common reaction.
   4. Hepatic and neurological toxicities are more common in fluoroquinolones.

TEST-TAKING HINT: Aminoglycosides cause kidney damage and loss of hearing. Levels are checked before and after dosing so that toxicity can be prevented.

9. 1. Vomiting is a side effect but is not related to the rate of infusion.
   2. Headache is not related to the rate of infusion.
   3. **"Red man syndrome" or "red neck syndrome" is flushing of the face, neck, and upper chest associated with too rapid an infusion of vancomycin. This can be prevented with infusing the vancomycin over 90 to 120 minutes and pretreating the patient with diphenhydramine (Benadryl) prior to the infusion.**
   4. Hypotension with shock can result from a histamine release from rapid infusion.

TEST-TAKING HINT: "Red man syndrome" is a side effect of too rapid an infusion of vancomycin.

10. 1. This response does not answer the parents' question.
    2. Growth hormone is available as a parenteral medication and is given intramuscularly or subcutaneously.
    3. **Growth hormone is approved for use only in children to treat a documented lack of growth hormone.**
    4. The nurse must first answer the parents' question about growth hormone.

TEST-TAKING HINT: Recall the reason for giving growth hormone.

11. 1. Abrupt withdrawal can cause severe side effects.
    2. **Abrupt cessation of long-term steroid therapy can cause acute adrenal insufficiency that could lead to death. Long-term steroid use can cause shrinkage of the adrenal glands, which decreases the production of the hormone.**

3. Central nervous system symptoms such as confusion and psychosis are adverse effects of steroids.
4. Gradual tapering of the dosages will prevent severe side effects and no blood work is required.

TEST-TAKING HINT: The test taker must know about abrupt withdrawal of steroids and the effects of steroids on the adrenal glands.

12. 1. The energy level takes much longer than 1 day to increase.
    2. **After starting therapy, peak levels of the drug may not be expected for many weeks to months. Clients need to know this to prevent them from stopping the medication because they think it is not working.**
    3. The drug works best when taken on an empty stomach; the patient should select a time each day when the stomach is empty. In children, just prior to bed may be the best time, as most children do not eat prior to bedtime.
    4. The drug works best when taken on an empty stomach. Taking it with milk is contraindicated.

TEST-TAKING HINT: Know the effects of levothyroxine and how to administer it.

13. 1. **The expected growth rate with growth hormone therapy is 3 to 5 inches in the first year.**
    2. Height and weight are measured monthly.
    3. Growth hormone is discontinued when optimal adult height is attained and fusion of the epiphyseal plates has occurred.
    4. Side effects include glucose intolerance, hypothyroidism, adrenocorticotropic hormone deficiency, hypercalciuria, renal calculi, gastrointestinal upset, and intracranial tumor growth.

TEST-TAKING HINT: Answer 2 is not correct as "must" is too strong. Answer 4 states "no side effects," and this is unrealistic. To choose the correct answer, the test taker must rely on knowledge of growth hormones.

14. 1. **Humalog insulin is rapid-acting and has an onset of 10 to 15 minutes.**
    2. Regular insulin has an onset of 30 minutes to 1 hour.
    3. NPH insulin has an onset of 1 to 2 hours and is intermediate-acting.

4. Ultralente insulin has an onset of 2 to 6 hours and is a long-acting insulin.

TEST-TAKING HINT: Review the onset, peak, and duration of all types of insulin.

15. 1. **Metoclopramide (Reglan) is a gastrointestinal stimulant that increases motility of the gastrointestinal tract, shortens gastric emptying time, and reduces the risk of the esophagus being exposed to gastric content.**
    2. Decreased tone in the esophageal sphincter increases the risk of gastric contents being regurgitated upward into the esophagus.
    3. There can be an increase in diarrhea because of the increase in gastrointestinal motility.
    4. Methyl scopolamine blocks effects of acetylcholine and relaxes sooth muscles.

TEST-TAKING HINT: Gastroesophageal reflux disease results in backward flow of gastric contents, so it is logical that a drug prescribed should promote forward movement of gastric content.

16. 1. **One of the side effects of high-dose steroids can be diabetes mellitus. The child needs to be evaluated so that prompt treatment can be initiated. The diabetes is self-limiting and after the steroids are discontinued should no longer be present. Other side effects include mood changes, hirsutism, trunk obesity, thin extremities, gastric bleeding, poor wound healing, hypertension, immunosuppression, insomnia, and increased appetite.**
    2. This is not a side effect of steroids. Deep vein thrombosis is related to clotting abnormalities.
    3. This is not a side effect of steroids.
    4. This is not a side effect of steroids.

TEST-TAKING HINT: Review side effects of high-dose steroid use.

17. 1. There should not be a change in potassium level, as the drug does not cause potassium loss.
    2. **Hemorrhagic cystitis is a major side effect of cyclophosphamide (Cytoxan); checking the urine for blood is an appropriate intervention.**
    3. Weights are obtained daily with clients receiving chemotherapy because of nausea and vomiting.
    4. There are no central nervous system side effects with cyclophosphamide (Cytoxan).

TEST-TAKING HINT: Review major side effects of cyclophosphamide.

18. 1. Mesna (Mesnex) is not a chemotherapeutic agent.
    2. Mesna (Mesnex) does not prevent arrhythmias.
    3. **Mesna (Mesnex) is a detoxifying agent used as a protectant against hemorrhagic cystitis induced by ifosfamide (Ifex) and cyclophosphamide (Cytoxan).**
    4. There is no medication that increases absorption of chemotherapy.

TEST-TAKING HINT: Review the action of mesna (Mesnex).

19. 1. Dalteparin sodium (Fragmin) is an anticoagulant used as prophylaxis for post-operative deep vein thrombosis.
    2. **Deferoxamine (Desferal) is an antidote for acute iron toxicity.**
    3. Diclofenac (Voltaren) is an anti-inflammatory drug.
    4. Diltiazem (Cardizem) is an antianginal agent for chronic stable angina.

TEST-TAKING HINT: Deferoxamine (Desferal) is used to prevent iron overload.

20. 1. Chemotherapy may cause anemia, which can compound the feeling of fatigue rather than reduce fatigue.
    2. The drug does not prevent infection, but it does increase the number of neutrophils.
    3. The drug may cause nausea and vomiting rather than reduce it.
    4. **The drug mobilizes stem cells to produce neutrophils.**

TEST-TAKING HINT: Recall the function of the neutrophils and how to stimulate them.

21. 1. Immunizations can be given when the child has a low-grade fever as long as the child is not ill appearing.
    2. Diagnose the problem before giving the vaccine. Just giving the acetaminophen (Tylenol) would not allow a diagnosis to be made, as it may mask symptoms.
    3. **Immunizations can be given when the child has a low-grade fever as long as the child is not ill appearing.**
    4. The nurse would not want to give an antibiotic until a bacterial infection was diagnosed.

TEST-TAKING HINT: Immunizations should not be given when a child has a high fever and appears ill.

22. 1. **Spinosad (Natroba) causes neuronal excitation leading to lice paralysis and death.**
2. Chlorhexidine (Hibiclens) is a skin cleanser. Clean gloves, not sterile gloves, should be used in treating lice.
3. Terbinafine (Lamisil) is an oral or nasal antifungal agent for the treatment of tinea infections.
4. Collagenase (Santyl) is an enzyme used in skin débriding.

TEST-TAKING HINT: Associate the nature of the parasite with the drug and application method.

23. 1. **The dose prescribed is too low.**
Strep throat is treated with amoxicillin at 50 mg/kg/day. Convert pounds to kilograms by dividing by 2.2 (2.2 lb = 1 kg)
42 lb ÷ 2.2 = 19.09 kg
Dosing parameters: 50 mg/kg/day × 19.09 = 954.5 mg/day
Ordered dose: 250 mg bid = 500 mg/day
2. The dose prescribed is too low.
3. The dose prescribed is too low.
4. The dose prescribed is too low.

TEST-TAKING HINT: First change pounds to kilograms. Calculate the ordered dose using the formula given in the question. Compare the order against the calculated appropriate dose.

24. 1. **0.25 mg.**
Convert pounds to kilograms by dividing by 2.2 (2.2 lb = 1 kg)
16 lb ÷ 2.2 = 7.27 kg
Calculate the dosage by weight: 0.07 mg/day × 7.27 = 0.5 mg/day
Divide the dose by 2 because it is to be given 2 times a day: 0.5 mg/day ÷ 2 doses = 0.25 mg for each dose
2. This dose is too high. Change the pounds to kilograms; the correct answer is 0.25 mg.
3. This is the total amount of drug for an entire day. Change the pounds to kilograms; the correct answer is 0.25 mg. Remember to divide by 2.
4. This dose is much too high. Change the pounds to kilograms; the correct answer is 0.25 mg.

TEST-TAKING HINT: Change the pounds to kilograms. The total amount is to be given twice a day, so calculate each dose.

25. 1. The formula to determine the correct answer is:
Desired over Available × Volume = amount to be given

2. The formula to determine the correct answer is:
Desired over Available × Volume = amount to be given
3. **Desired over Available × Volume = amount to be given**
300 mg/250 mg × 5 mL = 6 mL
4. The formula to determine the correct answer is:
Desired over Available × Volume = amount to be given

TEST-TAKING HINT: Use the formula to determine the correct answer.

26. 1. Digoxin (Lanoxin) should not be taken with food. Administer the medication 1 hour before or 2 hours after a meal.
2. The dose should not be repeated if the child vomits.
3. **The child's pulse should be monitored before each dose. The dose should be withheld according to the health-care provider's parameters.**
4. Checking weight is not related to the medication.

TEST-TAKING HINT: Know the principles of giving digoxin (Lanoxin). Knowing that the drug is given to decrease the heart rate and increase cardiac output should be a key to the answer involving checking pulse.

27. 1. Salicylic acid is used in the treatment of corns and warts.
2. **Benzoyl peroxide inhibits growth of *Propionibacterium acnes* (a gram-positive microorganism). It is effective against inflammatory and anti-inflammatory acne.**
3. Fluconazole (Diflucan) is an oral antifungal.
4. Clotrimazole (Lotrimin) is a topical antifungal.

TEST-TAKING HINT: The test taker needs to know the specific treatment for acne.

28. 1. The drug is not topical.
2. Dove Sensitive Soap is used for dry or easily irritated skin.
3. **It is mandatory to have a pregnancy test done before starting treatment because spontaneous abortions and/or fetal abnormalities have been associated in pregnancy with the use of isotretinoin (Accutane).**
4. Inflammation of the lips is a side effect of isotretinoin (Accutane), but moisture will not prevent the inflammation.

TEST-TAKING HINT: Consider birth defects associated with isotretinoin (Accutane).

29. 1. Dexamethasone (Decadron) is a corticosteroid used to decrease inflammation. Spinal cord–related spasms are not caused by inflammation.
2. **Baclofen (Lioresal) is used to treat the spasticity in cerebral palsy. It is a centrally acting muscle relaxant.**
3. Diclofenac (Voltaren) is a nonsteroidal anti-inflammatory drug.
4. Carbamazepine (Tegretol) is an antiepileptic used to treat seizures.

TEST-TAKING HINT: Spasticity affects the muscles.

30. 1. **The primary purpose of administrating an opioid analgesic is to relieve pain. The adverse effects that place the child at greatest risk are respiratory depression and decreased level of consciousness.**
2. Bowel sounds should be assessed because some opioids, such as morphine (Duramorph), can decrease gastric motility, but this is not as high a priority as a decrease in respirations.
3. Blood pressure could decrease and would be assessed, but it is not as high a priority as respirations. Decrease in blood pressure occurs after decrease in respiratory effort.
4. Oxygen saturation will decrease after a decrease in respiratory effort.

TEST-TAKING HINT: The critical word in this question is *priority*. The test taker should associate side effects from the drug that have the highest priority and will require nursing actions.

31. 1. Pull the pinna down and back for a child younger than age 3 years.
2. Placing the cotton in the ear tightly would be painful. The cotton could act as a wick and absorb the medication preventing its instillation. It will not help in the administration of the eardrops.
3. Having the child stay in an upright position after instillation does not affect administration of the eardrops.
4. **The correct way to administer eardrops in a child older than 3 years of age is to pull the pinna up and back, the same as for an adult.**

TEST-TAKING HINT: In infants, the ear canal is curved upward; therefore, the pinna should be pulled down and back. With children older than 3 years of age, the canal curves downward and forward; therefore, the pinna should be pulled up and back.

32. 1. **Amoxicillin is only given orally, so the order should be questioned.**
2. The dose cannot be given because the route is incorrect.
3. The dosing frequency is correct.
4. There is not enough information to determine if the dose is correct.

TEST-TAKING HINT: Focus on the route, dose, and frequency when administering a medication.

33. 1. This is correct, but it is not done first.
2. This is correct, but it is not done first.
3. This is correct, but it is not done first.
4. **The procedure for instilling eye ointment begins with washing hands followed by donning clean gloves.**

TEST-TAKING HINT: The key word in the question is *first*. Washing hands has the highest priority.

34. 1. **The medication should not be shared because of the risk of spreading the infection to another family member.**
2. The medication should be given only as prescribed. More frequent use could cause adverse reactions.
3. Inserting the dropper as far back as possible into the nasal canal could cause injury to the child.
4. Medications should not be saved for future illness, as the drug may not be appropriate.

TEST-TAKING HINT: The test taker must have specific knowledge of instillation of nasal drops.

35. 1. Trimethoprim/sulfamethoxazole (Septra, Bactrim) should be given on an empty stomach.
2. Trimethoprim/sulfamethoxazole (Septra, Bactrim) should be given on an empty stomach.
3. **Trimethoprim/sulfamethoxazole (Septra, Bactrim) should be administered with a full glass of water on an empty stomach. If nausea and vomiting occur, giving the drug with food may decrease gastric distress.**
4. Juice beverages should be avoided because they may irritate the bladder and are high in sugar content.

TEST-TAKING HINT: The test taker must know how to administer trimethoprim/sulfamethoxazole (Septra, Bactrim).

36. 1. First convert pounds to kilograms. The correct answer is 20 g.
2. **Convert pounds to kilograms: 2.2 lb = 1 kg**
Divide 22 pounds by 2.2
22 lb. ÷ 2.2 kg = 10 kg
Calculate the dose: 2 g/kg = 2 g × 10 kg = 20 g
3. First convert pounds to kilograms. The correct answer is 20 g.
4. First convert pounds to kilograms. The correct answer is 20 g.

TEST-TAKING HINT: Convert pounds to kilograms before starting any calculations.

37. 1. Hypertension is not associated with lindane (Kwell).
2. **Lindane (Kwell) with topical use is associated with seizures after absorption.**
3. Lindane (Kwell) is not associated with elevated liver functions.
4. Lindane (Kwell) does not cause alopecia.

TEST-TAKING HINT: Lindane (Kwell) is used as a second-line treatment for lice. Be aware of the reasons it should not be used a second time.

38. 1. Common adverse effects are headaches and abdominal complaints.
2. Albendazole (Albenza) is only effective against adult worms, so additional treatment is needed to kill the emerging parasites.
3. Albendazole (Albenza) is better absorbed when taken with a meal.
4. **As the first treatment kills the adult worms, a second treatment is done in 2 weeks to treat emerging parasites.**

TEST-TAKING HINT: Review medications used to treat pinworms and how they are administered.

39. 1. **Hydrocortisone cream should be used for brief periods because it can thin the skin and cause skin breakdown.**
2. Higher concentrations of hydrocortisone are contraindicated.
3. The drug does not lose its efficacy.
4. An antibiotic is inappropriate for the treatment of eczema.

TEST-TAKING HINT: Focus on the concentration of the hydrocortisone and the effects on the skin.

40. 1. This dose is too low.
2. **The dose is calculated by multiplying the weight by the milligrams. That result is divided by two doses. The milligrams are then used to determine the milliliters based on the concentration of the drug.**
40 mg × 15 kg = 600 mg/2 doses = 300 mg/dose
The concentration of the drug is 250 mg/5 mL. Use the formula "Desired over Available times Volume" to get the mL per dose.
300 mg/250 mg × 5 mL = 6 mL
3. This dose is too high.
4. This dose is too high.

TEST-TAKING HINT: Identify the key components of the question.

41. 1. First convert pounds to kilograms; multiplying 5 mg by weight gives the number of milligrams per 24 hours.
2. First convert pounds to kilograms; multiplying 5 mg by weight gives the number of milligrams per 24 hours.
3. **First convert 40 pounds to kilograms by dividing the pounds by 2.2 (2.2 lb = 1 kg)**
40 ÷ 2.2 = 18.18 kg
Multiplying 5 mg by the weight (18.18) gives the number of milligrams for 24 hours
18.18 kg × 5 mg = 90.9 mg/day
Divide the total milligrams (90.9 mg) by 4, as that is the number of doses
90.9 mg ÷ 4 = 22.73 mg per dose
4. First convert pounds to kilograms; multiplying 5 mg by weight gives the number of milligrams per 24 hours.

TEST-TAKING HINT: Convert pounds to kilograms and then identify the key components needed to determine the answer.

42. 1. **The onset of Lasix is 20 to 60 minutes. It peaks at 60 to 70 minutes, with a duration of 2 hours. By 24 hours, 50% is eliminated. Give the Lasix at 8:00 a.m. to avoid interruption of sleep with frequent urination.**
2. Noon is more appropriate than 6:00 p.m. and bedtime.
3. Because 50% remains in the body, a cumulative effect could disrupt the child's sleep-rest pattern.
4. An onset of 20 to 60 minutes results in a direct interruption of the sleep-rest pattern.

TEST-TAKING HINT: Knowledge of pharmacokinetics is necessary to determine the best time to administer Lasix. Knowing that the drug is a diuretic assists in determining a time that avoids disrupting the sleep-rest pattern.

43. 1. **The symptoms of an acute asthma attack are related to constriction of the airway, which leads to dyspnea and an increased respiratory rate. The albuterol (Proventil) is a beta-adrenergic agent that relaxes the smooth muscles of the bronchial tree, which will decrease wheezing.**
    2. The respiratory rate should return to normal.
    3. Hypertension is a side effect of albuterol (Proventil).
    4. Tachycardia is a side effect of albuterol (Proventil).

TEST-TAKING HINT: The test taker must know the primary outcome of the drug action.

44. 1. One side effect of albuterol (Proventil) is tachycardia, not bradycardia.
    2. Decreased blood pressure is not expected. Dizziness may occur from the tachycardia.
    3. **Potential side effects of this medication are stimulation of the central nervous system and cardiovascular system. Tachycardia is the most frequent side effect of albuterol (Proventil).**
    4. Increased blood pressure can occur, but the child will not experience lethargy until exhausted, which is a later effect.

TEST-TAKING HINT: Albuterol (Proventil) has a major side effect of tachycardia, which worsens with increased doses.

45. 1. The antibiotic should be given every 6 hours to maintain blood levels. This schedule means that the antibiotic would be given every 4 hours during the day, with 12 hours between the last night dose and the first morning dose.
    2. **Antibiotics should be scheduled to maintain therapeutic blood levels and not interfere with the child's sleep. This schedule allows for dosing every 6 hours during the day and allows the child to get 7 hours of uninterrupted sleep at night.**
    3. This is basically the same interval of dosing as answer 1.
    4. This is the same interval of dosing as answers 1 and 2.

TEST-TAKING HINT: Determine the best timing to maintain therapeutic drug levels and allow the patient to rest.

46. 1. The upper thigh is used for subcutaneous and intramuscular injections.
    2. The scapular area and back are used for allergy skin testing.
    3. The scapular area and back are used for allergy skin testing.
    4. **The ventral forearm is the preferred site for the tuberculin skin test.**

TEST-TAKING HINT: The test taker must know sites of administration of medications in children.

47. 1. **Desired over Available × Volume = Desired dose**
       75 mg/160 mg × 5 mL = 2.3 mL
    2. Desired over Available × Volume = Desired dose.
    3. Desired over Available × Volume = Desired dose.
    4. Desired over Available × Volume = Desired dose.

TEST-TAKING HINT: The test taker must know the correct formula and then use the information in the question to determine the answer.

48. 1. Weight gain is not a toxic reaction.
    2. Bradycardia is a side effect of digoxin (Lanoxin). Tachycardia is not.
    3. **Digoxin (Lanoxin) toxicity in infants and children may present with nausea, vomiting, anorexia, or a slow, irregular, apical heart rate.**
    4. Seizures are not a toxic reaction that occur with digoxin (Lanoxin).

TEST-TAKING HINT: The test taker must know common toxic effects of digoxin (Lanoxin), which is used frequently in children with heart defects.

49. 1. Use the child's weight × 10 mcg = the amount per kilogram per day. Divide this total by 2 to determine the amount per dose.
    2. **10 kg × 10 mcg/kg/day = 100 mcg ÷ 2 doses a day = 50 mcg/dose**
    3. Use the child's weight × 10 mcg = the amount per kilogram per day. Divide this total by 2 to determine the amount per dose.
    4. Use the child's weight × 10 mcg = the amount per kilogram per day. Divide this total by 2 to determine the amount per dose.

TEST-TAKING HINT: The test taker must know the correct formula to use.

50. 1. Preterm neonates with good renal function may receive indomethacin (Indocin), a prostaglandin inhibitor, to encourage patent ductus arteriosus closure.
2. Hypertension is a side effect of indomethacin (Indocin).
3. A prostaglandin inhibitor does not affect surfactant in the lungs.
4. The drug may cause nephrotoxicity.

TEST-TAKING HINT: Apply pathophysiology of the preterm neonate to the drug.

51. 1. Digoxin (Lanoxin) is given to treat congestive heart failure.
2. Antibiotics are used if there is an infection and prophylactically with invasive procedures.
3. **Prostaglandin E is necessary to maintain patency of the patent ductus arteriosus and improve systemic arterial flow in children with inadequate intracardiac mixing.**
4. Diuretics are given to treat congestive heart failure.

TEST-TAKING HINT: The test taker must know the pathophysiology of the defect and determine the most important treatment to improve cardiac function.

52. 1. This dose is too low. Determine the child's weight in kilograms; then multiply the child's weight by 25 mg.
2. This dose is too low. Determine the child's weight in kilograms; then multiply the child's weight by 25 mg.
3. **Determine the child's weight in kilograms by dividing 44 lb by 2.2 (2.2 lb = 1 kg). Then determine how many milligrams need to be given by multiplying the child's weight in kilograms by 25 mg.**
   44 lb ÷ 2.2 kg = 20 kg
   20 kg × 25 mg = 500 mg
   Use the formula Desired over Available × Volume = Desired dose
   500 mg/250 mg × 5 mL = 10 mL
4. This dose is too high. Determine the child's weight in kilograms; then multiply the child's weight by 25 mg.

TEST-TAKING HINT: The test taker must know the correct formula to use.

53. 1. Weight gain is not a side effect of erythromycin.
2. Diarrhea, not constipation, is an adverse reaction to erythromycin.
3. Mouth sores are not an adverse reaction.

4. **Common adverse reactions to erythromycin include nausea, vomiting, diarrhea, abdominal pain, and anorexia. Erythromycin should be given with a full glass of water and after meals. Because these gastrointestinal adverse reactions occur commonly, it may be necessary to give erythromycin with food.**

TEST-TAKING HINT: The test taker must know the major side effects of this drug are gastrointestinal.

54. 1. This rate is too low. Take the total volume and divide it by the number of hours.
2. **Take the total volume (300 mL) and divide it by the number of hours (12 hours)**
   300 mL ÷ 12 hours = 25 mL/hr
3. This rate is too high. Take the total volume and divide it by the number of hours.
4. This rate is too high. Take the total volume and divide it by the number of hours.

TEST-TAKING HINT: The test taker must know the correct formula to use and must not be distracted by additional information in the question.

55. 1. Take the dose of atropine times the child's weight in kilograms.
2. Take the dose of atropine times the child's weight in kilograms.
3. Take the dose of atropine times the child's weight in kilograms.
4. **Take the dose of atropine (0.02 mg/kg) times the child's weight (20 kg) 0.02 mg/kg × 20 kg = 0.4 mg**

TEST-TAKING HINT: Atropine is a medication given during a code situation, so the test taker must know how to calculate the dosing.

56. 1. **Atropine is an anticholinergic drug. It blocks vagal impulses to the myocardium and stimulates the cardioinhibitory center in the medulla. It increases heart rate and cardiac output.**
2. This is not the classification of atropine.
3. This is not the classification of atropine.
4. This is not the classification of atropine.

TEST-TAKING HINT: The test taker must know the classification of major drugs.

57. 1. There should be constipation, rather than diarrhea, because of decrease in smooth muscle contraction of the gastrointestinal tract.

2. There should be urinary retention due to decrease in smooth muscle contractions of the urinary tract.

3. **Atropine dries up secretions and also lessens the response of ciliary and iris sphincter muscles in the eye, causing mydriasis.**

4. Atropine usually causes paradoxical excitement in children, so lethargy should not occur.

TEST-TAKING HINT: The test taker must know the side effects based on the action of the drug and the age of the patient.

58. 1. The enzymes must be swallowed whole. Retention in the mouth may cause mucosal irritation and stomatitis.
    2. **When administrating enzymes to infants, the capsule may be opened and sprinkled over an acidic food, such as applesauce or mashed fruit.**
    3. The child should take the same amount of enzymes with each meal and half the dose with each snack.
    4. There is no need to refrigerate the medication.

TEST-TAKING HINT: By knowing that enzymes are capsules, the test taker should eliminate answer 1, as capsules are not chewed.

59. 1. There may be tachycardia but no hypertension.
    2. There is no sodium retention, so there will be no edema.
    3. **Common side effects are constipation and dry mouth as the oxybutynin (Ditropan) has an atropine-like effect.**
    4. Adverse effects from overdose may have some central nervous system effects such as nervousness that cause insomnia and hyperactivity.

TEST-TAKING HINT: Oxybutynin (Ditropan) has an atropine-like effect that causes vasoconstriction symptoms.

60. 1. Ribavirin (Virazole) is not given orally.
    2. Ribavirin (Virazole) is not given subcutaneously.
    3. Ribavirin (Virazole) is not given intramuscularly.
    4. **Ribavirin (Virazole) is an antiviral respiratory medication used in the hospital for children with severe respiratory syncytial virus. Administration is via nebulizer.**

TEST-TAKING HINT: The test taker must know that this medication is aerosolized.

61. 1. **The volume control chamber functions as a safety device. No more than 2 hours of solution is placed in the chamber at a time. If the pump should be programmed incorrectly, the child would get only 2 hours of fluids; then the pump would alarm. The nurse is thereby alerted that the pump was programmed incorrectly.**
    2. This is not a measure to prevent infection.
    3. The rationale for using a particular protocol for administration of intravenous fluids should not be based on convenience for the nurse, but rather on safety.
    4. Using a volume control chamber is more costly because it requires additional or different tubing.

TEST-TAKING HINT: The test taker must know safety issues for administration of intravenous fluids with children.

3

Growth and Development

KEYWORDS

The following words include English vocabulary, nursing/medical terminology, concepts, principles, or information relevant to content specifically addressed in the chapter or associated with topics presented in it. English dictionaries, your nursing textbooks, and medical dictionaries such as *Taber's Cyclopedic Medical Dictionary* are resources that can be used to expand your knowledge and understanding of these words and related information.

Anemia

Auscultate

Autonomy

Dehydration

Detachment

Gynecomastia

Hepatitis B

Industry

Inguinal hernia

Initiative

Palpate

ABBREVIATIONS

Atrial septal defect (ASD)

Emergency department (ED)

Face, legs, action, consolability, crying (FLACC)

Failure to thrive (FTT)

Intramuscular (IM)

Intravenous (IV)

Nothing by mouth (NPO)

Ounce (oz)

Pound (lb)

QUESTIONS

Infants

1. A 6-month-old male is at his well-child checkup. The nurse weighs him, and his mother asks if his weight is normal for his age. The nurse's best response is:
   1. "At 6 months, his weight should be approximately three times his birth weight."
   2. "Each child gains weight at his or her own pace."
   3. "At 6 months, his weight should be approximately twice his birth weight."
   4. "At 6 months, a child should weigh about 10 lb more than his or her birth weight."

2. How can the nurse best facilitate the trust relationship between infant and parents while the infant is hospitalized? The nurse should:
   1. Encourage the parents to remain at their child's bedside as much as possible.
   2. Keep parents informed about all aspects of their child's condition.
   3. Encourage the parents to hold their child as much as possible.
   4. Advise the parents to participate actively in their child's care.

3. The nurse is going to give a 6-month-old a dose of ceftriaxone (Rocephin) IM. What must the nurse do when the 1.5-mL dose arrives from the pharmacy?
1. Administer the injection into the deltoid muscle.
2. Divide the dose into two injections.
3. Administer the injection into the dorsogluteal muscle.
4. Give dose as a single injection into the vastus lateralis muscle.

4. Which statements by an infant's mother lead the nurse to believe that she needs further education about the nutritional needs of a 6-month-old? **Select all that apply.**
1. "I will continue to breastfeed my son and will give him oatmeal cereal two times a day."
2. "I will start my son on fruits and gradually introduce vegetables."
3. "I will start my son on carrots and will introduce one new vegetable every few days."
4. "I will not give my son any more than 4 to 6 ounces of baby juice per day."
5. "I will make sure my son gets cereal three times a day."

5. Which statement accurately describes the best method for assessing a 12-month-old?
1. The nurse should assess the child on the examining table.
2. The nurse should assess the child in a head-to-toe sequence.
3. The nurse should have the child's parent assist in holding her down.
4. The nurse should assess the child while she is in her parent's lap.

6. The nurse is instructing a new breastfeeding mother in the need to provide her premature infant with an adequate source of iron in her diet. Which statement reflects a need for further education of the new mother?
1. "I will use only breast milk or an iron-fortified formula as a source of milk for my baby until she is at least 12 months old."
2. "My baby will need to have iron supplements introduced when she is 4 months old."
3. "I will need to add iron supplements to my baby's diet when she is 2 months old."
4. "When my baby begins to eat solid foods, I should introduce iron-fortified cereals to her diet."

7. A first-time mother brings in her 5-day-old baby for a well-child visit. The nurse weighs the infant and reports a weight of 7 lb 5 oz to the mother. The mother looks concerned and tells the nurse that her baby weighed 7 lb 10 oz when she was discharged 4 days ago. The nurse's best response to the mother is:
1. "I will let the doctor know, and he will talk with you about possible causes of your infant's weight loss."
2. "A weight loss of a few ounces is common among newborns, especially for breastfeeding mothers."
3. "I can tell you are a first-time mother. Don't worry; we will find out why she is losing weight."
4. "Maybe she isn't getting enough milk. How often are you breastfeeding her?"

8. Which toy is the best choice for a 12-month-old?
1. Baby doll.
2. Musical rattle.
3. Board book.
4. Colorful beads.

9. The parents of a newborn are asking the nurse how to use the infant car seat and where it should be placed in their vehicle. Which is the most appropriate action by the nurse?
   1. Give the parents a pamphlet explaining how to install the car seat.
   2. Accompany the parents to the car and show them how to install the car seat.
   3. Contact the hospital's car-seat safety officer and ask the officer to accompany the parents to the car for car-seat installation.
   4. Show the parents a video on car-seat installation and safety and ask if they are comfortable with the information.

10. The mother of a newborn asks the nurse when the infant will receive the first hepatitis B immunization. Which is the nurse's best response?
    1. "Babies receive the hepatitis B vaccine only if their mother is hepatitis B–positive."
    2. "The first dose of the hepatitis B vaccine will be given prior to discharge today."
    3. "The first dose of hepatitis B vaccine is given at 1 year of age."
    4. "Babies receive their first hepatitis B vaccine at 6 months of age."

11. Which finding would the nurse consider abnormal when performing a physical assessment on a 6-month-old?
    1. Posterior fontanel is open.
    2. Anterior fontanel is open.
    3. Beginning signs of tooth eruption.
    4. Able to track and follow objects.

12. A mother requests that her child receive the varicella vaccine at the 9-month well-child checkup. The nurse tells the mother that:
    1. Children who are vaccinated will likely develop a mild case of the disease.
    2. The vaccine cannot be given at that visit.
    3. The vaccine will be administered after the physician examines the child.
    4. A booster vaccination will be needed at 18 months of age.

13. Which should the nurse teach the parents is one of the most common causes of injury and death for a 9-month-old infant?
    1. Poisoning.
    2. Child abuse.
    3. Aspiration.
    4. Dog bites.

14. An 8-day-old was admitted to the hospital with vomiting and dehydration. The newborn's heart rate is 170, respiratory rate is 44, blood pressure is 85/52, and temperature is 99°F (37.2°C). What is the nurse's best response to the parents who ask if the vital signs are normal?
    1. "The blood pressure is elevated, but the other vital signs are within normal limits."
    2. "The temperature is elevated, but the other vital signs are within normal limits."
    3. "The respiratory rate is elevated, but the other vital signs are within normal limits."
    4. "The heart rate is elevated, but the other vital signs are within normal limits."

15. The mother of an 11-month-old with iron-deficiency anemia tells the nurse that her infant is currently taking iron and a multivitamin. Which statement made by the mother should be of concern to the nurse?
    1. "I give the iron and multivitamin at the same time each morning."
    2. "I give the iron and multivitamin in the morning 6-oz bottle."
    3. "I give the iron and multivitamin 2 hours before I feed the morning bottle."
    4. "I give the iron and multivitamin in oral syringes toward the back of the cheek."

16. The nurse is using the FLACC scale to rate the pain level in a 9-month-old. Which is the nurse's best response to the father's question of what the FLACC scale is?
    1. "It estimates a child's level of pain utilizing vital sign information."
    2. "It estimates a child's level of pain based on parents' perception."
    3. "It estimates a child's level of pain utilizing behavioral and physical responses."
    4. "It estimates a child's level of pain utilizing a numeric scale from 0 to 5."

17. A 12-month-old boy weighed 8 lb 2 oz at birth. Understanding developmental milestones, what should the nurse caring for the child expect the current weight to be?
    1. 16 lb 4 oz
    2. 20 lb 5 oz
    3. 24 lb 6 oz
    4. 32 lb 8 oz

18. The nurse is assessing the pain level in an infant who just had surgery. The infant's parent asks which vital sign changes are expected in a child experiencing pain. The nurse's best response is:
    1. "We expect to see a child's heart rate decrease and respiratory rate increase."
    2. "We expect to see a child's heart rate and blood pressure decrease."
    3. "We expect to see a child's heart rate and blood pressure increase."
    4. "We expect to see a child's heart rate increase and blood pressure decrease."

Toddlers

19. Which statement by the mother of an 18-month-old would lead the nurse to believe that the child should be referred for further evaluation for developmental delay?
    1. "My child is able to stand but is not yet taking steps independently."
    2. "My child has a vocabulary of approximately 15 words."
    3. "My child is still sucking his thumb."
    4. "My child seems to be quite wary of strangers."

20. The mother of a child who is 2 years 6 months in age has arranged a play date with the neighbor and her child who is 2 years 9 months old. During the play date the two mothers should expect that the children will do which of the following?
    1. Share and trade their toys while playing.
    2. Play with one another with little or no conflict.
    3. Play alongside one another but not actively with one another.
    4. Only play with one or two items, ignoring most of the other toys.

21. Which foods would the nurse recommend to the mother of a 2-year-old with iron-deficiency anemia?
    1. 32 oz of whole cow's milk per day.
    2. Meats, eggs, and green vegetables.
    3. Fruits, whole grains, and rice.
    4. 8 oz of juice, three times per day.

22. A 2-year-old admitted to the hospital 2 days ago has been crying and is inconsolable much of the time. The nurse's best response to the child's parents who are concerned about this behavior is that the child is in the:
    1. Detachment phase of separation anxiety, which is normal for children during hospitalization.
    2. Despair stage of separation anxiety, which is normal for children during hospitalization.
    3. Bargaining stage of separation anxiety, which is normal for children during hospitalization.
    4. Protest stage of separation anxiety, which is normal for children during hospitalization.

23. Which should the nurse do to prevent separation anxiety in a hospitalized toddler?
    1. Assume the parental role when parents are not able to be at the bedside.
    2. Encourage the parents to always remain at the bedside.
    3. Establish a routine similar to that of the child's home.
    4. Rotate nursing staff so the child becomes comfortable with a variety of nurses.

24. According to developmental theories, which important event is essential to the development of the toddler?
    1. The child learns to feed self.
    2. The child develops friendships.
    3. The child learns to walk.
    4. The child participates in being potty-trained.

25. Which comment should the parent of a 2½-year-old expect from the toddler about a new baby brother?
    1. "When the baby takes a nap, will you play with me?"
    2. "Can I play with the baby?"
    3. "The baby is so cute. I love him."
    4. "It is time to put him away so we can play."

26. Which stressor is common in hospitalized toddlers? **Select all that apply.**
    1. Social isolation.
    2. Interrupted routine.
    3. Sleep disturbances.
    4. Self-concept disturbances.
    5. Fear of being hurt.

Preschooler

27. Which nursing action would help foster a hospitalized 3-year-old's sense of autonomy?
    1. Let the child choose what time to take the oral antibiotics.
    2. Allow the child to have a doll for medical play.
    3. Allow the child to administer her own dose of cephalexin (Keflex) via oral syringe.
    4. Let the child watch age-appropriate videos.

28. The best method to explain a procedure to a hospitalized preschool-age child is to:
    1. Show the child a pamphlet with pictures showing the procedure.
    2. Have the 5-year-old next door tell the 4-year-old about the experience.
    3. Demonstrate the procedure on a doll.
    4. Show the child a video of the procedure.

29. A 4-year-old is hospitalized for an ASD repair. The parents have decided to go home for a few hours to spend time with their other children. The child asks when her mommy and daddy will be back. The nurse's best response is:
    1. "Your mommy and daddy will be back after your nap."
    2. "Your mommy and daddy will be back at 6:00 p.m."
    3. "Your mommy and daddy will be back later this evening."
    4. "Your mommy and daddy will be back in 3 hours."

30. Which approach should the nurse use to gather information from a child brought to the ED for suspected child abuse?
    1. Promise the child that her parents will not know what she tells the nurse.
    2. Promise the child that she will not have to see the suspected abuser again.
    3. Use correct anatomical terms to discuss body parts.
    4. Tell the child that the abuse is not her fault and that she is a good person.

31. Which reaction would a nurse expect when giving a preschooler immunizations?
    1. The child remains silent and still.
    2. The child cries and tells the nurse that it hurts.
    3. The child tries to stall the nurse.
    4. The child remains still while telling the nurse that she is hurting him.

32. What can a nurse do to reinforce a 5-year-old's intellectual initiative when he asks about his upcoming surgery?
    1. Answer the child's questions about his upcoming surgery in simple terms.
    2. Provide the child with a book that has vivid illustrations about his surgery.
    3. Tell the child he should wait and ask the doctor his questions.
    4. Tell the child that she will answer his questions at a later time.

33. A 5-year-old boy has always been one of the shortest children in class. His mother tells the school nurse that her husband is 6′ tall and she is 5′7″. What should the nurse tell the child's mother?
    1. He is expected to grow about 2 inches every year from ages 6 to 9 years.
    2. He is expected to grow about 3 inches every year from ages 6 to 9 years.
    3. He should be seen by an endocrinologist for growth-hormone injections.
    4. His growth should be re-evaluated when he is 7 years old.

34. The nurse realizes that a 3½-year-old's mother needs further education about the Denver Developmental Screening Test when she states: **Select all that apply.**
    1. "It screens for gross motor skills."
    2. "It screens for fine motor skills."
    3. "It screens for intelligence level."
    4. "It screens for language development."
    5. "It screens for school readiness."

35. A 3-year-old admitted to the hospital with croup has the following vital signs: heart rate 90, respiratory rate 44, blood pressure 100/52, and temperature 98.8°F (37.1°C). The parents ask the nurse if these vital signs are normal. The nurse's best response is:
    1. "Your son's blood pressure is elevated, but the other vital signs are within the normal range."
    2. "Your son's temperature is elevated, but the other vital signs are within the normal range."
    3. "Your son's respiratory rate is elevated, but the other vital signs are within the normal range."
    4. "Your son's heart rate is elevated, but the other vital signs are within the normal range."

36. Which action is a developmentally appropriate method for eliciting a 4-year-old's cooperation in obtaining the blood pressure?
    1. Have the child's parents help put on the blood pressure cuff.
    2. Tell the child that if he sits still, the blood pressure machine will go quickly.
    3. Ask the child if he feels a squeezing of his arm.
    4. Tell the child that measuring the blood pressure will not hurt.

37. A 4-year-old hospitalized with FTT has orders for daily weights, strict intake and output, and calorie counts. Which action by the nurse would be a concern?
    1. The nurse weighs the child every morning after breakfast.
    2. The nurse weighs the child with no clothing except for undergarments.
    3. The nurse sits with the child while the child eats her meals.
    4. The nurse weighs the child using the same scale every morning.

38. A 3-year-old is attending her grandfather's funeral. Her parents told her that her grandfather is in heaven with God. Which statement describes a 3-year-old child's understanding of spirituality?
1. "The body is here with us on Earth, and the spirit is in heaven."
2. "He is in heaven. Is this heaven?"
3. "The spirit is no longer in his body."
4. "He won't need his body in heaven."

39. A 4-year-old boy has been hospitalized because he fell down the stairs. His mother is crying and states, "This is all my fault." Which is the nurse's best response?
1. "Accidents happen. You shouldn't blame yourself."
2. "Falls are one of the most common injuries in this age-group."
3. "It may be a good idea to put a gate on the stairs."
4. "Your son should be proficient at walking down the stairs by now."

School Age

40. Which nursing action is most appropriate to gain information about how a child is feeling?
1. Actively attempt to make friends with the child before asking about her feelings.
2. Ask the child's parents what feelings she has expressed in regard to her diagnosis.
3. Provide the child with some paper to draw a picture of how she is feeling.
4. Ask the child direct questions about how she is feeling.

41. Which statements would indicate to the nurse that a school-age child is not developmentally on track for age? **Select all that apply.**
1. The child is able to follow a four- to five-step command.
2. The child started wetting the bed on admission to the hospital.
3. The child has an imaginary friend named Kelly.
4. The child enjoys playing board games with her sister.
5. The child is not able to follow rules.

42. Which statement accurately describes how the nurse should approach an 11-year-old to do a physical assessment?
1. Ask the child's parents to remain in the room during the physical exam.
2. Auscultate the heart, lungs, and abdomen first.
3. Explain that the physical exam will not hurt.
4. Explain what the nurse will be doing in basic understandable terms.

43. Which is the best method of distraction for an 8-year-old who is having surgery later today to insert a central line and is NPO?
1. Use the telephone to call friends.
2. Watch television.
3. Play a board game.
4. Read the central-line pamphlet he was given.

44. Which activity can the nurse provide for a 9-year-old to encourage a sense of industry?
1. Allow the child to choose what time to take his medication.
2. Provide the child with the homework his teacher has sent.
3. Allow the child to assist with his bath.
4. Allow the child to help with his dressing change.

45. The mother of 10-year-old fraternal twins tells the nurse at their well-child checkup that she is concerned because her daughter has gained more weight and height than her twin brother. The mother is concerned that there is something wrong with her son. The nurse's best response is:
    1. "I understand your concern. I will talk with the physician, and we can draw some lab work."
    2. "Let me ask you whether your son has been ill lately."
    3. "It is normal for girls to grow a little taller and gain more weight than boys at this age."
    4. "It is normal for you to be concerned, but I am sure your son will catch up with your daughter eventually."

46. A 9-year-old girl builds a clubhouse in her backyard. She hangs a sign outside her clubhouse that has "No boys allowed" printed on it. The child's parents are concerned that she is excluding their neighbor's son, and they are upset. What should the school nurse tell the child's parents?
    1. Her behavior is cause for concern and should be addressed.
    2. Her behavior is common among school-age children.
    3. Her feelings about boys will subside within the next year.
    4. They should have their daughter speak with the school counselor.

47. What information should a school nurse include in a discussion on nutrition with a fourth-grade class?
    1. The number of calories that a fourth-grade child should consume in a day.
    2. A list of high-calorie foods that all fourth-graders should avoid.
    3. How to read food labels so that children know which foods are good for them.
    4. A list of nutritious foods with basic scientific information about how they affect the body organs and systems.

48. Which technique should the nurse suggest to the mother of an 8-year-old who does not want to complete her chores?
    1. Grounding.
    2. Time-out.
    3. Reward system.
    4. Spanking.

49. Which should the nurse recommend to the parents of a 9-year-old hospitalized following a bicycle injury? To prevent future injury, their child should:
    1. Wear safety equipment while riding bicycles.
    2. Read educational material on bicycle safety.
    3. Watch a video on bicycle safety.
    4. Ride his bike in the presence of adults.

Adolescent

50. A 16-year-old male is hospitalized for cystic fibrosis. He will be an inpatient for 2 weeks while he receives IV antibiotics. Which action taken by the nurse will most enhance his psychosocial development?
    1. Fax the teen's teacher and have her send in his homework.
    2. Encourage the teen's friends to visit him in the hospital.
    3. Encourage the teen's grandparents to visit frequently.
    4. Tell the teen he is free to use his phone to call or text friends.

51. To obtain an adolescent's health information, the nurse should:
    1. Interview the adolescent using direct questions.
    2. Gather information during a casual conversation.
    3. Interview the adolescent only in the presence of the parents.
    4. Gather information only from the parents.

52. Which method is the most effective way to present an educational program on abstinence to adolescents?
1. Use peer-led programs that emphasize the consequences of unprotected sexual contact.
2. Teach students methods to resist peer pressure.
3. Offer students the opportunity to care for a simulator infant for 1 week.
4. Offer statistics, pamphlets, and films discussing the consequences of unprotected sexual contact.

53. An 18-year-old with a rash and itching in the groin area is concerned that he has contracted a sexually transmitted disease and does not want his parents to find out. The nurse's best response is:
1. "We will need to contact your parents to let them know."
2. "We will not contact your parents regarding this visit."
3. "Who would you like us to contact about your visit here today?"
4. "We cannot promise that the hospital will not contact your parents."

54. A 13-year-old boy is hospitalized for a femur fracture. He was hit by a car while he and his friends were racing bikes near a major intersection. The child's parents are concerned about his judgment. The nurse should tell the parents that the behavior is:
1. Typical of young teens.
2. Related to hormonal surges during adolescence.
3. An isolated incident and will not likely happen again.
4. Related to teen rebellion.

55. A 16-year-old is having a discussion with the nurse about the teen's recent diagnosis of lupus. In explaining the child's prognosis, the nurse uses the knowledge that adolescents are:
1. Preoccupied with thoughts of the here and now.
2. Able to understand and imagine possibilities for the future.
3. Capable of thinking only in concrete terms.
4. Overly concerned with past events and relationships.

56. The mother of a 13-year-old girl tells the nurse that she is concerned because her daughter has gained 10 lb since she began puberty. The child's mother asks the nurse for advice about what to do about her daughter's weight gain. Which should the nurse do?
1. Provide the child's mother with some pamphlets on nutrition and healthy eating.
2. Provide the child's mother with information about a new exercise program for teens.
3. Inform the child's mother that it is common for teen girls to gain weight during puberty.
4. Inform the child's mother that her daughter will likely gain another 5 to 10 lb in the next year.

57. A 13-year-old tells the nurse that he is worried because his breasts are growing. They hurt, and he is embarrassed to take his shirt off during gym class. What should the nurse tell him?
1. "The pediatrician will draw some blood to find out why your breasts are growing."
2. "It is just a slight hormonal imbalance that can be easily corrected with medication."
3. "This is a normal condition of puberty that will resolve within a year or two."
4. "This is a rare finding that occurs in about 5% of boys during puberty."

58. An adolescent has a diagnosis of new-onset diabetes. What would most influence a teenager's food choices as he begins to make changes in his diet?
1. Parents and their dietary choices.
2. Cultural background.
3. Peers and their dietary choices.
4. Television and other forms of media influence.

59. The mother of a 15-year-old is frustrated because he spends much of his weekend time sleeping. Which is the nurse's best response to the mother's frustration?
1. "Your son may be trying to catch up on the sleep missed during the week."
2. "Developmental theorists believe that teens require more sleep as they begin to integrate new roles into their lives."
3. "Teens require more sleep because of the rapid physical growth that is occurring."
4. "Teens require more sleep because of the increase in their social obligations."

60. During an adolescent's initial physical assessment, the nurse notes signs and symptoms of nutritional deficit. Which assessment led the nurse to this initial conclusion?
1. Protein level within normal limits.
2. Blood pressure is 110/66.
3. Hair and nails are brittle and dry.
4. Teeth appear to be eroded.

61. The mother of an adolescent complains that he has had some recent behavioral changes. He comes home from school every day, closes his door, and refrains from interaction with his family. The nurse's best response to the mother is:
1. "You should speak with your son and ask him directly what is wrong with him."
2. "You should set limits with your son and tell him that this is unacceptable behavior."
3. "Your son's behavior is abnormal, and he is going to need a psychiatric referral."
4. "Your son's behavior is normal. You should listen to him without being judgmental."

ANSWERS AND RATIONALES

The correct answer number and rationale for why it is the correct answer are given in **boldface blue type**. Rationales for why the other possible answer options are incorrect also are given, but they are not in boldface type.

1. 1. At 6 months the weight should be approximately two times the birth weight.
   2. Infants gain weight at their own pace but should double the birth weight by 4 to 6 months.
   3. **Infants should double their birth weight by 4 to 6 months of age.**
   4. By 6 months an infant should have doubled the birth weight; 10 lb is a lot of weight to gain in 4 to 6 months.

   TEST-TAKING HINT: The test taker should have learned this specific physical developmental milestone.

2. 1. Having parents close to the child is important, but infants are most secure when they are being held, patted, and talked to.
   2. It is important that the nurse keep the parents informed about their child's condition, but it does not have any impact on the child's trust-versus-mistrust relationship with the parents.
   3. **Having parents hold their child while in the hospital is an excellent means of building the trust relationship. Infants are most secure when they are being held, patted, and spoken to.**
   4. Parents should be encouraged to learn their child's care, but it is not the best means of enhancing the trust relationship.

   TEST-TAKING HINT: The test taker must understand Erickson's stages, including the individual tasks that are met during each stage.

3. 1. The deltoid of a 6-month-old is not developed enough and should not be used for IM injections.
   2. **The nurse should not deliver more than 1 mL per IM injection to a 6-month-old.**
   3. The dorsogluteal muscle should not be used in children until they have been walking for at least 2 years.
   4. The vastus lateralis is the site of choice for an IM injection for a child 6 months old. However, the volume injected should not be more than 1 mL for a single injection.

   TEST-TAKING HINT: The test taker must have knowledge of IM injections sites and acceptable volumes for children of varying ages.

4. 2, 4, 5.
   1. Breastfeeding is the ideal nutrition for the first year of life. Cereal can be introduced between 4 and 6 months of age and offered twice a day.
   2. **Infants should be started on vegetables prior to fruits. The sweetness of fruits may inhibit infants from taking vegetables.**
   3. It is essential to introduce new foods one at a time to determine whether a child has any allergies.
   4. **Infants can be given fruit juice by 6 months of age, but it is recommended not to exceed 4 to 6 ounces per day.**
   5. **Infants need another source of iron by 4 to 6 months of age, so cereal is introduced twice a day.**

   TEST-TAKING HINT: The test taker must have knowledge of the iron needs of a normal infant.

5. 1. Children 12 months old are best assessed in proximity to their parents.
   2. The appropriate sequence for assessment with an infant is to auscultate first, palpate next, and assess ears, eyes, and mouth last. Least invasive procedures are recommended first.
   3. Infants do not like to be held down. This will likely cause the child distress. If the child needs to be held down, it is best to enlist the aid of another staff member.
   4. **Infants are most secure when in proximity to the parent. The parent's lap is an excellent place to assess the child.**

   TEST-TAKING HINT: Health-care professionals must use developmentally appropriate methods to approach children. The test taker must have knowledge of a child's psychosocial development. Answers 1 and 2 can be eliminated because these methods of assessment would be used on an older child.

6. 1. Breast milk or an iron-fortified formula is recommended as the primary source of nutrition for the first year of life.

2. Premature infants have iron stores from the mother that last approximately 2 months, so it is important to introduce an iron supplement by 2 months of age.

3. **Premature infants have iron stores from the mother that last approximately 2 months, so it is important to introduce an iron supplement by 2 months of age. Full-term infants have iron stores that last approximately 4 to 6 months.**

4. Iron-fortified cereals are a good source of iron once a child is old enough to consume solid foods.

TEST-TAKING HINT: The test taker must have knowledge of the recommended nutrition for an infant.

7. 1. A loss of a few ounces during the first few days of life is normal. There will be a reason for concern if the infant does not get back to birth weight in the first 2 weeks of life.

2. **Newborns can lose up to 10% of their birth weight without concern but should regain their birth weight by 2 weeks of age.**

3. The nurse should not make this comment. The mother will likely feel belittled, and she may be afraid to ask questions in the future.

4. A loss of a few ounces during the first few days of life is normal. Many times, infants of breastfeeding mothers lose weight initially because the mother's milk has not come in yet.

TEST-TAKING HINT: The test taker can eliminate answer 3. This is a nontherapeutic response. Remembering that newborns can lose up to 10% of their birth weight will help you choose the right response.

8. 1. The child can play with a small baby doll, but she will likely just put the doll in her mouth. She is not old enough to play appropriately with this toy.

2. **A musical rattle is the perfect toy for this child. Infants have short attention spans and enjoy auditory and visual stimulation.**

3. Reading to children is essential throughout childhood. However, the child will likely just chew on the book, so it is not the ideal choice.

4. Beads are not appropriate toys for infants because of the risk of choking.

TEST-TAKING HINT: The test taker must understand the developmental level of the child and know safety issues in order to choose the appropriate toy.

9. 1. Pamphlets may be a useful tool to reinforce teaching. However, a hands-on approach is best in this situation.

2. The nurse could accompany the parents if she is proficient in car-seat safety and installation.

3. **The car-seat safety officer is the best choice, as that individual would have the needed information and certification to help the family.**

4. A video may be a useful tool to reinforce teaching. However, a hands-on approach is best in this situation.

TEST-TAKING HINT: The question requires knowledge of the safety concerns involving proper car-seat installation. The question also requires the test taker to implement teaching and learning strategies for educating parents. Most people learn best with demonstration and return demonstration; therefore, the test taker can eliminate answers 1 and 4.

10. 1. Babies born to mothers positive for hepatitis B receive the first dose of hepatitis B vaccine within 12 hours of delivery.

2. **The first dose of hepatitis B vaccine is recommended between birth and 2 months. In most hospitals, newborns are given the vaccine prior to discharge.**

3. The first dose of hepatitis B vaccine is recommended between birth and 2 months. In most hospitals, newborns are given the vaccine prior to discharge.

4. The first dose of hepatitis B vaccine is recommended between birth and 2 months. In most hospitals, newborns are given the vaccine prior to discharge.

TEST-TAKING HINT: The test taker must have knowledge of vaccination schedules for children of varying ages.

11. 1. **The posterior fontanel should close between 6 and 8 weeks of age.**

2. The anterior fontanel usually closes between 12 and 18 months.

3. The infant usually has a first tooth erupt at about 6 months of age.

4. The infant should be able to track objects.

TEST-TAKING HINT: This is a specific physical developmental milestone that should be memorized.

12. 1. It is possible for children to develop a mild rash after receiving the varicella vaccine. However, the varicella vaccine is not usually administered prior to 1 year of age.

2. **The nurse should not give the vaccine. The varicella vaccine is not usually administered prior to 1 year of age unless there are extenuating circumstances.**
3. The varicella vaccine is not usually administered prior to 1 year of age.
4. The recommendation is that a second dose be administered at 4 to 6 years of age.

TEST-TAKING HINT: The test taker must understand basic immunization schedules to answer the question.

13. 1. Poisoning is more common among toddlers and preschoolers who are ambulating.
2. Child abuse is not one of the leading causes of injury and death in children. Accidents are the most common cause of injury and death.
3. **Aspiration is a common cause of injury and death among children of this age. These children often find small objects lying on the floor and place them in their mouth. Older siblings are often responsible for leaving small objects around.**
4. Dog bites are not a leading cause of injury or death in children.

TEST-TAKING HINT: The test taker must have knowledge of the primary safety concerns of infants. Answer 1 can be eliminated, as poisoning is more common among preschoolers. Child abuse and dog bites, answers 2 and 4, are not common causes of injury and death in infants.

14. 1. A normal systolic blood pressure for a child from birth to 1 month is 50 to 101. A normal diastolic blood pressure for a child from birth to 1 month is 42 to 64.
2. A normal temperature is 96.6°F to 100°F (35.8°C to 37.7°C).
3. A normal respiratory rate for a child from birth to 1 month is 30 to 60.
4. **A normal heart rate for a child from birth to 1 month is 90 to 160.**

TEST-TAKING HINT: Normal vital signs for each age-group should be memorized in order to understand abnormalities that occur with different disease processes.

15. 1. It is always a good idea for parents to administer medications at the same time each day.
2. **Medications should never be mixed in a large amount of food or formula because the parent cannot be sure that the child will take the entire feeding. Formula decreases the absorption of iron.**

3. Giving medications in a nipple is an acceptable method of administering liquid oral medications to infants.
4. An oral syringe is a good method of administering oral medications. The syringe should be placed in the back side of the cheek. Small amounts of the medication should be given at a time.

TEST-TAKING HINT: The test taker must have knowledge of medication administration. Answers 1, 3, and 4 can be eliminated as they are all appropriate methods for administering medications to infants.

16. 1. Vital signs are not considered when measuring pain using the FLACC scale.
2. The parents' perception of their child's pain level is not considered when using the FLACC scale.
3. **The FLACC scale utilizes behavioral and physical responses of the child to measure the child's level of pain. The scale utilizes facial expression, leg position, activity, intensity of cry, and level of consolability.**
4. The FLACC scale assigns a numeric value to a child's pain level, which is rated from 0 to 10.

TEST-TAKING HINT: The test taker must have knowledge of pain rating scales used to measure the pain of nonverbal children.

17. 1. Children should double their birth weight by 6 months of age.
2. Children should triple their birth weight by 12 months of age.
3. **Children should triple their birth weight by 12 months of age.**
4. Children should triple their birth weight by 12 months of age.

TEST-TAKING HINT: This is a specific physical developmental milestone that should be memorized.

18. 1. When a child is experiencing pain, the normal physiological response is for the heart rate and respiratory rate to increase.
2. When a child is experiencing pain, the normal physiological response is for the heart rate and blood pressure to increase.
3. **When a child is experiencing pain, the normal physiological response is for the heart rate, respiratory rate, and blood pressure to increase.**
4. When a child is experiencing pain, the normal physiological response is for the heart rate, respiratory rate, and blood pressure to increase.

TEST-TAKING HINT: The test taker must have knowledge of vital sign changes that occur when a child is in pain.

19. 1. **The child should be walking independently by 15 to 18 months. Because this toddler is 18 months and not walking, a referral should be made for a developmental consult.**
    2. The vocabulary of an 18-month-old should be 10 words or more.
    3. Thumb-sucking is still common for 18-month-olds and may actually be at its peak at that age.
    4. It is very common for a child of 18 months to exhibit stranger anxiety.

TEST-TAKING HINT: The age of the child is essential to answering this question. The test taker needs to know basic developmental milestones in order to choose the appropriate intervention.

20. 1. Toddlers do not share their possessions well. One of their favorite words is "mine."
    2. Because toddlers do not share well, they are often in conflict with one another during play.
    3. **Toddlers engage in parallel play. They often play alongside another child, but they rarely engage in activities with the other child.**
    4. Toddlers have very short attention spans and commonly play with various items for short periods.

TEST-TAKING HINT: The age of the child is essential to answering this question. The test taker needs to know the developmental level of the child in order to choose the appropriate form of play.

21. 1. One of the primary reasons toddlers develop iron-deficiency anemia is because they are consuming too much milk, which is limiting their intake of iron-rich foods. Milk is a poor source of iron and should be limited to 24 ounces per day.
    2. **Meat, eggs, and green vegetables are excellent sources of iron.**
    3. Iron-enriched cereals are a good choice for children, but this list of foods does not contain the most iron-rich foods.
    4. Increasing the amount of juice the child consumes will not provide needed iron. Instead, the focus is on providing the child with the most iron-rich foods.

TEST-TAKING HINT: The test taker must have knowledge of the recommended nutrition for children and which foods are high in iron such as eggs, meats, and fortified cereals.

22. 1. During the detachment phase of separation anxiety, children are usually fairly cheerful, and they often lack a preference for their parents.
    2. During the despair stage of separation anxiety, children usually have a loss of appetite, altered sleep patterns, and a lack of much interest in play.
    3. The bargaining stage is not a stage of separation anxiety; it is one of the stages of grief.
    4. **During the protest stage of separation anxiety, children are often inconsolable and often cry more than they do when they are at home. These children also frequently ask to go home.**

TEST-TAKING HINT: The test taker must know the stages of separation anxiety to answer the question.

23. 1. The nurse should try to comfort the child and be friendly, but should not try to replace the parent.
    2. Parents should be encouraged to be with their child as much as possible. However, parents may feel guilty if they leave knowing the staff believes the parents should always be at the bedside.
    3. **It is very important to try to maintain a child's home routine both when parents are present and when they have to leave the hospital. This will increase the child's sense of security and decrease anxiety.**
    4. Providing consistent nursing care is important, not rotating staff. The child needs consistent care to decrease anxiety.

TEST-TAKING HINT: The test taker must have knowledge of the stages of separation anxiety. Answer 1 can be ruled out because the nurse should never assume a parental role with a child. Answer 4 can be eliminated because it is essential that children be provided with continuity of care.

24. 1. Toddlers are in a stage of life in which they like to do for themselves. However, developmental theorists such as Erickson and Freud believe that toilet training is the essential event that must be mastered by the toddler.

2. Toddlers engage in more parallel play. Building friendships is not common until school age and adolescence.
3. Walking should be mastered by 18 months of age.
4. **Developmental theorists such as Erickson and Freud believe that toilet training is the essential event that must be mastered by the toddler.**

TEST-TAKING HINT: The test taker must be able to apply the developmental theories of Freud and Erickson.

25. 1. Toddlers are egocentric and are not yet capable of delayed gratification. It is unlikely that the child will wait to play with her parent until the baby sleeps.
2. Toddlers do not usually engage in play with others. They are generally involved in parallel play.
3. Toddlers usually initially resent the presence of new siblings because they take away some of the parents' time and attention.
4. **This is a typical statement that would be made by a toddler. Toddlers are very egocentric and do not consider the needs of the other child.**

TEST-TAKING HINT: The age of the child is essential to answering this question. The test taker must know the psychosocial development of the toddler in order to choose the appropriate statement.

26. **2, 3, 5.**
1. Social isolation is a stressor of the hospitalized teen.
2. **Common stressors of the hospitalized toddler include interrupted routine, sleep pattern disturbances, and fear of being hurt.**
3. **Common stressors of the hospitalized toddler include interrupted routine, sleep pattern disturbances, and fear of being hurt.**
4. Self-concept disturbance is a stressor of the hospitalized teen.
5. **Common stressors of the hospitalized toddler include interrupted routine, sleep pattern disturbances, and fear of being hurt.**

TEST-TAKING HINT: The age of the child is essential to answering this question. The test taker must know the developmental level of the child and common stressors that affect hospitalization to choose the appropriate intervention.

27. 1. Medication administration times must be adhered to. A preschooler should not be allowed to choose administration times.
2. A doll for medical play is an excellent method for teaching children about medical procedures, but it will not enhance her sense of autonomy.
3. **Allowing preschoolers to participate in actions of which they are capable is an excellent way to enhance their autonomy.**
4. Age-appropriate videos are a good way to occupy the child during hospitalization, but they will not enhance her autonomy.

TEST-TAKING HINT: The test taker must understand the meaning of the word "autonomy" and know Erickson's stages of development to answer this question. The test taker also needs to consider safe nursing care. Answers 1 and 4 could be detrimental to the welfare of the child.

28. 1. The child is too young to understand the procedure using pamphlets.
2. Four-year-old children are egocentric and will not relate other children's experiences to their own.
3. **A 4-year-old child understands in very concrete and simple terms. Therefore, medical play is an excellent method for helping to understand the procedure.**
4. Showing a video of the procedure to a preschooler would be very inappropriate. The preschooler is a concrete thinker and would not understand the video.

TEST-TAKING HINT: The age of the child is essential to answering this question. The test taker must understand the developmental level of the child to choose the appropriate intervention. Most 4-year-olds are unable to read, so answer 1 can be eliminated.

29. 1. **Preschoolers understand time in relation to events.**
2. Preschoolers cannot tell time.
3. Preschoolers want concrete information, and the words "this evening" are not meaningful to them.
4. Preschoolers have no concept of how long an hour is.

TEST-TAKING HINT: The age of the child is essential to answering this question. The test taker must have knowledge of a child's understanding of the concept of time. Answers 2, 3, and 4 can be eliminated because they provide choices for time measurement that would only be understandable to children of school age or older.

30. 1. The nurse should always be honest with the child to develop a level of trust. The nurse should not promise not to tell.
    2. The nurse should not make a promise that cannot be kept. Once again, the trust relationship could be jeopardized if the child feels the nurse lied.
    3. The nurse should discuss body parts in relation to the child's vocabulary.
    4. **Many young children believe abuse or illness is their fault, so they should be reminded they are not to blame. Many children this age believe they have acquired a disease or have been abused because they are bad people.**

    TEST-TAKING HINT: The safety and security of the child is paramount. The child needs to know she is safe and she did not cause the abuse. Answers 1 and 2 can be eliminated because of the word "promise." The nurse needs to build a trusting relationship with the child and should never make a promise that cannot be kept.

31. 1. Teens are more likely to be stoic and remain still and silent during injections.
    2. **The common response of a 5-year-old is to cry and protest during an immunization.**
    3. School-age children are most likely to try to stall the nurse.
    4. Teens usually remain still, and they may calmly tell the nurse that they are feeling pain during the injection.

    TEST-TAKING HINT: The age of the child is essential to answering this question. The test taker must understand the child's psychosocial development in order to choose the appropriate response.

32. 1. **The child is taking the initiative to ask questions, as all preschoolers do, and the nurse should always answer those questions as appropriately and accurately as possible.**
    2. A book illustrating what will happen to the child may help him, but it will not encourage his intellectual initiative.
    3. By not answering the child's questions, the nurse may actually be stifling his sense of initiative.
    4. By not answering the child's questions, the nurse may actually be stifling his sense of initiative.

TEST-TAKING HINT: The test taker must understand the cognitive level of the child in order to choose the appropriate intervention. Answers 3 and 4 can be eliminated because the nurse is avoiding the child's questions.

33. 1. **During the school-age years, a child grows approximately 2 inches per year.**
    2. During the school-age years, a child grows approximately 2 inches per year.
    3. This is not the appropriate time to have the child evaluated. His mother needs to reserve her concerns until he is older. He will likely begin to catch up with his peers within the next year.
    4. The child should continue to see his pediatrician for annual visits, but there is no need for a special visit to re-evaluate his growth at this time.

    TEST-TAKING HINT: This is a specific physical developmental milestone that should be memorized.

34. **3, 5.**
    1. The Denver Developmental Screening Test evaluates children from 1 month to 6 years of age and is used to screen gross motor skills, fine motor skills, language development, and personal/social development.
    2. The Denver Developmental Screening Test evaluates children from 1 month to 6 years and is used to screen gross motor skills, fine motor skills, language development, and personal/social development.
    3. **The Denver Developmental Screening Test does not test a child's level of intelligence.**
    4. The Denver Developmental Screening Test evaluates children from 1 month to 6 years and is used to screen gross motor skills, fine motor skills, language development, and personal/social development.
    5. **The Denver Developmental Screening Test evaluates children from 1 month to 6 years and is used to screen gross motor skills, fine motor skills, language development, and personal/social development not school readiness.**

    TEST-TAKING HINT: The test taker must know the Denver Developmental Screening Test and what it screens for.

35. 1. A normal systolic blood pressure for a child from 3 to 6 years is 78 to 111. A normal diastolic blood pressure for a child from 3 to 6 years is 42 to 70.

2. A normal temperature is 96.6°F to 100°F (35.8°C to 37.7°C).

3. **A normal respiratory rate for a child from 3 to 6 years is 20 to 30 breaths per minute.**

4. A normal heart rate for a child from 3 to 6 years is 75 to 120.

TEST-TAKING HINT: Normal vital signs for each age-group should be memorized in order to understand abnormalities that occur with different disease processes.

36. 1. Preschool children like to do things for themselves and will not likely behave any better for the parents than for the nurse.

2. The nurse should not promise the child that the procedure will go quickly. The nurse needs to develop a trusting relationship with the child; therefore, only promises that can be kept should be made.

3. **Preschool children enjoy games, and it is a good way to elicit their assistance and cooperation during a procedure.**

4. The nurse should not promise the child that the procedure will not hurt. Each child's perception of pain is individual. The nurse needs to develop a trusting relationship with the child; therefore, only promises that can be kept should be made.

TEST-TAKING HINT: The test taker needs to understand the psychosocial and cognitive development of a preschooler in order to choose the appropriate intervention. Answers 2 and 4 can be eliminated because nurses should never make promises to children that they may not be able to keep. It is difficult to build a trusting relationship with children unless the nurse is completely honest.

37. 1. **The child should be weighed every day on the same scale before eating. Her weight will not be an accurate reflection if she is fed prior to being weighed.**

2. The child should be weighed only in undergarments. The weight of clothing must not be included.

3. The nurse should remain in the room while the child eats in order to accurately record a calorie count.

4. The child should be weighed on the same scale every time. All scales are not equally accurate, so it is important to use the same scale in order to obtain an accurate trend.

TEST-TAKING HINT: The test taker must have knowledge of a child's nutrition and how to obtain an accurate weight.

38. 1. Three-year-old children do not understand the difference between body and spirit. Their understanding of spirituality is literal in nature.

2. **Three-year-old children are literal thinkers. The child's parents told her that Grandpa was in heaven. She sees his body, so she thinks they are all in heaven.**

3. Three-year-old children do not understand the difference between body and spirit. Their understanding of spirituality is literal in nature.

4. Three-year-old children think of spirituality in literal terms and do not understand the concept of heaven.

TEST-TAKING HINT: The age of the child is essential to answering this question. The test taker must understand the cognitive development of the child in order to choose the appropriate response. Answers 1, 3, and 4 can be eliminated because they demonstrate the understanding of an older, school-age child.

39. 1. This comment will not make the mother feel any better. The mother is going to blame herself regardless of where the blame lies. The nurse would do better to just listen than to make this sort of comment.

2. **Falls are one of the most common injuries, and it may make the parent feel better to know that this is common.**

3. It may be a good idea to put up a gate, but in this situation the nurse's comment may be interpreted as judgmental.

4. Children walk, climb stairs, and run without paying attention to what might be in their way and can fall easily.

TEST-TAKING HINT: The test taker must understand the psychological state of the parent. Most parents blame themselves whenever their children are injured, so answer 1 can be eliminated. Answer 3 implies that the injury is the parent's fault, so it too can be eliminated.

40. 1. The nurse should not attempt to make friends with the child too quickly. The child should be given the opportunity to observe the nurse working in order to increase her comfort level with the nurse.

2. The child's parents are a good source of information, but the child may not have expressed all of her feelings to her parents.

3. **Often children will include much more detail about their feelings in drawings. They will often express things in pictures they are unable to verbalize.**

4. School-age children do not often share all of their feelings verbally, especially to people with whom they are not familiar.

TEST-TAKING HINT: The age of the child is essential to answering this question. The test taker must also have knowledge of the psychosocial development of the school-age child.

41. **3, 5.**
1. School-age children should be able to follow a four- to five-step command, so this does not indicate that the child has a developmental delay.
2. The child was potty-trained before entering the hospital, and bedwetting is a common form of regression seen in hospitalized children. The child will likely return to her normal toileting habits when she returns home.
3. **Most school-age children do not have imaginary friends. This is much more common for children of 3 and 4 years of age.**
4. Most school-age children do enjoy playing board games.
5. **Most school-age children like rules and understand the consequences of not obeying them.**

TEST-TAKING HINT: The test taker must understand the stressors that affect school-age children who are hospitalized and how they react to those stressors based on their developmental level.

42. 1. Privacy is very important to school-age children. The child should be given the choice of having his parents present for the exam.
2. School-age children can be assessed in a head-to-toe sequence.
3. The nurse should not promise that the exam will not hurt.
4. **School-age children are capable of understanding basic functions of the body and can understand what the nurse will be doing if explained in basic terms.**

TEST-TAKING HINT: Health-care professionals must approach children using developmentally appropriate methods. The test taker must have knowledge of a child's psychosocial development. Answers 1 and 2 can be eliminated because they are methods of assessment used for younger children.

43. 1. Talking to friends may distract the child for some time. However, the conversation could revert to a discussion about the upcoming surgery.
2. Watching television may distract the child for some time, but he may still be thinking about his surgery.
3. **A board game is the optimal choice because school-age children enjoy being engaged in an activity with others that will require some skill and challenge.**
4. Reading material about the surgery will only increase his thoughts about the surgery.

TEST-TAKING HINT: The age of the child is essential to answering this question. The test taker must utilize the cognitive developmental level of the child to choose the appropriate method of distraction.

44. 1. Giving the child choices while in the hospital is important. However, medications should be kept on schedule. It is essential to give them at the prescribed time.
2. **The school-age child is focused on academic performance; therefore, the child can achieve a sense of industry by completing his homework and staying on track with his classmates.**
3. The child should have already mastered bathing. It is not likely to give him a sense of accomplishment.
4. The child may enjoy assisting with his dressing change, but it is not the best example of industry.

TEST-TAKING HINT: The test taker must have knowledge of Erickson's stages of development. Answer 1 can be eliminated because it could be detrimental to children to allow them to choose medication times. Answers 3 and 4 can be eliminated because they are not activities that help the child achieve a sense of industry.

45. 1. This is not an appropriate response. The nurse should be aware that it is normal for girls to grow taller and gain more weight than boys near the end of middle childhood.
2. This is not an appropriate response. The nurse should be aware that it is normal for girls to grow taller and gain more weight than boys near the end of middle childhood.
3. **This is the appropriate response. The nurse understands that it is normal for girls to grow taller and gain more weight than boys near the end of middle childhood.**

4. This is not the best response. The boy will likely surpass his sister when he reaches adolescence.

TEST-TAKING HINT: This is a specific physical developmental milestone that should be memorized.

46. 1. The child's behavior is normal. Girls of 9 and 10 generally prefer to have friends who are of the same gender.
    2. **This is common behavior. Girls of 9 and 10 generally prefer to have friends who are of the same gender.**
    3. Girls of 9 and 10 generally prefer to have friends who are of the same gender. The child will likely have the same feelings next year.
    4. There is no need for the child to see the counselor. Girls of 9 and 10 generally prefer to have friends who are of the same gender.

TEST-TAKING HINT: The age of the child is essential to answering this question. The test taker understands the psychosocial development of the child in order to choose the appropriate behavior. Answer 3 can be eliminated because it is too absolute. There is no way to determine exactly how long the child will have these feelings about boys.

47. 1. School-age children do not engage in calorie counting. This is an adult activity.
    2. Children may not want to hear this information, as most of them enjoy consuming high-calorie foods that taste good.
    3. School-age children do not engage in calorie counting. This is an adult activity.
    4. **Reviewing nutritious choices keeps the lesson on a positive note, and school-age children are very interested in how food affects their bodies. They are capable of understanding basic medical terminology.**

TEST-TAKING HINT: The test taker must have knowledge of school-age children's cognitive level and their ability to process and understand information.

48. 1. Grounding is a technique that generally works well with adolescents.
    2. Time-out is a technique that is primarily used for toddler and preschool children.
    3. **School-age children usually respond very well to a reward system and often enjoy the rewards so much that they will continue chores without continual reminders.**
    4. Spanking is a suggestion that should never be given to families.

TEST-TAKING HINT: The age of the child is essential to answering this question. The test taker must understand the psychosocial development of the child in order to choose the appropriate intervention. Answer 4 can be eliminated because physical punishment should never be suggested. Answer 1 can be eliminated because it is a technique that works best with adolescents. Answer 2 can be eliminated because it is a technique that works best with toddlers and preschool children.

49. 1. **Safety equipment is essential for bicycling, skateboarding, and participating in contact sports. Most injuries occur during the school-age years, when children are more active and participate in contact sports.**
    2. Educational material is a good way to reinforce the use of safety equipment, but the parents must insist that the child use his safety equipment.
    3. Video material is a good way to reinforce the use of safety equipment, but the parents must insist that the child use his safety equipment.
    4. The child's parents may not always be present when he rides his bike, so the use of safety equipment is the primary concern.

TEST-TAKING HINT: This is a question focusing on safety. The test taker must understand that educational material may reinforce a child's knowledge of safety. However, in order to avoid injury, the best thing a parent can do is insist on the use of safety equipment.

50. 1. The teen may want to continue his schoolwork while in the hospital, but it is not the best means of enhancing his psychosocial development.
    2. **Teens are most concerned about being like their peers. Having the teen's friends visit will help him feel he is still part of the school and social environment.**
    3. The teen may want to see his grandparents, but they are not the primary focus in his life.
    4. Calling or texting friends is a good means of remaining in contact with peers. However, having direct contact with friends is a better means of maintaining social contact.

TEST-TAKING HINT: The age of the child is essential to answering this question. The test taker must understand that peers are central to an adolescent's life.

51. 1. Teens may not speak as freely when asked direct questions.
2. **Frequently adolescents will share more information when it is gathered during a casual conversation.**
3. Teens may share more information when they are not in the presence of their parents. It is important to interview the teen first. Parent information can be obtained following the interview with the teen.
4. It is important to gather information from both the teen and the parent first, then the teen alone.

TEST-TAKING HINT: The age of the child is essential to answering this question. Answers 3 and 4 contain the word "only." There are rare instances in nursing when the word "only" would apply. These answers can usually be eliminated.

52. 1. **Adolescents are most concerned with what their peers think and feel. They are most receptive to information that comes from another adolescent.**
2. It is very difficult for teens to resist peer pressure even with the appropriate tools of resistance.
3. Infant simulators are useful, but they are very expensive and often difficult to obtain.
4. Pamphlets are helpful aids in relaying information to teens, but hearing the information firsthand from a peer is the most effective method of education.

TEST-TAKING HINT: The test taker must understand the psychosocial development of an adolescent in order to choose the appropriate intervention. Adolescents focus on their relationships with peers and are much more influenced by peers than by multimedia information or by information provided by an adult.

53. 1. An adolescent has a right to privacy; if he does not want his parents contacted and as long as no harm has come to him, they do not need to be contacted.
2. **An adolescent has every right to privacy as long as the situation is not life threatening.**
3. The nurse can ask if the patient would like the nurse to contact someone; again, if the teen says no, that is his or her right.
4. An adolescent has every right to privacy as long as the situation is not life threatening. Therefore, the hospital can promise not to contact the parents.

TEST-TAKING HINT: The test taker must have knowledge of the psychosocial development of an adolescent and what the state law says about privacy.

54. 1. **The brains of young teens are not completely developed, which often leads to poor judgment and impulse control.**
2. Hormonal changes in teens play a primary role in the development of secondary sex characteristics.
3. The child may be prone to other lapses in judgment. The brains of young teens are not completely developed, which often leads to poor judgment and low impulse control.
4. The child's behavior had nothing to do with rebellion.

TEST-TAKING HINT: The age of the child is essential to answering this question. The test taker must understand the psychosocial and cognitive development of the adolescent in order to choose the appropriate intervention.

55. 1. Adolescents are becoming abstract thinkers and are able to imagine possibilities for the future.
2. **Adolescents are becoming abstract thinkers and are able to imagine possibilities for the future.**
3. Preschool and school-age children think in concrete terms. Adolescents are beginning to think in abstract terms.
4. Adolescents are becoming abstract thinkers and are able to imagine possibilities for the future. They are not preoccupied with past events.

TEST-TAKING HINT: The test taker must understand the cognitive level of an adolescent in order to choose the appropriate answer.

56. 1. The child's mother may be interested in information relating to proper nutrition and exercise. However, the most important thing is for the nurse to let the child's mother know that this is a normal finding in teenage girls as they enter puberty.
2. The child's mother may be interested in information relating to proper nutrition and exercise. However, the most important thing is for the nurse to let the mother know that this is a normal finding in teenage girls as they enter puberty.
3. **The nurse should tell the child's mother that this is a normal finding in teenage girls as they enter puberty.**

4. The nurse knows that it is normal for girls to gain weight during puberty but has no idea how much weight the child will gain or if she will gain any more.

TEST-TAKING HINT: The test taker must have knowledge of the physical development of adolescent girls.

57. 1. Gynecomastia and breast tenderness are common for about a third of boys during middle puberty. Gynecomastia usually resolves in 2 years.
2. Gynecomastia and breast tenderness are common for about a third of boys during middle puberty. Gynecomastia usually resolves in 2 years.
3. **Gynecomastia and breast tenderness are common for about a third of boys during middle puberty. Gynecomastia usually resolves in 2 years.**
4. Gynecomastia and breast tenderness are common for about a third of boys during middle puberty. Gynecomastia usually resolves in 2 years.

TEST-TAKING HINT: The test taker must have knowledge about the physical development of adolescent boys.

58. 1. The child's family does have some influence on his dietary choices, but teens are more focused on being like their peers.
2. The child's culture does affect his food choices. However, teens are more likely to choose "junk foods" and foods that their peers are eating.
3. **As a teen, the child is most influenced by his peers. Teens long to be like others around them.**
4. Television does affect personal food choices, but the peer group still has the most prevalent impact in a teen's life.

TEST-TAKING HINT: The age of the child is essential to answering this question. The test taker must understand that peers are central to an adolescent's life.

59. 1. Teens require more sleep because of the rapid physical growth that occurs during adolescence.
2. Teens are trying to integrate new roles into their lives. However, that has no impact on their need for increased sleep.
3. **Teens require more sleep because of the rapid physical growth that occurs during adolescence.**
4. Teens are generally more social and may be staying out late. However, their increased requirement for sleep is related to their rapid growth during adolescence.

TEST-TAKING HINT: The test taker must have knowledge of the physical growth and development of adolescents.

60. 1. A low protein level could indicate a nutritional deficit. However, this would not be an indication that the nurse sees on an initial assessment. Laboratory work would be required to have this information.
2. This is a normal blood pressure for a teen.
3. **Dry and brittle hair and nails are common among people who have a nutritional deficit.**
4. Eroded teeth are common in those who have frequent vomiting. The acidic nature of the vomitus causes the enamel of the teeth to deteriorate, causing erosion. Eroded teeth may be seen in teens with bulimia; however, by itself, this is not a sign of nutritional deficit.

TEST-TAKING HINT: The test taker must have knowledge of the nutritional needs of an adolescent. Answer 1 can be eliminated because it states that the value is normal. Answer 2 can be eliminated because it is a normal blood pressure. Answer 4 can be eliminated because it relates more to bulimia than to nutritional deficit alone.

61. 1. If the child's parents confront him, he may feel as though they are being judgmental, and he will likely not want to communicate with them. When parents begin a dialogue with their child early on in life, they are more capable of approaching the child when they do notice behavioral changes.
2. Setting limits is always a good thing to do with children. However, the child's parents are not addressing the reason for his behavioral changes.
3. The child's behavior is typical of a teen's response to developmental and psychosocial changes of adolescence. He does not need a psychological referral at this time.
4. **The child's behavior is typical of a teen's response to developmental and psychosocial changes of adolescence.**

TEST-TAKING HINT: The age of the child is essential to answering this question. The test taker must understand the psychosocial development of an adolescent in order to choose the appropriate answer. Adolescents focus on their relationships with peers and are much more influenced by peers than by parents. Adolescents also want privacy, so the best thing parents can do is listen to their teens.

Pediatric Health Issues 4

KEYWORDS

The following words include English vocabulary, nursing/medical terminology, concepts, principles, or information relevant to content specifically addressed in the chapter or associated with topics presented in it. English dictionaries, your nursing textbooks, and medical dictionaries such as *Taber's Cyclopedic Medical Dictionary* are resources that can be used to expand your knowledge and understanding of these words and related information.

100% Oxygen via non-rebreather mask
Activated charcoal
Alcohol poisoning
Anticipatory guidance
Assessment
Bacterial meningitis
Carbon monoxide poisoning
Cervical spine precautions
Child abuse
Childproofing measures
Concussion
Congenital hypothyroidism
Contact precautions
Cystic fibrosis
Digoxin (Lanoxin)
Droplet (airborne) precautions
Early intervention services
Epinephrine 1 : 1000 subcutaneous injection
Erythema infectiosum (fifth disease)
Exanthema subitum (roseola)
Galactosemia
Genetic counseling
Hepatitis B antigen
Hepatitis B immune globulin
Hepatitis B vaccine

Immunizations
Initial neurological assessment
Jaw thrust maneuver
Kawasaki disease
Lead poisoning
Low-phenylalanine diet
Maple syrup urine disease
Munchausen syndrome by proxy
Near-drowning
Newborn assessment
Normal growth and development
Poisoning
Renal diet
Respiratory precautions
Rheumatic fever
Rotovirus vaccine
Serial neurological assessments
Sexual abuse
Shaken baby syndrome
Spinal cord injuries
Tay-Sachs disease
Tuberculosis
Vaccine information statement
Varicella (chickenpox)
Varicella vaccine

ABBREVIATIONS

Diphtheria, tetanus toxoid, and acellular pertussis (DTaP)
Haemophilus influenza type B (Hib)
Human immunodeficiency virus (HIV)

Inactivated polio vaccine (IPV)
Measles, mumps, rubella (MMR)
Phenylketonuria (PKU)

QUESTIONS

1. The mother of a 3-week-old infant tells the nurse she is residing in a homeless shelter and is concerned about her baby's mild cough, poor appetite, low-grade fever, weight loss, and fussiness over the past 2 weeks. Which nursing intervention would be the nurse's highest priority?
   1. Weigh the baby to have an accurate weight using standard precautions.
   2. Reassure the mother that the baby may only have a cold, which can last a few weeks.
   3. Immediately initiate droplet face-mask precautions and isolate the infant.
   4. Take a rectal temperature while completing the assessment using standard precautions.

2. Which would be the priority nursing intervention for a newly admitted child with Kawasaki disease?
   1. Continuous cardiovascular and oxygen-saturation monitoring.
   2. Vital signs every 4 hours until stable.
   3. Strict intake and output monitoring hourly.
   4. Begin aspirin therapy after fever has resolved.

3. Which clinical assessment of a neonate with bacterial meningitis would warrant immediate intervention?
   1. Irritability.
   2. Rectal temperature of 100.6°F (38.1°C).
   3. Quieter than usual.
   4. Respiratory rate of 24 breaths per minute.

4. An 18-month-old is discharged from the hospital after having a febrile seizure secondary to exanthem subitum (roseola). On discharge, the mother asks the nurse if her 6-year-old twins will get sick. Which teaching about the transmission of roseola would be most accurate?
   1. The child should be isolated in the home until the vesicles have dried.
   2. The child does not need to be isolated from the older siblings.
   3. Administer acetaminophen to the older siblings to prevent seizures.
   4. Monitor older children for seizure development.

5. The pregnant mother of a child diagnosed with erythema infectiosum (fifth disease) is crying, and says, "I am afraid. Will my unborn baby die? I have a planned cesarean section next week." Which statement would be the most therapeutic response?
   1. "Let me get the physician to come and talk with you."
   2. "I understand. I would be afraid, too."
   3. "Would you like me to call your obstetrician to have you seen as soon as possible?"
   4. "I understand you are afraid. Can we can talk about your concerns?"

6. Which would be the priority intervention for a child suspected of having varicella (chickenpox)?
   1. Contact precautions.
   2. Contact and droplet respiratory precautions.
   3. Droplet respiratory precautions.
   4. Universal precautions and standard precautions.

7. Which would be the priority intervention for a child diagnosed with chickenpox (varicella) who was prescribed diphenhydramine (Benadryl) for itching?
   1. Give a warm bath with mild soap before lotion application.
   2. Avoid Caladryl lotion while taking diphenhydramine (Benadryl).
   3. Apply Caladryl lotion generously to decrease itching.
   4. Give a cool shower with mild soap to decrease itching.

8. Which signs and symptoms would the nurse expect to assess in a child with rheumatic fever?
   1. Ankle and knee joint pain.
   2. Negative group A beta streptococcal culture.
   3. Large red "bulls eye"–appearing rash.
   4. Stiff neck with photophobia.

9. The parents of a 12-month-old with HIV are concerned about his receiving routine immunizations. What will the nurse tell them about immunizations?
   1. "You are concerned about your child receiving immunizations. Let me explain why your child will not receive routine immunizations today."
   2. "Your child will receive the recommended vaccines today."
   3. "Your child is not severely immunocompromised, but I would still be concerned about his receiving routine immunizations."
   4. "Your child may develop infections if he gets his routine immunizations. Your child will not be immunized today."

10. After airway, breathing, and circulation have been assessed and stabilized, which intervention should the nurse implement for a child diagnosed with encephalitis?
    1. Assist with a lumbar puncture and give reassurance.
    2. Obtain a throat culture, then begin antibiotics.
    3. Perform initial and serial neurological assessments.
    4. Administer antibiotics and antipyretics.

11. Expected nursing assessments of a newborn with suspected cystic fibrosis would include which of the following? **Select all that apply.**
    1. Observe frequency and nature of stools.
    2. Provide chest physical therapy.
    3. Observe for weight gain.
    4. Assess parents' compliance with fluid restrictions.
    5. Assess respiratory system frequently.

12. Which treatment would the nurse anticipate for a 2-week-old boy diagnosed with PKU?
    1. There is no treatment or special diet.
    2. A high-phenylalanine diet.
    3. A low-phenylalanine diet.
    4. The mother would be advised not to breastfeed the infant.

13. Which teaching would be important to discuss with the family of a newborn with PKU?
    1. Studies have shown that children with PKU outgrow the disease.
    2. Consumption of decreased amounts of protein and dairy products is advised.
    3. High-protein and high-dairy products consumption must be maintained.
    4. Exclusive breastfeeding is encouraged for maximal nutrition for the child.

14. Which teaching is most important for a child with PKU?
    1. The child is able to eat a quarter-pound hamburger and drink a milkshake daily.
    2. If the child wants soda, diet soda is preferred over milk or dairy products.
    3. The child may have ice cream in an unlimited quantity once a week.
    4. Diet soda or anything with the sweetener aspartame should be avoided.

15. Which intervention should the nurse implement for a newborn diagnosed with galactosemia?
    1. Eliminate all milk and lactose-containing foods.
    2. Encourage breastfeeding as long as possible.
    3. Encourage lactose-containing formulas.
    4. Avoid feeding soy-protein formula to the newborn.

16. Which statement by the parent of a newborn diagnosed with galactosemia demonstrates successful teaching?
1. "This is a rare disorder that usually does not affect future children."
2. "Our newborn looks normal; he may not have galactosemia."
3. "Our newborn may need to take penicillin and other medications to prevent infection."
4. "Penicillin and other drugs that contain lactose as fillers need to be avoided."

17. Which signs and symptoms would the nurse expect to assess in a newborn with congenital hypothyroidism?
1. Preterm, diarrhea, and tachycardia.
2. Post-term, constipation, and bradycardia.
3. High-pitched cry, colicky, and jittery.
4. Lethargy, diarrhea, and tachycardia.

18. Which families would be appropriate to refer for genetic counseling?
1. Parents with macrosomic infant.
2. Parents with neonatal abstinence syndrome infant.
3. Couple with a history of planned abortions.
4. Couple with a history of multiple miscarriages.

19. Which statement from parents of a newborn diagnosed with Tay-Sachs disease indicates successful understanding of the long-term prognosis?
1. "If we give our baby a proper diet, early intervention, and physical therapy, he can live to adulthood."
2. "He will have normal development for about 6 months before progressive developmental delays occur."
3. "With intense physical therapy and early intervention, we can prevent developmental delays."
4. "If we give our baby a lactose-free diet for life, we can minimize developmental delays and learning disabilities."

20. Which intervention might the nurse anticipate in a 2-day-old infant diagnosed with maple syrup urine disease?
1. High-protein, high–amino acid diet.
2. Low-protein, limited–amino acid diet.
3. Low-protein, low-sodium diet.
4. Phenylalanine-restricted diet.

21. What would be the priority nursing action on finding the varicella vaccine at room temperature on the shelf in the medication room?
1. Ensure the varicella vaccine's integrity is intact; if intact, follow the five rights of medication administration.
2. Do not administer this batch of vaccine.
3. Ensure the varicella vaccine's integrity is intact; if intact, give the vaccine after verifying proper physician orders.
4. Ask the mother if the child has had any prior reactions to varicella.

22. Which would be the most therapeutic response for the mother of a 6-month-old who tells the nurse she does not want her infant to have the DTaP vaccine because the infant had localized redness the last time she received the vaccine?
1. "I will let the physician know, and we will not administer the DTaP vaccination today."
2. "Every child has that allergic reaction, and your child will still get the DTaP today."
3. "I will let the physician know that you refuse further immunizations for your daughter."
4. "Would you mind if we discussed your concerns?"

23. Which nursing intervention should take place prior to all vaccination administrations?
    1. Document the vaccination to be administered on the immunization record and medical record.
    2. Provide the vaccine information statement handout and answer all questions.
    3. Administer the most painful vaccination first, and then alternate injection sites.
    4. Refer to the vaccination as "baby shots" so that the parent understands the baby will be receiving an injection.

24. Which would be the nurse's best response if a mother asks if her baby still needs the Hib vaccine because he already had Hib?
    1. "Yes, it is recommended that the baby still get the Hib vaccine."
    2. "No, if he has had Hib, he will not need to receive the vaccine."
    3. "Let me take a nasal swab first; if it is negative, he will receive the Hib vaccine."
    4. "The physician will order a blood test, and depending on results, your child may need the vaccine."

25. What would be the nurse's best response if the foster mother of a 15-month-old with an unknown immunization history comes to the clinic requesting immunizations?
    1. "Your foster child will not receive any immunizations today."
    2. "Your foster child will receive the MMR, Hib, IPV, and hepatitis B vaccines."
    3. "Your foster child could have harmful effects if we revaccinate with prior vaccines."
    4. "Your foster child will receive only the Hib and DTaP vaccines today."

26. Which medication is most important to have available in all clinics and offices if immunizations are administered?
    1. Diphenhydramine (Benadryl) injection.
    2. Diphenhydramine (Benadryl) liquid.
    3. Epinephrine 1 : 1000 injection.
    4. Epinephrine 1 : 10,000 injection.

27. Which is the nurse's best response to the mother of a 2-month-old who is going to get IPV immunization when the mother tells the nurse the older brother is immunocompromised?
    1. "Your baby should not be immunized because your immunocompromised son could develop polio."
    2. "Your baby should receive the oral poliovirus vaccine instead so that your immunocompromised son does not get sick."
    3. "You should separate your 2-month-old child from the immunocompromised son for 7 to 14 days after the IPV."
    4. "Your baby can be immunized with the IPV; he will not be contagious."

28. Which would be the priority intervention for the newborn of a mother positive for hepatitis antigen?
    1. The newborn should be given the first dose of hepatitis B vaccine by 2 months of age.
    2. The newborn should receive the hepatitis B vaccine and hepatitis B immune globulin within 12 hours of birth.
    3. The newborn should receive the hepatitis B vaccine and hepatitis B immune globulin within 24 hours of birth.
    4. The newborn should receive hepatitis B immune globulin within 12 hours of birth.

29. Which instruction would be of highest priority for the mother of an infant receiving his first oral rotavirus vaccine?
    1. "Call the physician if he develops fever or cough."
    2. "Call the physician if he develops fever, redness, or swelling at the injection site."
    3. "Call the physician if he develops a bloody stool or diarrhea."
    4. "Call the physician if he develops constipation and irritability."

30. What would be the best plan of care for a newborn whose mother's hepatitis B antigen status is unknown?
    1. Give the infant the hepatitis B vaccine within 12 hours of birth.
    2. Give the infant the hepatitis B vaccine and hepatitis B immune globulin within 12 hours of birth.
    3. Give the infant the hepatitis B vaccine within 24 hours of birth.
    4. Give the infant the hepatitis B vaccine and hepatitis B immune globulin within 24 hours of birth.

31. When discharging a newborn, which injury prevention instruction would be of highest priority to tell the parents?
    1. "Place safety locks on all medicine cabinets and household cleaning supplies."
    2. "Transport the infant in the front seat when driving alone so that you can see the baby."
    3. "Never leave the baby unattended on a raised, unguarded area."
    4. "Place safety guards in front of any heating appliance, stove, fireplace, or radiator."

32. A 10-month-old is carried into the emergency department by her parents after she fell down 15 stairs in her walker. Which would be your highest priority nursing intervention?
    1. Assess airway while simultaneously maintaining cervical spine precautions.
    2. Assess airway, breathing, and circulation simultaneously.
    3. Prepare for diagnostic radiological testing to check for any injuries.
    4. Obtain venous access and draw blood for testing.

33. Which would be the most appropriate discharge instructions for a child with a right wrist sprain 3 hours ago?
    1. "You should rest, elevate the wrist above the heart, apply heat wrapped in a towel, and use the sling when walking."
    2. "You can use the wrist, but stop if it hurts; elevate the wrist when not in use and use the sling when walking."
    3. "You should rest, apply ice wrapped in a towel, elevate the wrist above the heart, and use the sling when walking."
    4. "You do not have to take any special precautions; do not use any movements that cause pain and apply alternate heat and ice, each wrapped in a towel."

34. A child with a newly applied left leg cast initially feels fine, then starts to cry and tells his mother his leg hurts. Which assessment would be the nurse's first priority?
    1. Cast integrity.
    2. Neurovascular integrity.
    3. Musculoskeletal integrity.
    4. Soft tissue integrity.

35. Which would be the most appropriate injury prevention/safety teaching for an adolescent?
    1. Inquire which are the favorite sports, discuss the teen's knowledge and application of appropriate safety principles.
    2. Tell the teen to be careful performing sports activities because every sport has the potential for injury.
    3. Tell the teen not to let friends encourage drinking, smoking, or taking drugs.
    4. Ask the mother what sports the teen plays and if a helmet is worn with contact sports.

36. Which assessment is most important after any injury in a child?
    1. History of loss of consciousness and length of time unconscious.
    2. Serial assessments of level of consciousness.
    3. Initial neurological assessment.
    4. Initial vital signs and oxygen saturation level.

37. Which is the most appropriate nursing intervention when caring for a child newly admitted with a mild head concussion and no cervical spine injury?
    1. Keep head of bed flat, side rails up, and safety measures in place.
    2. Elevate head of bed, side rails up, and safety measures in place.
    3. Observe for drainage from any orifice and notify physician immediately.
    4. Continually stimulate the child to keep awake to check neurological status.

38. Which is the most appropriate teaching to the parents of a child in the emergency department after a near-drowning if the child is awake, alert, and has no respiratory distress?
    1. "Your child will most likely be discharged, and you should watch for any cough or trouble breathing."
    2. "Your child will need to have a preventive tube for breathing and ventilation to ensure the lungs are clear."
    3. "Your child will be fine, but sometimes antibiotics are started as a preventive."
    4. "Your child will most likely be admitted for at least 24 hours and observed for respiratory distress or any swelling of the brain."

39. What would be the most appropriate advice to give to the parent of a child with slight visual blurring after being hit in the face with a basketball?
    1. "Apply ice, observe for any further eye complaints, and bring him back if he has increased pain."
    2. "Take him to the emergency department to ensure that he does not have any internal eye damage."
    3. "Call your pediatrician if he starts vomiting, is hard to wake up, or has worsening of eye blurring."
    4. "Observe for any further eye complaints, headaches, dizziness, or vomiting, and if worsening occurs, take him to your pediatrician."

40. Which would be the best response to the mother of a 13-year-old who continues to ask to ride his 16-year-old cousin's all-terrain vehicle?
    1. Emphasize the wearing of safety apparel and adult supervision.
    2. Explain that he is developing increased physical skills; if he wears safety apparel and shows maturity, it should be fine.
    3. All-terrain vehicles are not recommended for those younger than 16 years of age.
    4. This is a stage at which the child is seeking independence and should be allowed to participate in new physical activities.

41. Which response about safety measures is the most appropriate advice for the 2-year-old's mother who had her older home remodeled to reduce the lead level? **Select all that apply.**
    1. "Wash and dry the child's hands and face before he eats."
    2. "Remodeling the home to remove the lead is all you need to do."
    3. "It is best to use cold water to prepare the child's food to decrease the lead."
    4. "Diet does not matter in reducing lead levels in the child."
    5. "Drinking two cups of milk per day helps to decrease lead levels."

42. Which intervention would be most appropriate for a 3-year-old who has just ingested dish detergent?
    1. Discuss childproofing measures in the home in a nonthreatening manner.
    2. Inquire about the circumstances of the ingestion.
    3. Discuss having ipecac and the Poison Control phone number in the home.
    4. Tell the mother you will be giving the boy medicine to make him throw up.

43. Which would be the most appropriate intervention for a 4-year-old brought to the emergency department after ingesting a small watch battery?
    1. No treatment would be needed; assess and monitor airway, breathing, circulation, and abdominal pain.
    2. Ask the mother the time of the ingestion; if it was more than 2 hours ago, it will probably pass in his bowel movement.
    3. Assess and monitor airway, breathing, circulation, and abdominal pain; anticipate admission and prepare for surgical intervention.
    4. Discuss childproofing measures needed in the home with a 4-year-old child; provide anticipatory guidance concerning other possible poisonous ingestions.

44. Which nursing intervention would be of highest priority for a 2-year-old suspected of digoxin ingestion?
    1. Provide supplemental oxygen.
    2. Establish intravenous access.
    3. Draw blood for a STAT digoxin level.
    4. Provide continuous cardiac monitoring.

45. Which would be the priority nursing intervention for a child with carbon monoxide poisoning?
    1. Provide supplemental 100% oxygen.
    2. Provide continuous oxygen saturation monitoring.
    3. Establish intravenous access.
    4. Draw blood for a STAT carbon monoxide level.

46. Which would be appropriate anticipatory guidance during the well-care visit of a 17-year-old?
    1. Discuss alcohol use and potential for alcohol poisoning.
    2. Discuss secondary sex characteristics that will develop.
    3. Teach about anger management and safe sex.
    4. Teach about peer pressure and desire for independence.

47. Which would be the best response to a 10-year-old who asks if she can take acetaminophen (Tylenol) daily if she gets aches and pains?
    1. Tell her it is better not to take medication if she gets aches and pains; she should check with a parent before taking any medication.
    2. Teach her that nonprescription drugs such as acetaminophen (Tylenol) can be a poisoning hazard if too many are taken; it is best for her to check with a parent.
    3. Encourage her to keep a log of when she takes acetaminophen (Tylenol) to try to establish what is causing her aches and pains.
    4. Sometimes it is okay to take acetaminophen (Tylenol) daily, but it depends on why she has aches and pains.

48. What would be the nurse's best advice to a mother who says her 3-year-old ingested Visine eye solution?
    1. "Initiate vomiting immediately."
    2. "Call the Poison Control Center."
    3. "Call the pediatrician right away."
    4. "Dilute with milk 1 : 1 volume of suspected ingestion."

49. What would be the best response to a mother who tells the nurse that the only way she can get her 2-year-old to take medicine is to call it candy?
    1. Tell her that is fine as long as the child takes all of the medicine.
    2. Discuss the importance of not calling medicine candy to prevent accidental drug ingestion.
    3. Discuss with the mother that the child does not have to take the medicine if she does not want it.
    4. Tell the mother her child will have to go to "time-out" if she does not take her medicine.

50. Which nursing plan would be most successful if the nurse has to administer activated charcoal to a 5-year-old?
    1. Have the parents tell the child he has to drink it while providing a movie to distract him.
    2. Tell child it is candy, it tastes good, do not let him look at it, and he will get a toy after he takes it all down.
    3. Mix it with a sweet flavoring, provide a straw, and give it in an opaque cup with a cover.
    4. Have the child's parent take some first to show the boy it does not taste too bad, and then administer it to him quickly.

51. Which statement most accurately describes child abuse?
    1. Physical abuse and neglect, usually carried out by a known adult.
    2. Intentional and unintentional physical and emotional abuse and neglect.
    3. Sexual abuse of children, usually by an adult.
    4. Intentional physical, emotional, and/or sexual abuse and/or neglect.

52. What is the most likely cause of a child's illness if it is unexplained, prolonged, recurrent, and extremely rare and usually occurs when the caregiver is present?
    1. Genetic disorder.
    2. Munchausen syndrome by proxy.
    3. Duchenne muscular dystrophy.
    4. Syndrome of inappropriate antidiuretic hormone.

53. Which statement would be most therapeutic to a child the nurse suspects has been abused?
    1. "Who did this to you? This is not right."
    2. "This is wrong that your parents did not protect you."
    3. "This is not your fault; you are not to blame for this."
    4. "I will not tell anyone."

54. The mother of a 6-month-old states that since yesterday, the infant cries when anyone touches her arm. Which would be the priority assessment after the airway, breathing, and circulation had been assessed and found stable?
    1. Ask the mother if she knows what happened.
    2. Assess infant for other signs of potential physical abuse.
    3. Prepare for radiological diagnostic studies.
    4. Establish intravenous access and draw blood for diagnostic testing.

55. Which assessment of an 18-month-old with burns on his feet would cause suspicion of child abuse?
    1. Splash marks on his right lower leg.
    2. Burns noted on right arm.
    3. Symmetrical burns on both feet.
    4. Burns mainly noted on right foot.

56. Which would be the nurse's priority intervention if a 7-year-old's mother tells the nurse she has noticed excessive masturbation?
    1. Tell her it is normal development for children of this age.
    2. Ask the mother if anyone is abusing the child.
    3. Talk with the child and find out why she is touching herself down there.
    4. Investigate thoroughly the circumstances in which she masturbates.

57. Which statement by the mother would lead the nurse to suspect sexual abuse in a 4-year-old?
    1. "She has just started masturbating."
    2. "She has lots more temper tantrums."
    3. "She now has an invisible friend."
    4. "She wants to spend time with her sister."

58. What would be the priority intervention when a 10-year-old comes to the school nurse's office because of a headache, and the nurse notices various stages of bruising on the inner aspects of the upper arms? **Select all that apply.**
    1. Call the child's parent and ask if acetaminophen (Tylenol) can be given for the headache.
    2. Call the child's parent and ask about the arm bruises.
    3. Ask the child what happened to her arms and have her describe the headache.
    4. Inquire about the child's headache and bruising on her arms; file mandatory reporting forms.
    5. Call the child's parent to pick her up from school, and complete required school nurse visit forms.

59. Which statement is true of abused children?
    1. They will tell the truth if asked about their injuries.
    2. They will repeat the same story that their parents tell.
    3. They usually are not noted to have any changes in behavior.
    4. They will have outgoing personalities and be active in school activities.

60. Which statement is true of shaken baby syndrome? **Select all that apply.**
    1. There may be absence of external signs of injury.
    2. Multiple reports of the baby crying for long periods of time.
    3. Shaken babies usually do not have retinal hemorrhage.
    4. Shaken babies usually have signs of a subdural hematoma.
    5. Shaken babies have signs of external head injury.

61. What would be the best response if the mother of a child on kidney dialysis tells the nurse he has no appetite and eats only bananas?
    1. "Right now his stomach is upset, and as long as he is eating something to give him strength, it is fine."
    2. "Let's talk about your son and his diet."
    3. "Bananas are good to eat; they are rich in needed nutrients."
    4. "Did you try asking him what else he may want to eat?"

The correct answer number and rationale for why it is the correct answer are given in **boldface blue type.** Rationales for why the other possible answer options are incorrect also are given, but they are not in boldface type.

1. 1. Weighing the child would be important but would not be the priority when concerned about an infectious cause. Initiating droplet precautions to prevent infecting others would be a priority, then weighing the infant.
   2. The symptoms are not suggestive of a cold but of something more serious. Infants do not usually lose weight, nor are they irritable with a simple cold, but they can be fussy.
   3. **Children with tuberculosis may have a history of living in a crowded home or could be homeless. Other symptoms may include a cough, cold symptoms, low-grade fever, fussiness, poor appetite, and exposure to a person with tuberculosis. Initiation of droplet precautions and isolation of the infant would be warranted in this situation.**
   4. Taking the infant's temperature is important, but initiating droplet precautions would be the priority.

   TEST-TAKING HINT: The test taker should be highly suspicious of tuberculosis given the family and patient history. Health-care personnel need to be vigilant to contain and prevent further spread of communicable diseases. This child could have meningitis, which would also require isolation and respiratory precautions.

2. 1. **Cardiovascular manifestations of Kawasaki disease are the major complications in pediatric clients. Continuous cardiac monitoring is required to alert the nurse of any cardiovascular complications. Decreased oxygen saturation and respiratory changes have been shown to be early indicators of potential complications.**
   2. Vital signs would be taken every 1 to 2 hours until stable on a new admission with Kawasaki disease.
   3. Strict intake and output monitoring is very important, but because the major complications with Kawasaki disease are cardiovascular, continuous cardiac monitoring is the priority.

4. High-dose aspirin therapy is begun and continued until the child has been afebrile for 48 to 72 hours; then the child is placed on low-dose therapy.

TEST-TAKING HINT: The test taker should understand that cardiovascular manifestations of Kawasaki disease are the major complications in pediatric clients.

3. 1. With the diagnosis of suspected bacterial meningitis, the neonate is expected to be irritable, which frequently accompanies increased intracranial pressure.
   2. A rectal temperature of 38.1°C or 100.6°F indicates a low-grade fever and is not as concerning as the slower-than-normal respiratory rate of 24.
   3. The fact the infant is quieter than normal is in response to the slow respiratory rate and sepsis the neonate is experiencing.
   4. **A normal neonate's respiratory rate is 30 to 60 breaths per minute. Neonates' respiratory systems are immature, and the rate may initially double in response to illness. If no immediate interventions are begun when there is respiratory distress, a neonate's respiratory rate will slow down, respiratory distress will worsen, and, eventually, respiratory arrest will occur. Neonates with slower- or faster-than-normal respiratory rates are true emergency cases; they require identification of the cause of distress.**

TEST-TAKING HINT: The test taker needs to know the normal range of vital signs and when to be concerned to help answer the question.

4. 1. The rash is pink and maculopapular, not vesicular. The incubation period is 5 to 15 days and more commonly seen in children 6 months to 3 years of age. Isolating the siblings is not necessary.
   2. **The route of roseola transmission is unknown, and the disease is more commonly seen in children 6 months to 3 years of age, so siblings do not need to be isolated.**
   3. Because the siblings have no history of seizures, it is not necessary to administer acetaminophen to prevent seizures.

4. Febrile seizures are not usually seen in children older than 6 years, and because they have no history of seizures, it is not necessary to monitor them for seizure development.

TEST-TAKING HINT: The test taker should understand that the route of exanthema subitum (roseola) transmission is unknown, and the disease is usually limited to children 6 months to 3 years of age; isolation is not necessary.

5. 1. Having the physician come back and talk with the pregnant mother of a child with fifth disease is appropriate, but these are certainly concerns the nurse can address by using therapeutic communication.
2. Acknowledging the mother's fear is therapeutic, and it is appropriate to intervene.
3. Informing the obstetrician would be appropriate after dealing therapeutically with the mother's concerns.
4. **There is less risk of fetal death in the second half of the pregnancy. It is more therapeutic to acknowledge a client's fears. After acknowledging her fears, the appropriate response would be to discuss concerns and clarify any misconceptions.**

TEST-TAKING HINT: The test taker should understand there is a 10% risk of fetal death if a mother is exposed to erythema infectiosum (fifth disease) during the first half of her pregnancy.

6. 1. The primary source of transmission is secretions from the respiratory tract (droplet) of infected persons (airborne). Transmission occurs by direct contact, skin lesions to a lesser extent, and contaminated objects.
2. **Varicella (chickenpox) is highly contagious. Contact and droplet respiratory precautions should be started immediately because the primary source of transmission is secretions of the respiratory tract (droplet) and also by contaminated objects.**
3. Droplet precaution is very important because that is the primary source of transmission. Transmission also occurs by direct contact and contaminated objects.
4. Standard precautions (formerly, universal precautions) should always be maintained; the term refers to protecting oneself from patient's blood or body fluids.

TEST-TAKING HINT: The test taker understands that the primary source of transmission of varicella (chickenpox) is secretions of the respiratory tract of infected persons (airborne). Transmission occurs by direct contact, skin lesions to a lesser extent, and contaminated objects.

7. 1. To help decrease itching, a cool bath is a better option. Soap and warm water can cause more itching.
2. **Caladryl lotion contains diphenhydramine (Benadryl), and the child would be at risk for toxicity if the Caladryl is applied to open lesions.**
3. Caladryl lotion is applied in an amount to cover the lesions.
4. A cool shower can be soothing and decrease itching. Mild soap is drying to the lesions and can cause more itching.

TEST-TAKING HINT: The test taker should understand that Caladryl lotion contains diphenhydramine (Benadryl).

8. 1. **Joint pain or arthritis is the most common symptom of acute rheumatic fever (60% to 80% of first attacks). The joint pain usually occurs in two or more large joints (ankle, knee, wrist, or elbow).**
2. Rheumatic fever usually follows group A streptococcal infection, and the culture is usually positive.
3. Large red "bull's-eye" lesions are more characteristic of Lyme disease. The rash associated with rheumatic fever is erythematous with a demarcated border.
4. A stiff neck with photophobia is more indicative of meningitis.

TEST-TAKING HINT: The test taker should remember the major and minor criteria of rheumatic fever to answer this question.

9. 1. **The nurse acknowledges a client's fears and then discusses the concerns to clarify any misconceptions. Immunizations and influenza vaccine are recommended to prevent infection. Immunocompromised HIV-infected children should not receive the varicella and MMR live vaccines.**
2. Recommended immunizations for a 12-month-old include varicella and MMR (live vaccines), which are not administered to an immunocompromised child.
3. Recommended vaccines will not be administered because the child is immunocompromised.

4. The recommendation is for the child to receive routine immunizations unless the child is immunocompromised.

TEST-TAKING HINT: The test taker should know that families and patients who are HIV-positive should be taught ways to prevent infections, including the administration of immunizations.

10. 1. Airway, breathing, and circulation are part of the primary patient assessment. Neurological assessment is the next assessment to perform.
    2. The child has been diagnosed with encephalitis. Unless there is a concern about the child's having strep throat, a throat culture would not be obtained.
    3. **Initial and serial neurological assessments would be a priority nursing intervention in a child with a neurological problem. These assessments monitor for changes in neurological status.**
    4. Encephalitis is usually caused by a virus; therefore, antibiotics are not ordered. Antipyretics may be used to help control fevers.

TEST-TAKING HINT: The test taker should understand that the primary assessment includes ensuring patent airway, breathing, circulation, and intact neurological status. In a child with a neurological problem, continue monitoring for changes in neurological status.

11. 1, 3.
    1. **Cystic fibrosis is inherited as an autosomal-recessive trait, causing exocrine gland dysfunction. About 7% to 10% of newborns with cystic fibrosis present with meconium ileus, so assessing stool frequency and consistency is important.**
    2. Chest physical therapy would not be initiated in a newborn without a definitive diagnosis.
    3. **Assessing weight is important in newborns because they can lose up to 10% of their birth weight, and it can take up to 2 weeks for them to regain their birth weight.**
    4. The newborn would not be placed on fluid restriction even if diagnosed with cystic fibrosis.
    5. The newborn's respiratory system would be monitored as often as other infants if the newborn has no respiratory symptoms.

TEST-TAKING HINT: The test taker should understand that cystic fibrosis is inherited as an autosomal-recessive trait that causes exocrine gland dysfunction and affects the respiratory, gastrointestinal, and reproductive systems.

12. 1. PKU is inherited as an autosomal-recessive trait. The enzyme phenylalanine hydroxylase controlling the conversion of phenylalanine to tyrosine is missing. A low-phenylalanine diet is the treatment to prevent brain damage.
    2. PKU is inherited as an autosomal-recessive trait. The enzyme phenylalanine hydroxylase controlling the conversion of phenylalanine to tyrosine is missing. A low-phenylalanine diet is the treatment to prevent brain damage.
    3. **PKU is inherited as an autosomal-recessive trait. The enzyme phenylalanine hydroxylase controlling the conversion of phenylalanine to tyrosine is missing. A low-phenylalanine diet is the treatment to prevent brain damage.**
    4. Breast milk has low amounts of phenylalanine, so the mother can breastfeed as long as the infant's level of phenylalanine is monitored.

TEST-TAKING HINT: The test taker should understand that PKU is a genetic inherited autosomal-recessive trait caused by a missing enzyme. This enzyme is needed to metabolize the essential amino acid phenylalanine.

13. 1. PKU is a genetic autosomal-recessive inherited trait. Phenylalanine is an essential amino acid, which makes it impossible to remove totally from the diet. Treatment is a low-phenylalanine diet. Individuals do not outgrow PKU.
    2. **Many high-protein foods such as meats and dairy products are restricted or eliminated from the diet because of their high phenylalanine content.**
    3. High-protein foods such as meat and dairy products are restricted to small amounts or eliminated because of their high phenylalanine content.
    4. Breast milk contains PKU, and if the mother wanted to breastfeed, the infant would need careful monitoring of PKU levels.

TEST-TAKING HINT: The test taker should understand that PKU is a genetic autosomal-recessive inherited trait. Strict, lifelong dietary restrictions and monitoring are required. Diet management includes meeting the child's nutritional and growth needs while maintaining phenylalanine levels within a safe range.

14. 1. High-protein foods such as meats and dairy products are restricted because of their high phenylalanine content.
2. The sweetener aspartame (NutraSweet, Equal) should be avoided because it is converted to phenylalanine in the body.
3. Because of their high-protein content, dairy products are limited or eliminated from the diet.
4. **The artificial sweetener aspartame (NutraSweet, Equal) should be avoided because it is converted to phenylalanine in the body.**

TEST-TAKING HINT: The test taker should understand how PKU is treated to successfully answer this question.

15. 1. **Galactosemia is a rare autosomal-recessive disorder involving an inborn error of carbohydrate metabolism. The hepatic enzyme galactose-1-phosphate uridyl transferase is absent, causing the failure of galactose to be converted into glucose. Glucose builds up in the bloodstream, which can result in liver failure, cataracts, and renal tubular problems. Treatment of galactosemia involves eliminating all milk and lactose-containing foods, including breast milk and formulas.**
2. Galactosemia is a rare autosomal-recessive disorder involving an inborn error of carbohydrate metabolism and requires that all milk and lactose-containing foods, including breast milk and formulas, are eliminated.
3. Galactosemia is a rare autosomal-recessive disorder involving an inborn error of carbohydrate metabolism and requires that all milk and lactose-containing foods, including breast milk and formulas, be eliminated.
4. Galactosemia is a rare autosomal-recessive disorder involving an inborn error of carbohydrate metabolism and requires that all milk and lactose-containing foods, including breast milk and formulas, be eliminated. Soy protein is the preferred formula.

TEST-TAKING HINT: The test taker should understand that galactosemia is a rare autosomal-recessive disorder involving an inborn error of carbohydrate metabolism.

16. 1. Galactosemia is a rare genetic autosomal-recessive disorder involving an inborn error of carbohydrate metabolism that may affect future children.
2. Infants usually appear normal at birth, but within a few days of ingesting milk begin to vomit and lose weight.
3. Many drugs, such as penicillin, contain unlabeled lactose as filler and need to be avoided.
4. **Many drugs, such as penicillin, contain unlabeled lactose as filler and need to be avoided.**

TEST-TAKING HINT: The test taker should understand that galactosemia is a rare genetic autosomal-recessive disorder involving an inborn error of carbohydrate metabolism that may affect future children.

17. 1. Congenital hypothyroidism clinical manifestations may include bradycardia, constipation, poor feeding, lethargy, jaundice prolonged for more than 2 weeks, cyanosis, respiratory difficulties, hoarse cry, large anterior/posterior fontanels, post-term, birth weight greater than 4000 g.
2. **Congenital hypothyroidism clinical manifestations may include bradycardia, constipation, poor feeding, lethargy, jaundice prolonged for more than 2 weeks, cyanosis, respiratory difficulties, hoarse cry, large anterior/posterior fontanels, post-term, and birth weight greater than 4000 g.**
3. Having a high-pitched cry and being colicky and jittery usually indicate drug withdrawal or a neurological problem.
4. Congenital hypothyroidism clinical manifestations may include bradycardia, constipation, poor feeding, lethargy, jaundice prolonged for more than 2 weeks, cyanosis, respiratory difficulties, hoarse cry, large anterior/posterior fontanels, post-term, and birth weight greater than 4000 g.

TEST-TAKING HINT: The test taker needs to know clinical manifestations of hypothyroidism to answer this question.

18. 1. Macrosomia (large for gestational age) does not require genetic counseling.
2. Neonatal abstinence syndrome is a term used to describe a set of symptoms displayed by infants exposed to chemicals in utero.

3. Couples with planned abortions would not need genetic counseling unless there were genetic problems with children and/or adults in their families.
4. **Couples with a history of multiple miscarriages, stillbirths, or infertility should be referred for genetic counseling to try to determine the cause of their problems with maintaining a pregnancy.**

TEST-TAKING HINT: The test taker should understand that couples with multiple miscarriages, stillbirths, or infertility should be referred to genetic counseling to assist in a successful pregnancy.

19. 1. Tay-Sachs disease is a genetic disorder in which the infant has normal development for the first 6 months. After 6 months, developmental delays and neurological worsening occur. Dietary restriction or providing physical therapy does not change the outcome.
2. **Tay-Sachs disease is a genetic disorder in which the infant has normal development for the first 6 months. After 6 months, developmental delays and neurological worsening occur. Dietary restriction or providing physical therapy does not change the outcome.**
3. Tay-Sachs disease is a genetic disorder in which the infant has normal development for the first 6 months. After 6 months, developmental delays and neurological worsening occur. Dietary restriction or providing physical therapy does not change the outcome.
4. Tay-Sachs disease is a genetic disorder in which the infant has normal development for the first 6 months. After 6 months, developmental delays and neurological worsening occur. Dietary restriction or providing physical therapy does not change the outcome.

TEST-TAKING HINT: The test taker should understand that Tay-Sachs disease is a genetic disorder in which the infant dies in childhood.

20. 1. Maple syrup urine disease is a genetic inborn error of metabolism. It is a deficiency of decarboxylase, which is needed to degrade some amino acids. If left untreated, altered tone, seizures, and death can occur.
2. **A child with maple syrup urine disease will be on a low-protein, limited–amino acid diet for life. Patients need a diet high in thiamine.**

3. A child with maple syrup urine disease will be on a low-protein, limited–amino acid diet for life. Sodium is not restricted. Patients need a diet high in thiamine.
4. A child with maple syrup urine disease will be on a low-protein, limited–amino acid diet for life. Phenylalanine is not restricted. Patients need a diet high in thiamine.

TEST-TAKING HINT: Maple syrup urine disease is a genetic disorder with restricted branched-chain amino acids, for example, valine, leucine, and isoleucine.

21. 1. Varicella vaccine should be kept frozen in the lyophilized form. After reconstitution, the varicella vaccine should be given within 30 minutes to ensure viral potency. The five rights of patient medication should always be followed prior to administration.
2. **The varicella vaccine integrity cannot be assured if the vaccine is at room temperature, so do not administer.**
3. Varicella vaccine should be kept frozen in the lyophilized form. After reconstitution, the varicella vaccine should be given within 30 minutes to ensure viral potency. If the vaccine is not frozen, do not administer.
4. This is an important question to ask the mother but does not address the questions of the nurse finding the varicella vaccine at room temperature.

TEST-TAKING HINT: Varicella vaccine should be kept frozen in the lyophilized form. The vaccine diluents can be kept at room temperature.

22. 1. A common reaction to the DTaP vaccine is local swelling and redness at the injection site, which disappears in a few days. The nurse should not speak for the physician.
2. This local reaction is not considered an allergic reaction or an indication the child should not receive this immunization again.
3. The nurse is interpreting what the mother has stated to include refusal of all vaccines.
4. **This is the therapeutic response—discussing the mother's concerns about the immunizations and local reactions.**

TEST-TAKING HINT: The test taker needs to know common local reactions to immunizations.

23. 1. Written information about the vaccine should always be given prior to any immunization administered as well as allowing time for questions. Accurate documentation should always occur after immunizations are given.

2. **Written information about the vaccine should always be given prior to any immunization administered as well as allowing time for questions.**
3. Administer the most painful immunization last.
4. The word "shots" has a negative connotation to parents and should be avoided.

TEST-TAKING HINT: The test taker should understand that the vaccine information statement must be given and discussed with the parent before administering the vaccine.

24. 1. **The infant needs the Hib vaccine to ensure protection against many serious infections caused by Hib, such as bacterial meningitis, bacterial pneumonia, epiglottitis, septic arthritis, and sepsis.**
2. The infant needs the Hib vaccine to ensure protection against many serious infections caused by Hib, such as bacterial meningitis, bacterial pneumonia, epiglottitis, septic arthritis, and sepsis.
3. A nasal swab is used to diagnose a respiratory syncytial virus (RSV) infection, which is unrelated to a Hib infection.
4. A blood test does not diagnose previous Hib infection in a healthy child.

TEST-TAKING HINT: The test taker should understand that the Hib vaccine protects against serious infections.

25. 1. The option is to try to determine immunization status by contacting previous health-care providers for a record of vaccines received. If previous providers are unknown, then the child will receive recommended immunizations for age.
2. MMR, Hib, IPV, or hepatitis B vaccines would not routinely be due at this visit.
3. There are usually no harmful effects to a child with unknown immunization status if revaccinated.
4. **Vaccines routinely due at 15 months include Hib and DTaP. To catch up missed immunizations, the nurse would need the child's immunization record to verify what he has received.**

TEST-TAKING HINT: The test taker would need to know what to do when the child's immunization status is unknown.

26. 1. It's important to have diphenhydramine (Benadryl) available but not as important as having epinephrine.
2. Diphenhydramine (Benadryl) liquid is important to have available also, but it is not as important as having epinephrine available.

3. **Epinephrine 1 : 1000 injection would be the drug of choice for subcutaneous injection if a severe allergic reaction occurs in an office or clinic setting.**
4. Epinephrine 1 : 10,000 injection should be given intravenously only. Most children in a clinic or office setting receive immunizations during their well-child visit and do not have intravenous catheters in place for immediate access.

TEST-TAKING HINT: The test taker understands that in all offices and clinics offering immunizations, epinephrine is the most important medication to have on hand in the event of an allergic reaction. Epinephrine's usual dose is 0.01 mg/kg of 1 : 1000 subcutaneous solution.

27. 1. IPV does not contain live poliovirus, so the virus cannot be transmitted to the immunocompromised sibling.
2. The oral polio vaccine contains weakened poliovirus; rarely, the virus can be transmitted to someone immunocompromised. The virus is shed in the stool.
3. There is no need to isolate the sibling from the child receiving the inactive poliovirus vaccine because the virus cannot be transmitted.
4. **The infant should be immunized as recommended and will not shed the poliovirus.**

TEST-TAKING HINT: The test taker understands that household contacts and siblings of immunocompromised children are able to receive the IPV. They should not receive the oral poliovirus vaccine because there is a rare risk of vaccine-associated polio paralysis.

28. 1. The newborn should receive both hepatitis B vaccine and hepatitis B immune globulin within 12 hours of birth to prevent hepatitis B infection.
2. **The newborn should receive both hepatitis B vaccine and hepatitis B immune globulin within 12 hours of birth to prevent hepatitis B infection.**
3. The newborn should receive both hepatitis B vaccine and hepatitis B immune globulin within 12 hours of birth to prevent hepatitis B infection.
4. The newborn should receive both hepatitis B vaccine and hepatitis B immune globulin within 12 hours of birth to prevent hepatitis B infection.

TEST-TAKING HINT: The test taker should understand that infants born to mothers who test positive for hepatitis B antigen should receive hepatitis B vaccine and hepatitis B immune globulin within 12 hours of birth to prevent infection.

29. 1. There is a very small incidence of infants developing intussusception, signaled by the onset of bloody stool or diarrhea, after receiving oral rotovirus vaccine. Cough is not associated with this vaccine.
    2. This is an oral vaccine, not an injectable vaccine.
    3. **There is a very small incidence of infants developing intussusception, signaled by the onset of bloody stools or diarrhea after receiving oral rotavirus vaccine.**
    4. There is a very small incidence of infants developing intussusception, signaled by the onset of bloody stool or diarrhea after receiving oral rotavirus vaccine.

    TEST-TAKING HINT: The test taker should know potential adverse effects from the oral rotavirus vaccine.

30. 1. Infants born to mothers of unknown hepatitis B antigen status should be given the hepatitis B immune globulin and hepatitis B vaccine within 12 hours of birth.
    2. **Infants born to mothers of unknown hepatitis B antigen status should be given the hepatitis B immune globulin and hepatitis B vaccine within 12 hours of birth.**
    3. Infants born to mothers of unknown hepatitis B antigen status should be given the hepatitis B immune globulin and hepatitis B vaccine within 12 hours of birth.
    4. Infants born to mothers of unknown hepatitis B antigen status should be given the hepatitis B immune globulin and hepatitis B vaccine within 12 hours of birth.

    TEST-TAKING HINT: The test taker should understand that infants born to mothers with unknown hepatitis B antigen status should be given the hepatitis B immune globulin and hepatitis B vaccine within 12 hours of birth.

31. 1. The priority is to prevent the infant from rolling off a raised surface. Placing safety locks is done when the infant is a few months old.
    2. The infant should be transported in the middle of the back seat of the vehicle, which is considered the safest place.

3. **The highest priority in newborn injury prevention is never to leave the baby unattended on a raised, unguarded surface. Involuntary reflexes may cause the infant to move and fall.**
4. Placing safety guards is the priority when the infant is a few months old and mobile.

TEST-TAKING HINT: The test taker knows developmentally appropriate injury prevention and then discusses it with the parent.

32. 1. **Priority nursing intervention with pediatric trauma patients is airway assessment while maintaining cervical spine precautions. If the airway is compromised, immediate corrective action should be taken prior to assessment of breathing.**
    2. Assessing airway, breathing, and circulation will be done in that order, not simultaneously.
    3. Diagnostic radiological testing is done after the child is stabilized.
    4. Venous access and blood draws are done after airway, breathing, and circulation have been assessed.

    TEST-TAKING HINT: The test taker should understand that pediatric trauma patients can also have spinal cord injuries and what the priorities are in those situations.

33. 1. For the first 24 hours, rest, ice, compression, and elevation (RICE) are recommended for acute injury. The wrist should be kept immobile and elevated.
    2. The wrist should be kept immobile and elevated.
    3. **For the first 24 hours, rest, ice, compression, and elevation (RICE) are recommended for acute injury.**
    4. For the first 24 hours, rest, ice, compression, and elevation are recommended for acute injury.

    TEST-TAKING HINT: The test taker should remember the acronym RICE (rest, ice, compression, and elevation) or ICES (ice, compression, elevation, support).

34. 1. Neurovascular integrity should be assessed first and frequently because neurovascular compromise may cause serious consequences. Neurovascular integrity should be assessed using the 5 Ps: increased Pain out of proportion with injury, Pallor of extremity, Paresthesia, Pulselessness at distal part of extremity, and Paralysis post cast application. Cast integrity would be assessed, but neurovascular integrity is the highest priority.

2. **Neurovascular integrity should be assessed first and frequently because neurovascular compromise may cause serious consequences. Neurovascular integrity should be assessed using the 5 Ps: increased Pain out of proportion with injury, Pallor of extremity, Paresthesia, Pulselessness at distal part of extremity, and Paralysis post cast application.**

3. Neurovascular integrity should be assessed first and frequently because neurovascular compromise may cause serious consequences. Neurovascular integrity should be assessed using the 5 Ps: increased Pain out of proportion with injury, Pallor of extremity, Paresthesia, Pulselessness at distal part of extremity, and Paralysis post cast application. Musculoskeletal integrity would be assessed after neurovascular integrity.

4. Neurovascular integrity should be assessed first and frequently because neurovascular compromise may cause serious consequences. Neurovascular integrity should be assessed using the 5 Ps: increased Pain out of proportion with injury, Pallor of extremity, Paresthesia, Pulselessness at distal part of extremity, and Paralysis post cast application Soft tissue integrity is assessed last.

TEST-TAKING HINT: The test taker should understand that neurovascular integrity should be assessed first.

35. 1. **Adolescence is a time of need for independence and learning to make appropriate decisions. Safety is always a concern, and tying a safety discussion to the teen's interest in sports will help keep him safe. The nurse needs to inquire about and build on the teen's interests and knowledge.**

2. Lecturing to an adolescent would not be appropriate; the nurse needs to determine what the teen knows about safety measures for that sport and then build on that information.

3. Determining whether the teen drinks, smokes, or uses drugs and what he thinks about those activities is the first step. Lecturing is never appropriate.

4. The teen should be addressed directly.

TEST-TAKING HINT: The test taker should understand that age and developmentally appropriate injury prevention teachings are most effective.

36. 1. History of loss of consciousness and length of time unconscious is important information, but serial assessments give current information.

2. **Serial assessments of level of consciousness are the most important observations of a child after any injury. That information tells you if the child's condition is changing.**

3. Initial neurological assessments are important but provide only a baseline.

4. Initial vital signs and oxygen saturation level give a baseline and help when looking at serial assessments.

TEST-TAKING HINT: The test taker should understand that serial observations of the child's level of consciousness are the most important nursing observations.

37. 1. The head of the bed should be elevated to decrease intracranial pressure. Side rails should be up to help ensure the child stays in bed, and age-appropriate safety measures should be instituted.

2. **The head of the bed should be elevated to decrease intracranial pressure. Side rails should be up to help ensure the child stays in bed, and age-appropriate safety measures should be instituted.**

3. Drainage from the nose or ear would indicate more severe head injury and would be reported to the physician. The priority would be elevating the head of the bed to decrease intracranial pressure.

4. The child may sleep, but frequent assessments will be made, and the child will be awakened often.

TEST-TAKING HINT: The test taker should understand that the appropriate nursing intervention would be to elevate the head of the bed to decrease intracranial pressure.

38. 1. Any child who has had a near-drowning experience should be admitted for observation. Even if a child does not appear to have any injury from the event, complications can occur within 24 hours. Respiratory compromise and cerebral edema can be delayed complications.

2. A ventilation tube would not be inserted unless the child needs it as determined by blood gases, x-rays, and clinical picture.

3. Any child who has had a near-drowning experience should be admitted for observation. Even if a child does not appear to have any injury from the event, complications can occur within 24 hours. Respiratory compromise and cerebral edema can be delayed complications.

4. **Any child who has had a near-drowning experience should be admitted for observation. Even if a child does not appear to have any injury from the event, complications can occur within 24 hours after the event. Respiratory compromise and cerebral edema can be delayed complications.**

TEST-TAKING HINT: The test taker should understand that respiratory compromise and cerebral edema may occur 24 hours after near-drowning. This means that children with a near-drowning event should be admitted.

39. 1. Trauma to the eyes and surrounding structures is the leading cause of blindness in children. This incident would be considered blunt force trauma to the eyes, and the child should receive immediate medical attention.

2. **This type of eye injury is considered blunt force trauma to the eyes, and the child should be evaluated medically for assessment and prevention of eye damage. Slight blurring could indicate eye injuries, such as detached retina and hyphema, which need immediate medical intervention.**

3. This type of eye injury is considered blunt force trauma to the eyes, and the child should be evaluated medically for assessment and prevention of eye damage. Slight blurring could indicate eye injuries, such as detached retina and hyphema, which need immediate medical intervention.

4. This type of eye injury is considered blunt force trauma to the eyes, and the child should be evaluated medically for assessment and prevention of eye damage. Slight blurring could indicate eye injuries, such as detached retina and hyphema, which need immediate medical intervention.

TEST-TAKING HINT: The test taker should understand that trauma to the eyes and supporting structures are the leading cause of blindness in children.

40. 1. The teen may be at the developmental stage of seeking independence, but adolescents do not yet have the emotional or physical development to operate all-terrain vehicles. The American Academy of Pediatrics states that those younger than 16 years should not operate all-terrain vehicles. Wearing safety apparel is important in all sports.

2. The teen may be at the developmental stage of seeking independence, but adolescents do not yet have the emotional or physical development to operate all-terrain vehicles. The American Academy of Pediatrics states that those younger than 16 years should not operate all-terrain vehicles.

3. **The teen may be at the developmental stage of seeking independence, but adolescents do not yet have the emotional or physical development to operate all-terrain vehicles. The American Academy of Pediatrics states that those younger than 16 years should not operate all-terrain vehicles.**

4. The teen may be at the developmental stage of seeking independence, but adolescents do not yet have the emotional or physical development to operate all-terrain vehicles. The American Academy of Pediatrics states that those younger than 16 years should not operate all-terrain vehicles.

TEST-TAKING HINT: The test taker should understand that in early adolescence the teen does not have the physical or emotional development to handle all-terrain vehicles.

41. 1, 3.
1. **Washing and drying hands and face, especially before eating, decreases lead ingestion.**
2. Other measures can be taken to decrease ingestion of lead, such as washing hands and face before eating.
3. **Hot water absorbs lead more readily than cold water.**
4. Diet does matter; regular meals, adequate iron and calcium, and less fat help the child absorb less lead.
5. Drinking two cups of milk per day is important for children but does not help decrease lead levels.

TEST-TAKING HINT: The test taker should understand lead poisoning usually occurs with hand-to-mouth activity in toddlers.

42. 1. This is not the time to teach about childproofing the home. The parent will feel guilty, and anxiety would prevent the parent from remembering the advice.
2. **The most therapeutic approach is to inquire about the circumstances of the ingestion in a nonjudgmental manner.**
3. Ipecac is no longer recommended to be kept in the home because of the increasing number of medications where its use is contraindicated. All households should have the Poison Control number beside a telephone or on speed-dial.
4. Do not give the child an emetic medication unless instructed to do so by Poison Control or a health-care provider.

TEST-TAKING HINT: The test taker needs knowledge of therapeutic communication to answer this question.

43. 1. A battery is considered a corrosive poison, and medical attention should be sought.
2. Determining the time of ingestion is important, but treatment should be started when a battery is ingested.
3. **Batteries are considered corrosives; the child will be admitted, and surgery may be necessary for removal.**
4. This is not the time to discuss childproofing measures. The parent would be anxious and feel guilty about the ingestion.

TEST-TAKING HINT: The test taker should understand that a battery is considered a poison and that medical attention is required.

44. 1. Continuous cardiac monitoring would be the priority because of the bradycardia and dysrhythmias that can occur with digoxin toxicity. Oxygen may be needed if there is enough bradycardia to cause a decrease in oxygen saturation.
2. The priority is to establish continuous cardiac monitoring. If it is determined that venous access is necessary, then that can be established.
3. The digoxin level would be good to know, but that is not the priority.
4. **Bradycardia and cardiac dysrhythmias are common signs of digoxin toxicity in children. Continuous cardiac monitoring is the highest priority to detect dysrhythmias before they became lethal.**

TEST-TAKING HINT: The test taker should understand that bradycardia and cardiac dysrhythmia are common signs of digoxin toxicity in children.

45. 1. **Provide 100% oxygen via non-rebreather mask as quickly as possible if carbon monoxide poisoning is suspected because the signs and symptoms of carbon monoxide poisoning are related to tissue hypoxia.**
2. When carbon monoxide enters the blood, it readily combines with hemoglobin to form carboxyhemoglobin. Tissue hypoxia reaches dangerous levels because carbon monoxide does not release easily. Oxygen saturation obtained by oximetry will be normal because oxygen saturation monitoring does not measure dysfunctional hemoglobin.
3. The priority is to provide supplemental oxygen, then establish intravenous access.
4. Although a carbon monoxide level may be ordered, the highest priority nursing intervention is to administer oxygen.

TEST-TAKING HINT: The test taker should understand that 100% oxygen via non-rebreather mask is given as quickly as possible if carbon monoxide poisoning is suspected.

46. 1. **Developmentally appropriate anticipatory guidance for a 17-year-old is to discuss alcohol use and potential for alcohol poisoning.**
2. The development of secondary sex characteristics would be discussed with a younger adolescent.
3. Discussing their thoughts about anger management and safe sex would be initiated with younger teens.
4. Discussions about peer pressure would be done with younger teens when it is more prominent.

TEST-TAKING HINT: The test taker should understand that alcohol poisoning can occur with binge drinking and should be discussed during older adolescent well visits.

47. 1. Tell the child occasional use of acetaminophen (Tylenol) for aches and pains is recommended. Daily use can cause rebound so that when she stops taking the medication, her aches and pains will be worse. At this age, her parents should be involved in her over-the-counter drug use.
2. Too much acetaminophen (Tylenol) can cause liver damage; she should check with her parent before taking it.
3. Keeping a log can be helpful in determining what triggers her aches and pains. The priority would be to recommend that she not take pain medication daily.

4. **If she needs pain medication daily, a cause needs to be determined.**

TEST-TAKING HINT: The test taker needs to know what would be considered therapeutic management of the child's pain.

48. 1. Vomiting is contraindicated with this medication; the best advice is to call Poison Control first. Visine (topical sympathomimetic) can cause serious or fatal consequences if even a little is ingested.
   2. **Calling Poison Control is the first step for ingestion of any known or unknown substance. Visine (topical sympathomimetic) can cause serious or fatal consequences if even a little is ingested.**
   3. The parents of any child who has had an unintentional ingestion should be counseled to call Poison Control to determine treatment. Visine (topical sympathomimetic) can cause serious or fatal consequences if even a little is ingested.
   4. Overdoses are not treated with diluted milk unless indicated.

TEST-TAKING HINT: The test taker should understand that in cases of drug poisonings, Poison Control should be called immediately.

49. 1. Medications should never be called candy to prevent the accidental ingestion of medication by children who think it is candy.
   2. **Medications should never be called candy to prevent the accidental ingestion of medication by children who think it is candy.**
   3. This is one of those instances when the toddler has to do something he may not want to do.
   4. The medication has to be taken, and the toddler is not given an option. Going to "time-out" delays the administration of the medication.

TEST-TAKING HINT: The test taker should understand that medication should never be called candy to prevent accidental ingestion.

50. 1. Charcoal is odorless and tasteless, but the black color should be masked. Providing a movie is a good distraction but is not the best answer.
   2. Never tell a child that medicine is candy in order to prevent accidental overdose.
   3. **Mixing charcoal with a sweetening agent may help the child ingest it. Children usually like sweeter drinks. Hiding the black color in an opaque container with a lid may also make it more palatable.**

4. A parent can help by tasting the charcoal first, but getting the child to drink it quickly probably will not happen.

TEST-TAKING HINT: The test taker should understand that masking the taste and black color will make the activated charcoal more tolerable.

51. 1. Child abuse is intentional physical, emotional, and/or sexual abuse and/or neglect.
   2. Child abuse is intentional physical, emotional, and/or sexual abuse and/or neglect.
   3. Child abuse is intentional physical, emotional, and/or sexual abuse and/or neglect.
   4. **Child abuse is intentional physical, emotional, and/or sexual abuse and/or neglect.**

TEST-TAKING HINT: The test taker needs to know the definition.

52. 1. Genetic disorders can usually be explained by specific testing. Munchausen syndrome by proxy may be the cause of unexplained, prolonged, rare, recurrent illnesses. It usually occurs when the caregiver is present.
   2. **Munchausen syndrome by proxy may be the cause of unexplained, prolonged, rare, recurrent illnesses. It usually occurs when the caregiver is present.**
   3. Duchenne muscular dystrophy is a genetic disorder characterized by muscle weakness usually appearing in the third year of life.
   4. Syndrome of inappropriate antidiuretic hormone results from hypothalamic dysfunction and is not unexplained.

TEST-TAKING HINT: The test taker needs to know the definition of Munchausen syndrome by proxy or else eliminate other options and make an educated guess.

53. 1. Immediately asking, "Who did this?" is not therapeutic.
   2. Blaming the parents for not protecting the child is inappropriate.
   3. **When communicating with a child you think may have been abused, it is the most therapeutic to tell the child it is not the child's fault.**
   4. Someone has to be told; lying to the child is not appropriate or therapeutic.

TEST-TAKING HINT: The test taker should understand that if someone verbalizes abuse, therapeutic communication is extremely important to use.

54. 1. **The health-care provider's highest priority should be to try to get the child's history information from the parent.**
2. Assess the child for other signs of potential physical abuse after you have determined the child is stable. Children who are physically abused may have other injuries in various stages of healing.
3. Radiological studies will be ordered, but more information as to what may have caused the injury is important information to obtain.
4. Intravenous access and blood tests may not be indicated.

TEST-TAKING HINT: The test taker should understand that history information is very important in trying to determine the cause of the arm pain.

55. 1. Burns on both feet are more indicative of a child being held in hot water, thus indicating abuse.
2. Burns on the arm may or may not indicate abuse. History information is important to determine that.
3. **Physical abuse has certain characteristics. Symmetrical burns on both feet indicate abuse.**
4. Burns mainly on the right foot might indicate the child got into a tub of hot water and then got out without putting the other foot in, which would not indicate abuse.

TEST-TAKING HINT: The test taker should understand that physical signs suggestive of abuse are symmetrical burns with absence of splash marks.

56. 1. Masturbation is most common in 4-year-olds and during adolescence.
2. **Masturbation may indicate sexual abuse. It is imperative that the nurses do a thorough investigation if a parent is concerned about a child's masturbation.**
3. Talking with the child to find out why she is masturbating would be one component of a thorough investigation. Children do not have insight into their behaviors, however, so she may not be able to state why.
4. Masturbation may indicate sexual abuse. It is imperative that the nurse do a thorough investigation if a parent is concerned about a child's masturbation.

TEST-TAKING HINT: The test taker should understand that masturbation may indicate sexual abuse.

57. 1. Sexual exploration may be more prominent during this stage.
2. **Increased temper tantrums, increased sleep disorders, and depression may indicate sexual abuse.**
3. Children develop invisible friends about this time and this is a normal part of development.
4. Wanting to spend more time with a sibling is a part of normal development at this age.

TEST-TAKING HINT: The test taker should understand that increased temper tantrums, increased sleep disorders, and depression may indicate sexual abuse.

58. 2, 3.
1. The priority at this time is to ensure the child's safety. Coming to the school nurse may be a cry for help.
2. **The priority is the child's safety and asking about the arm bruises.**
3. **Her safety should be ensured first, then discuss physical complaints. School nurses are mandatory reporters of any suspected child abuse.**
4. Ensuring the child's safety is the highest priority when a health-care professional suspects child abuse.
5. Ensuring the child's safety is the highest priority when a health-care professional suspects child abuse.

TEST-TAKING HINT: Accurate assessment, description, and documentation should be recorded by the nurse. Child protective personnel should be notified of suspected abuse.

59. 1. Abused children frequently lie about their injuries from fear about what will happen to them.
2. **Abused children frequently repeat the same story that their parents tell.**
3. Changes in behavior may suggest abuse.
4. Children who are abused may become withdrawn and not participate in school activities.

TEST-TAKING HINT: The test taker should understand that abused children commonly repeat the same story that their parents tell to avoid being punished.

60. 1, 3, 4.
1. **There may be absence of external signs of injury in shaken baby syndrome because the injury can cause retinal hemorrhage and subdural hematoma.**
2. The baby crying often is not an indication of abuse.

3. Retinal hemorrhage is indicative of shaken baby syndrome in an infant without external signs of injury.
4. Subdural hematoma is indicative of shaken baby syndrome in an infant without external signs of injury.
5. Infants with shaken baby syndrome do not usually have signs of external head injury.

TEST-TAKING HINT: The test taker should understand that there may be an absence of external signs of injury in shaken baby syndrome.

61. 1. It would be most therapeutic to discuss with the mother and child the best foods to eat and to avoid on a renal diet. Bananas should be limited because of their high potassium content. Potassium is excreted in the urine.

2. It would be most therapeutic to discuss with the mother and child the best foods to eat and to avoid on a renal diet. Bananas should be limited because of their high potassium content.
3. Bananas are high in potassium, so the number consumed needs to be limited.
4. It would be most therapeutic to discuss with the mother and child the best foods to eat and to avoid on a renal diet. Bananas should be limited because of their high potassium content.

TEST-TAKING HINT: The test taker should know dietary restrictions for a child with chronic kidney disease.

Respiratory Disorders

5

KEYWORDS

The following words include English vocabulary, nursing/medical terminology, concepts, principles, or information relevant to content specifically addressed in the chapter or associated with topics presented in it. English dictionaries, your nursing textbooks, and medical dictionaries such as *Taber's Cyclopedic Medical Dictionary* are resources that can be used to expand your knowledge and understanding of these words and related information.

Albuterol

Antipyretic

Aspirated

Autosomal-dominant

Azotorrhea

Bradycardia

Bronchiectasis

Bronchoscopy

Constipation

Croup

Dysphagia

Edema

Epiglottitis

Eustachian tube

Fluticasone (Flovent)

Heimlich maneuver

Montelukast (Singulair)

Otitis media

Palivizumab (Synagis)

Pharyngitis

Polyethylene glycol 3350 (MiraLAX)

Prednisone

Steatorrhea

Stridor

Subglottic

Tachycardia

Tachypnea

Tonsillectomy

Tracheostomy

Trendelenburg position

Wheezing

ABBREVIATIONS

Arterial blood gas (ABG)

As needed (PRN)

Blood urea nitrogen (BUN)

Chest physiotherapy (CPT)

Complete blood count (CBC)

Cystic fibrosis (CF)

Emergency department (ED)

Hydrogen ion concentration (pH)

Laryngotracheobronchitis (LTB)

Metered dose inhaler (MDI)

Partial thromboplastin time (PTT)

Respiratory syncytial virus (RSV)

Upper respiratory infection (URI)

QUESTIONS

1. How does the nurse interpret the laboratory analysis of a stool sample containing excessive amounts of azotorrhea and steatorrhea in a child with cystic fibrosis (CF)? The values indicate the child is:
   1. Not compliant with taking her vitamins.
   2. Not compliant with taking her enzymes.
   3. Eating too many foods high in fat.
   4. Eating too many foods high in fiber.

2. Which would the nurse explain to parents about the inheritance of cystic fibrosis?
   1. CF is an autosomal-dominant trait passed on from the child's mother.
   2. CF is an autosomal-dominant trait passed on from the child's father.
   3. The child of parents who are both carriers of the gene for CF has a 50% chance of acquiring CF.
   4. The child of a mother who has CF and a father who is a carrier of the gene for CF has a 50% chance of acquiring CF.

3. The parent of a 4-month-old with cystic fibrosis (CF) asks the nurse what time to begin the child's first chest physiotherapy (CPT) each day. Which is the nurse's best response?
   1. "Thirty minutes before feeding the child breakfast."
   2. "After deep-suctioning the child each morning."
   3. "Thirty minutes after feeding the child breakfast."
   4. "Only when the child has congestion or coughing."

4. The parent of an infant with cystic fibrosis (CF) asks the nurse how to meet the child's increased nutritional needs. Which is the nurse's best suggestion?
   1. "You may need to increase the number of fresh fruits and vegetables you give your infant."
   2. "You may need to advance your infant's diet to whole cow's milk because it is higher in fat than formula."
   3. "You may need to change your infant to a higher-calorie formula."
   4. "You may need to increase your infant's carbohydrate intake."

5. The parent of a child with cystic fibrosis (CF) is excited about the possibility of the child receiving a double lung transplant. What should the parent understand?
   1. The transplant will cure the child of CF and allow the child to lead a long and healthy life.
   2. The transplant will not cure the child of CF but will allow the child to have a longer life.
   3. The transplant will help to reverse the multisystem damage that has been caused by CF.
   4. The transplant will be the child's only chance at surviving long enough to graduate from college.

6. A 2-year-old has just been diagnosed with cystic fibrosis (CF). The parents ask the nurse what early respiratory symptoms they should expect to see in their child. Which is the nurse's best response?
   1. "You can expect your child to develop a barrel-shaped chest."
   2. "You can expect your child to develop a chronic productive cough."
   3. "You can expect your child to develop bronchiectasis."
   4. "You can expect your child to develop wheezing respirations."

7. The parent of a child with cystic fibrosis (CF) asks the nurse what will be done to relieve the child's constipation. Which is the nurse's best response?
   1. "Your child likely has an obstruction and will require surgery."
   2. "Your child will likely be given IV fluids."
   3. "Your child will likely be given MiraLAX."
   4. "Your child will be placed on a clear liquid diet."

8. The parents of a 5-week-old have just been told that their child has cystic fibrosis (CF). The mother had a sister who died of CF when she was 19 years of age. The parents are sad and ask the nurse about their child's projected life expectancy. What is the nurse's best response?
   1. "The life expectancy for CF patients has improved significantly in recent years."
   2. "Your child might not follow the same course that the mother's sister did."
   3. "The health-care provider will come to speak to you about treatment options."
   4. The nurse answers their questions briefly, listens to their concerns, and is available later after they've processed the information.

9. A 7-month-old has a low-grade fever, nasal congestion, and a mild cough. What should the nursing care management of this child include? **Select all that apply.**
   1. Maintaining strict bedrest.
   2. Avoiding contact with family members.
   3. Instilling saline nose drops and bulb suctioning.
   4. Keeping the head of the bed flat.
   5. Providing humidity, and propping the head of the bed up.

10. A school-age child has been diagnosed with nasopharyngitis. The parent is concerned because the child has had little or no appetite for the last 24 hours. Which is the nurse's best response?
    1. "Do not be concerned; it is common for children to have a decreased appetite during a respiratory illness."
    2. "Be sure your child is taking an adequate amount of fluids. The appetite should return soon."
    3. "Try offering the child some favorite foods. Maybe that will improve the appetite."
    4. "You need to force your child to eat whatever you can; adequate nutrition is essential."

11. A child's parent asks the nurse what treatment the child will need for the diagnosis of strep throat. Which is the nurse's best response?
    1. "Your child will be sent home on bedrest and should recover in a few days without any intervention."
    2. "Your child will need to have the tonsils removed to prevent future strep infections."
    3. "Your child will need oral penicillin for 10 days and should feel better in a few days."
    4. "Your child will need to be admitted to the hospital for 5 days of intravenous antibiotics."

12. A child is complaining of throat pain. Which statement by the mother indicates that she needs more education regarding the care and treatment of her child's pharyngitis?
    1. "I will have my child gargle with salt water three times a day."
    2. "I will offer my child ice chips several times a day."
    3. "I will give my child Tylenol every 4 to 6 hours as needed."
    4. "I will ask the nurse practitioner for some amoxicillin."

13. A school-age child has been diagnosed with strep throat. The parent asks the nurse when the child can return to school. Which is the nurse's best response?
    1. "Forty-eight hours after the first documented normal temperature."
    2. "Twenty-four hours after the first dose of antibiotics."
    3. "Forty-eight hours after the first dose of antibiotics."
    4. "Twenty-four hours after the first documented normal temperature."

14. A school-age child is admitted to the hospital for a tonsillectomy. During the nurse's postoperative assessment, the child's parent tells the nurse that the child is in pain. Which of the following observations would be of most concern to the nurse?
    1. The child's heart rate and blood pressure are elevated.
    2. The child complains of having a sore throat.
    3. The child is refusing to eat solid foods.
    4. The child is swallowing excessively.

15. The nurse is reviewing discharge instructions with the parents of a child who had a tonsillectomy a few hours ago. The parents tell the nurse that the child is a big eater, and they want to know what foods to give the child for the next 24 hours. What is the nurse's best response?
    1. "The child's diet should not be restricted at all."
    2. "The child's diet should be restricted to clear liquids."
    3. "The child's diet should be restricted to ice cream and cold liquids."
    4. "The child's diet should be restricted to soft foods."

16. Which laboratory result will provide the most important information regarding the respiratory status of a child with an acute asthma exacerbation?
    1. CBC.
    2. ABG.
    3. BUN.
    4. PTT.

17. What is the most important piece of information that the nurse must ask the parent of a child in status asthmaticus?
    1. "What time did your child eat last?"
    2. "Has your child been exposed to any of the usual asthma triggers?"
    3. "When was your child last admitted to the hospital for asthma?"
    4. "When was your child's last dose of medication?"

18. Which is the nurse's best response to parents who ask what impact asthma will have on the child's future in sports?
    1. "As long as your child takes prescribed asthma medication, the child will be fine."
    2. "The earlier a child is diagnosed with asthma, the more significant the symptoms."
    3. "The earlier a child is diagnosed with asthma, the better the chance the child has of growing out of the disease."
    4. "Your child should avoid playing contact sports and sports that require a lot of running."

19. Which statement by the parent of a child using an albuterol inhaler leads the nurse to believe that further education is needed on how to administer the medication?
    1. "I should administer two quick puffs of the albuterol inhaler using a spacer."
    2. "I should always use a spacer when administering the albuterol inhaler."
    3. "I should be sure that my child is in an upright position when administering the inhaler."
    4. "I should always shake the inhaler before administering a dose."

20. Which should the nurse administer to provide quick relief to a child with asthma who is coughing, wheezing, and having difficulty catching her breath?
    1. Prednisone.
    2. Montelukast (Singulair).
    3. Albuterol.
    4. Fluticasone (Flovent).

21. Which child with asthma should the nurse see first?
    1. A 12-month-old who has a mild cry, is pale in color, has diminished breath sounds, and has an oxygen saturation of 93%.
    2. A 5-year-old who is speaking in complete sentences, is pink in color, is wheezing bilaterally, and has an oxygen saturation of 93%.
    3. A 9-year-old who is quiet, is pale in color, and is wheezing bilaterally with an oxygen saturation of 92%.
    4. A 16-year-old who is speaking in short sentences, is wheezing, is sitting upright, and has an oxygen saturation of 93%.

22. Which breathing exercises should the nurse have an asthmatic 3-year-old child do to increase her expiratory phase?
    1. Use an incentive spirometer.
    2. Breathe into a paper bag.
    3. Blow a pinwheel.
    4. Take several deep breaths.

23. The parents of a 6-year-old who has a new diagnosis of asthma ask the nurse what to do to make their home a more allergy-free environment. Which is the nurse's best response?
    1. "Use a humidifier in your child's room."
    2. "Have your carpet cleaned chemically once a month."
    3. "Wash household pets weekly."
    4. "Avoid purchasing upholstered furniture."

24. A parent asks how to care for a child at home who has the diagnosis of viral tonsillitis. Which is the nurse's best response?
    1. "You will need to give your child a prescribed antibiotic for 10 days."
    2. "You will need to schedule a follow-up appointment in 2 weeks."
    3. "You can give your child acetaminophen (Tylenol) every 4 to 6 hours as needed for pain."
    4. "You can place warm towels around your child's neck for comfort."

25. Which would be an early sign of respiratory distress in a 2-month-old?
    1. Breathing shallowly.
    2. Tachypnea.
    3. Tachycardia.
    4. Bradycardia.

26. Which would be appropriate nursing care management of a child with the diagnosis of mononucleosis?
    1. Only family visitors.
    2. Bedrest.
    3. Clear liquids.
    4. Limited daily fluid intake.

27. Which should the nurse instruct children to do to stop the spread of influenza in the classroom? **Select all that apply.**
    1. Stay home if they have a runny nose and cough.
    2. Wash their hands after using the restroom.
    3. Wash their hands after sneezing.
    4. Have a flu shot annually.
    5. Drink lots of water during the day.

28. Who is at the highest priority to receive the flu vaccine?
    1. A healthy 8-month-old who attends day care.
    2. A 3-year-old who is undergoing chemotherapy.
    3. A healthy 7-year-old who attends public school.
    4. An 18-year-old who is living in a college dormitory.

29. The parent of a child with influenza asks the nurse when the child is most
    infectious. Which is the nurse's best response?
    1. "Twenty-four hours before and after the onset of symptoms."
    2. "Twenty-four hours after the onset of symptoms."
    3. "One week after the onset of symptoms."
    4. "One week before the onset of symptoms."

30. A 6-week-old is admitted to the hospital with influenza. The child is crying, and the
    father tells the nurse that his son is hungry. The nurse explains that the baby is not
    to have anything by mouth. The parent does not understand why the child cannot
    eat. Which is the nurse's best response to the parent?
    1. "We are giving your child intravenous fluids, so there is no need for anything by
       mouth."
    2. "The shorter and narrower airway of infants increases their chances of aspiration
       so your child should not have anything to eat now."
    3. "When your child eats, he burns too many calories; we want to conserve the
       child's energy."
    4. "Your child has too much nasal congestion; if we feed the child by mouth, the
       distress will likely increase."

31. Which statement by the parents of a toddler with repeated otitis media indicates
    they need additional teaching?
    1. "If I quit smoking, my child may have a decreased chance of getting an ear
       infection."
    2. "As my child gets older, he should have fewer ear infections, because his immune
       system will be more developed."
    3. "My child will have fewer ear infections if he has his tonsils removed."
    4. "My child may need a speech evaluation."

32. Which is the nurse's best response to a parent who asks what can be done at home
    to help an infant with upper respiratory infection (URI) symptoms and a fever get
    better?
    1. "Give your child small amounts of fluid every hour to prevent dehydration."
    2. "Give your child Robitussin at night to reduce his cough and help him sleep."
    3. "Give your child a baby aspirin every 4 to 6 hours to help reduce the fever."
    4. "Give your child an over-the-counter cold medicine at night."

33. Which should be included in instructions to the parent of a child prescribed
    amoxicillin to treat an ear infection?
    1. "Continue the amoxicillin until the child's symptoms subside."
    2. "Administer an over-the-counter antihistamine with the antibiotic."
    3. "Administer the amoxicillin until all the medication is gone."
    4. "Allow your child to administer his own dose of amoxicillin."

34. The parent of a child with frequent ear infections asks the nurse if there is anything
    that can be done to help avoid future ear infections. Which is the nurse's best
    response?
    1. "Your child should be put on a daily dose of montelukast (Singulair)."
    2. "Your child should be kept away from tobacco smoke."
    3. "Your child should be kept away from other children with otitis media."
    4. "Your child should always wear a hat when outside in the cold."

35. Which child would benefit most from having ear tubes placed? **Select all that apply.**
    1. A 9-month-old who has had one ear infection.
    2. A 13-month old with recurrent ear infections.
    3. A 2-year-old who has had five previous ear infections.
    4. A 3-year-old whose sibling has had four ear infections.
    5. A 7-year-old who has had two ear infections this year.

36. Which is the nurse's best response to the parent of an infant diagnosed with the first otitis media who wonders about long-term effects?
    1. "The child could suffer hearing loss."
    2. "The child could suffer some speech delays."
    3. "The child could suffer recurrent ear infections."
    4. "The child could require ear tubes."

37. An infant is not sleeping well, is crying frequently, has yellow drainage from the ear, and is diagnosed with an ear infection. Which nursing objective is the priority for the family?
    1. Educating the parents about signs and symptoms of an ear infection.
    2. Providing emotional support for the parents.
    3. Providing pain relief for the child.
    4. Promoting the flow of drainage from the ear.

38. A parent asks the nurse how it will be determined whether their child has respiratory syncytial virus (RSV). Which is the nurse's best response?
    1. "We will do a simple blood test to determine whether your child has RSV."
    2. "There is no specific test for RSV. The diagnosis is made based on the child's symptoms."
    3. "We will swab your child's nose and send that specimen for testing."
    4. "We will have to send a viral culture to an outside lab for testing."

39. Which statement indicates the parent needs further teaching on how to prevent his other children from contracting respiratory syncytial virus (RSV)?
    1. "I should make sure that both my children receive palivizumab (Synagis) injections for the remainder of this year."
    2. "I should be sure to keep my infected child away from his brother until he has recovered."
    3. "I should insist that all people who come in contact with my children thoroughly wash their hands before playing with them."
    4. "I should insist that anyone with a respiratory illness avoid contact with my children until well."

40. Which child is at highest risk for requiring hospitalization to treat respiratory syncytial virus (RSV)?
    1. A 2-month-old who was born at 32 weeks.
    2. A 16-month-old with a tracheostomy.
    3. A 3-year-old with a congenital heart defect.
    4. A 4-year-old who was born at 30 weeks.

41. Which physical findings would be of most concern in an infant with respiratory distress?
    1. Tachypnea.
    2. Mild retractions.
    3. Wheezing.
    4. Grunting.

42. How will a child with respiratory distress and stridor who is diagnosed with RSV be treated?
    1. Intravenous antibiotics.
    2. Intravenous steroids.
    3. Nebulized racemic epinephrine.
    4. Alternating doses of acetaminophen (Tylenol) and ibuprofen (Motrin).

43. What would the nurse advise the parent of a child with a barky cough that gets worse at night?
    1. Take the child outside into the more humid night air for 15 minutes.
    2. Take the child to the ED immediately.
    3. Give the child an over-the-counter cough suppressant.
    4. Give the child warm liquids to soothe the throat.

44. Which child is in the greatest need of emergency medical treatment?
    1. A 3-year-old who has a barky cough, is afebrile, and has mild intercostal retractions.
    2. A 6-year-old who has high fever, no spontaneous cough, and frog-like croaking.
    3. A 7-year-old who has abrupt onset of moderate respiratory distress, a mild fever, and a barky cough.
    4. A 13-year-old who has a high fever, stridor, and purulent secretions.

45. What information should the nurse provide the parent of a child diagnosed with nasopharyngitis?
    1. Complete the entire prescription of antibiotics.
    2. Avoid sending the child to day care.
    3. Use comfort measures for the child.
    4. Restrict the child to clear liquids for 24 hours.

46. Which assessment is of greatest concern in a 15-month-old?
    1. The child is lying down and has moderate retractions, low-grade fever, and nasal congestion.
    2. The child is in the tripod position and has diminished breath sounds and a muffled cough.
    3. The child is sitting up and has coarse breath sounds, coughing, and fussiness.
    4. The child is restless and crying, has bilateral wheezes, and is feeding poorly.

47. Which is diagnostic for epiglottitis?
    1. Blood test.
    2. Throat swab.
    3. Lateral neck x-ray of the soft tissue.
    4. Signs and symptoms.

48. What should be the nurse's first action with a child who has a high fever, dysphagia, drooling, tachycardia, and tachypnea?
    1. Immediate IV placement.
    2. Immediate respiratory treatment.
    3. Thorough physical assessment.
    4. Lateral neck radiographs.

49. Which is the nurse's best response to the parent of a child diagnosed with epiglottitis who asks what the treatment will be?
    1. Complete a course of intravenous antibiotics.
    2. Surgery to remove the tonsils.
    3. 10 days of aerosolized ribavirin.
    4. No intervention.

50. A mother is crying and tells the nurse that she should have brought her son in yesterday when he said his throat was sore. Which is the nurse's best response to this parent whose child is diagnosed with epiglottitis and is in severe distress and in need of intubation?
    1. "Children this age rarely get epiglottitis; you should not blame yourself."
    2. "It is always better to have your child evaluated at the first sign of illness rather than wait until symptoms worsen."
    3. "Epiglottitis is slowly progressive, so early intervention may have decreased the extent of your son's symptoms."
    4. "Epiglottitis is rapidly progressive; you could not have predicted his symptoms would worsen so quickly."

51. The parent of a child with croup tells the nurse that her other child just had croup and it cleared up in a couple of days without intervention. She asks the nurse why this child is exhibiting worse symptoms and needs to be hospitalized. Which is the nurse's best response?
    1. "Some children just react differently to viruses. It is best to treat each child as an individual."
    2. "Younger children have wider airways that make it easier for bacteria to enter and colonize."
    3. "Younger children have short and wide eustachian tubes, making them more susceptible to respiratory infections."
    4. "Children younger than 3 years usually exhibit worse symptoms because their immune systems are not as developed."

52. A 5-year-old is brought to the ED with a temperature of 99.5°F (37.5°C), a barky cough, stridor, and hoarseness. Which nursing intervention should the nurse prepare for?
    1. Immediate IV placement.
    2. Respiratory treatment of racemic epinephrine.
    3. A tracheostomy set at the bedside.
    4. Informing the child's parents about a tonsillectomy.

53. Which intervention is most appropriate to teach the mother of a child diagnosed with a URI and a dry, hacking cough that prevents him from sleeping?
    1. Give cough suppressants at night.
    2. Give an expectorant every 4 hours.
    3. Give cold and flu medication every 8 hours.
    4. Give ½ teaspoon of honey four to five times per day.

54. Which statement about pneumonia is accurate?
    1. Pneumonia is most frequently caused by bacterial agents.
    2. Children with bacterial pneumonia are usually sicker than children with viral pneumonia.
    3. Children with viral pneumonia are usually sicker than those with bacterial pneumonia.
    4. Children with viral pneumonia must be treated with a complete course of antibiotics.

55. Which child diagnosed with pneumonia would benefit most from hospitalization?
    1. A 13-year-old who is coughing, has coarse breath sounds, and is not sleeping well.
    2. A 14-year-old with a fever of 38.6°C (101.5°F), rapid breathing, and a decreased appetite.
    3. A 15-year-old who has been vomiting for 3 days and has a fever of 38.5°C (101.3°F).
    4. A 16-year-old who has a cough, chills, fever of 38.5°C (101.3°F), and wheezing.

56. Which position would be most comfortable for a child with left-sided pneumonia?
1. Trendelenburg.
2. Left side.
3. Right side.
4. Supine.

57. A child with severe cerebral palsy is admitted to the hospital with aspiration pneumonia. What is the most beneficial educational information that the nurse can provide to the parents?
1. The signs and symptoms of aspiration pneumonia.
2. The treatment plan for aspiration pneumonia.
3. The risks associated with recurrent aspiration pneumonia.
4. The prevention of aspiration pneumonia.

58. A 3-year-old is brought to the ED with coughing and gagging. The parent reports that the child was eating carrots when she began to gag. Which diagnostic evaluation will be used to determine whether the child has aspirated carrots?
1. Chest x-ray.
2. Bronchoscopy.
3. Arterial blood gas (ABG).
4. Sputum culture.

59. The parent of a 9-month-old calls the ED because his child is choking on a marble. The parent asks how to help his child while awaiting Emergency Medical Services. Which is the nurse's best response?
1. "You should administer five abdominal thrusts followed by five back blows."
2. "You should try to retrieve the object by inserting your finger in your child's mouth."
3. "You should perform the Heimlich maneuver."
4. "You should administer five back blows followed by five chest thrusts."

60. Which information will be most helpful in teaching parents about the primary prevention of foreign body aspiration?
1. Signs and symptoms of foreign body aspiration.
2. Therapeutic management of foreign body aspiration.
3. Most common objects that toddlers aspirate.
4. Risks associated with foreign body aspiration.

61. What does the therapeutic management of cystic fibrosis (CF) patients include?
Select all that apply.
1. Providing a high-protein, high-calorie diet.
2. Providing a high-fat, high-carbohydrate diet.
3. Encouraging exercise.
4. Minimizing pulmonary complications.
5. Encouraging medication compliance.

62. A chloride level greater than _____ is a positive diagnostic indicator of cystic fibrosis (CF).

ANSWERS AND RATIONALES

The correct answer number and rationale for why it is the correct answer are given in **boldface blue type.** Rationales for why the other possible answer options are incorrect also are given, but they are not in boldface type.

1. 1. The child's compliance with vitamins would not be reflected in a laboratory result of azotorrhea and steatorrhea. If the client were not taking daily vitamin supplements, there might be a deficiency in those vitamins.
   2. **If the child were not taking enzymes, the result would be a large amount of undigested food, azotorrhea, and steatorrhea in the stool. Pancreatic ducts in CF clients become clogged with thick mucus that blocks the flow of digestive enzymes from the pancreas to the duodenum. Therefore, clients must take digestive enzymes with all meals and snacks to aid in absorption of nutrients. Often, teens are noncompliant with their medication regimen because they want to be like their peers.**
   3. Steatorrhea is an increased amount of fat in the stool. However, in CF patients, it is not a result of eating too many fatty foods.
   4. Azotorrhea is an increased amount of protein in the stool. Steatorrhea is an increased amount of fat in the stool. Neither is a result of eating too many foods high in fiber.

   TEST-TAKING HINT: The test taker needs to understand the pathophysiology of CF and the impact it has on the gastrointestinal system. The test taker also must be familiar with the conditions azotorrhea and steatorrhea.

2. 1. CF is inherited as an autosomal-recessive trait. Both parents must be carriers of the gene in order for their child to inherit the disease. If both parents are carriers of the CF gene, each child they have has a 25% chance of acquiring the disease and a 50% chance of being a carrier of the disease. If a child is born to a parent with CF and the other parent is a carrier, the child has a 50% chance of acquiring the disease and a 50% chance of being a carrier of the disease.
   2. CF is inherited as an autosomal-recessive trait. Both parents must be carriers of the gene in order for their child to inherit the gene. If a child is born to parents who are both carriers of the CF gene, the child has a 25% chance of acquiring the disease and a 50% chance of being a carrier of the disease. If the child is born to a parent with CF and the other parent is a carrier, the child has a 50% chance of acquiring the disease and a 50% chance of being a carrier of the disease.
   3. If a child is born to parents who are both carriers of the CF gene, the child has a 25% chance of acquiring the disease and a 50% chance of being a carrier of the disease.
   4. **If the child is born to a parent with CF and the other parent is a carrier, the child has a 50% chance of acquiring the disease and a 50% chance of being a carrier of the disease.**

   TEST-TAKING HINT: Answers 1 and 2 can be eliminated with knowledge of the genetic inheritance of CF. CF is inherited as an autosomal-recessive trait.

3. 1. **CPT should be done in the morning prior to feeding to avoid the risk of the child vomiting.**
   2. Infants with CF are not routinely deep-suctioned. Occasionally, if they have a weak cough reflex, infants may be suctioned following CPT to stimulate them to cough.
   3. If CPT is done following feeding, it increases the likelihood that the child may vomit.
   4. CPT should be done as a daily regimen with all CF patients. CPT helps to break up the secretions in the lungs and makes it easier for the patient to clear those secretions.

   TEST-TAKING HINT: Answer 4 can be eliminated because of the word "only." There are very few times in health care when an answer will be "only." Answer 3 can be eliminated when one considers the risk of vomiting and aspiration that may occur if percussion is performed following eating.

4. 1. Children with CF have difficulty absorbing nutrients because of the blockage of the pancreatic duct. Pancreatic enzymes cannot reach the duodenum to aid in digestion of food. These children often require up to 150% of the caloric intake of their peers. The nutritional recommendation for CF patients is high-calorie and high-protein.
2. Whole cow's milk is a good source of fat but is not an increased source of protein that is recommended for CF patients. Another consideration here is that whole cow's milk is not recommended until 12 months of age.
3. **Often infants with CF need to have a higher-calorie formula to meet their nutritional needs. Infants may also be placed on hydrolysate formulas that contain medium-chain triglycerides.**
4. An increase in carbohydrate intake is not usually necessary. The nutritional recommendation for CF patients is high-calorie and high-protein.

TEST-TAKING HINT: Answers 1, 2, and 4 can be eliminated with understanding of the nutritional needs of the child with CF. Answer 2 can also be eliminated because whole cow's milk is not recommended until 12 months of age.

5. 1. A lung transplant does not cure CF, but the transplanted lungs do not contain the CF genes. Although the new lungs do not contain CF, the sinuses, pancreas, intestines, sweat glands, and reproductive tract do. The new lungs are more susceptible to infection because of the immunosuppressive therapy that must be given post-transplant. Immunosuppressive drugs make it difficult for the body to fight infection, which can lead to lung damage.
2. **A lung transplant does not cure CF, but it does offer the client an opportunity to live a longer life. The concerns are that, after the lung transplant, the child is at risk for rejection of the new organ and for development of secondary infections because of the immunosuppressive therapy.**
3. The lung transplant does not reverse the damage that has been done to the child's other organs, but it does offer a chance of a longer life.
4. The average life span of a client with CF has risen over the years with the daily regimens of CPT, exercise, medications, and high-calorie, high-protein diets.

TEST-TAKING HINT: Answer 4 can be eliminated because of the word "only." There are very few times in health care when an answer will be "only." Answers 1 and 3 can be eliminated if the test taker has a basic knowledge of the pathophysiology of CF.

6. 1. A barrel-shaped chest is a long-term respiratory problem that occurs as a result of recurrent hyperinflation of alveoli.
2. A chronic productive cough is common as pulmonary damage increases.
3. Bronchiectasis develops in advanced stages of CF.
4. **Wheezing respirations and a dry, nonproductive cough are common early symptoms in CF.**

TEST-TAKING HINT: Answer 2 can be eliminated because of the word "chronic." "Chronic" implies that the disease process is advanced rather than in the initial stages. Answers 1 and 3 can be eliminated if the test taker has knowledge of signs and symptoms of advanced lung disease.

7. 1. CF clients who present with constipation usually do not require surgery. They commonly receive a stool softener or an osmotic solution orally to relieve their constipation.
2. IV fluids may be ordered if the client is NPO for any reason. However, IV fluids do not help relieve the client's constipation. CF clients with constipation commonly receive a stool softener or an osmotic solution orally to relieve their constipation.
3. **CF clients with constipation commonly receive a stool softener or an osmotic solution such as polyethylene glycol 3350 (MiraLAX) orally to relieve their constipation.**
4. CF clients are not placed on a clear liquid diet to relieve the constipation. CF clients with constipation commonly receive a stool softener or an osmotic solution orally to relieve their constipation. Once the constipation is relieved, the client will likely be placed on a low-fat diet and a stool softener.

TEST-TAKING HINT: Answers 1 and 2 can be eliminated because surgery and IV fluids are not indicated for constipation.

8. 1. The parents are devastated by the new diagnosis and are likely not ready to hear about the current life expectancy for CF patients. They are in shock and are trying to deal with the new diagnosis, so any additional information will just add to their stress level.
   2. The mother had a negative experience with CF in her own family and will likely continue to focus on her past experience with the disease. It may be more effective to give her time to consider her child's diagnosis and present her with information about current treatments and life span in a few days.
   3. Having the health-care provider return with additional information will not help these parents at this time. They need time before they are given additional information.
   4. **The nurse's best intervention is to listen as the parents express their concerns and fears. The nurse's answers should be brief, knowing that the parents are not able to process information right now. The nurse should be available later if the parents have any other concerns or questions or if they just need someone with whom to talk.**

   TEST-TAKING HINT: When parents are given information that their child has a chronic life-threatening disease, they are not capable of processing all the information right away; they need time. Parents are routinely given more information than they can possibly understand and often just need someone to listen to their concerns and needs.

9. 3, 5.
   1. Strict bedrest is not necessary. Children with respiratory illnesses usually self-limit their activity. Parents just need to ensure that their children are getting adequate rest.
   2. It is not necessary to avoid contact with family members. Nasopharyngitis is spread by contact with the secretions, so hand washing is the key to limiting the spread of the virus.
   3. **Infants are nose breathers and often have increased difficulty when they are congested. Nasal saline drops and gentle suctioning with a bulb syringe are often recommended.**
   4. The head of the bed should be elevated in order to help with the drainage of secretions.

5. **Other helpful suggestions for infants with colds are to provide humidity with a cool mist humidifier or take them into a steamy bathroom; in addition, raising the head of the bed helps with drainage of secretions.**

TEST-TAKING HINT: The test taker can eliminate answer 4 given a basic understanding of interventions to improve respiratory function.

10. 1. It is common for children to have a decreased appetite when they have a respiratory illness. However, the nurse needs to instruct the parent to offer fluids to ensure the child stays hydrated.
   2. **It is common for children to have a decreased appetite when they have a respiratory illness. The nurse is appropriately instructing the parent that the child will be fine by taking in an adequate amount of fluid which will keep the child hydrated.**
   3. The child may want to eat some favorite foods; however, the child will be fine if an adequate amount of fluid is maintained.
   4. The parent should not force the child to eat; the child's appetite should return in a couple of days.

TEST-TAKING HINT: Answer 4 can be eliminated because one should not force the child to eat. If the word "encourage" had been used, answer 4 would have been a better choice, although still not the best answer. Answer 1 can be eliminated because the nurse did not inform the parent of the importance of maintaining adequate fluid intake.

11. 1. The child may need bedrest. However, the child does need antibiotics to treat the strep infection.
   2. The child does not need the tonsils removed; the child has strep throat. Surgical removal of the tonsils is done only following recurrent bouts of infection.
   3. **The child will need a 10-day course of penicillin/amoxicillin to treat the strep infection. It is essential that the nurse always tell the family that, although the child will feel better in a few days, the entire course of antibiotics must be completed.**
   4. Strep throat can be treated at home with oral penicillin/amoxicillin and does not require IV antibiotics and hospitalization.

TEST-TAKING HINT: Answer 2 can be eliminated because it is a treatment for recurrent tonsillitis, not strep throat. Answer 1 can be eliminated if the test taker understands that bacterial infections need to be treated with antibiotics.

12. 1. Gargling with warm salt water is a recommended treatment to relieve some of the discomfort associated with pharyngitis.
    2. Encouraging ice chips is a recommended treatment to relieve some of the discomfort associated with pharyngitis.
    3. Acetaminophen (Tylenol) is a suggested treatment for relief of discomfort related to pharyngitis.
    4. **Pharyngitis is a self-limiting viral illness that does not require antibiotic therapy. Pharyngitis should be treated with rest and comfort measures, including acetaminophen (Tylenol), throat sprays, cold liquids, and Popsicles.**

TEST-TAKING HINT: Answers 1, 2, and 3 are comfort measures. The question requires that the student have knowledge regarding pharyngitis.

13. 1. School systems require that children remain home for 24 hours after having a documented fever. However, in this question the child has been diagnosed with strep throat. Even if the child is fever-free, the child must have completed a 24-hour course of antibiotics before returning to school. Children with strep throat are no longer contagious 24 hours after initiation of antibiotic therapy.
    2. **Children with strep throat are no longer contagious 24 hours after initiation of antibiotic therapy.**
    3. Children with strep throat are no longer contagious 24 hours after initiation of antibiotic therapy.
    4. School systems require that children remain home for 24 hours after having a documented fever. However, in this question the child has been diagnosed with strep throat. Even if the child is fever-free, the child must have completed a 24-hour course of antibiotics before returning to school. Children with strep throat are no longer contagious 24 hours after initiation of antibiotic therapy.

TEST-TAKING HINT: The test taker can eliminate answers 1 and 4 given knowledge of the communicability of strep throat.

14. 1. The patient is complaining of pain so it is not unusual that there is an elevated heart rate and blood pressure. The nurse should address the pain by giving any PRN pain medications ordered or calling the health-care provider for an order.
    2. Most children will complain after a tonsillectomy. This is expected.
    3. Oral intake is usually limited to Popsicles, ice chips, and cold liquids following a tonsillectomy. The child is in pain and should not be expected to be eating solid foods 8 hours after surgery.
    4. **Excessive swallowing is a sign that the child is swallowing blood. This should be considered a medical emergency, and the health-care provider should be contacted immediately. The child is likely bleeding and will need to return to surgery.**

TEST-TAKING HINT: Answer 1 can be eliminated if the test taker understands the common vital-sign changes that occur when a person is experiencing pain.

15. 1. A child should be restricted to soft foods for the first couple of days postoperatively. Soft foods are recommended because the child will have a sore throat for several days following surgery. Soft foods will decrease the risk of bleeding.
    2. Most children self-limit their food intake postoperatively. Children can have solids, but soft foods are recommended for the first several postoperative days.
    3. Most children prefer to eat cold foods, but they are not restricted to them.
    4. **Soft foods are recommended to limit the child's pain and to decrease the risk for bleeding.**

TEST-TAKING HINT: The test taker can eliminate answer 1 by knowing there are usually some dietary restrictions following any surgical procedure.

16. 1. The CBC gives the health-care team information about the child's red and white blood cell count and hemoglobin and hematocrit levels. The CBC indicates if the child has or is developing an infection, but it reveals nothing about the child's current respiratory status.
    2. **The ABG gives the health-care team valuable information about the child's respiratory status: level of oxygenation, carbon dioxide, and blood pH.**

3. The BUN provides information about the patient's kidney function, but it reveals nothing regarding the patient's respiratory status.
4. The PTT provides information about how long it takes the patient's blood to clot, but it reveals nothing about the patient's respiratory status.

TEST-TAKING HINT: The test taker can eliminate answers 1, 3, and 4 with a knowledge of common laboratory tests.

17. 1. The nurse needs to know when the child ate last in the event that the child may need to be intubated for severe respiratory distress, but it is not the most vital piece of information to best treat the child for the current state of distress.
    2. The nurse needs to know if the child was exposed to anything that usually triggers the asthma, but that is not the most important information for treating the child's immediate need.
    3. Knowing when the child was admitted last will give the nurse an idea of the severity of the child's asthma, but that is not the most important information for treating the child's immediate need.
    4. **The nurse needs to know what medication the child had last and when the child took it in order to know how to begin treatment for the current asthmatic condition.**

TEST-TAKING HINT: Whereas all of the information here is essential, answer 4 gives the most important information. The test taker can eliminate answers 2 and 3 because the responses to these inquiries have no direct impact on the immediate treatment of the child. These two answers give information about the severity of the child's illness, but they do not affect the immediate treatment plan. Answer 4 is essential to deciding what medication should be given the child to relieve the current symptoms.

18. 1. It is essential that the child take all of the scheduled asthma medications, but there is no guarantee the child will be fine and be able to play all sports.
    2. **When a child is diagnosed with asthma at an early age, the child is more likely to have significant symptoms on aging.**
    3. Children diagnosed at an early age usually exhibit worse symptoms than those diagnosed later in life.

4. Children with asthma are encouraged to participate in sports.

TEST-TAKING HINT: The test taker can eliminate answer 4 because not all asthmatics also have exercise-induced asthma.

19. 1. **The parent of an asthmatic child should always give one puff at a time and wait 1 minute before administering the second puff.**
    2. A spacer is recommended when administering medications by metered dose inhaler (MDI) to children.
    3. The child should be in an upright position when medications are administered by MDI.
    4. The inhaler should always be shaken before administering a dose of the medication.

TEST-TAKING HINT: The test taker evaluates how the parents administer the MDI.

20. 1. Prednisone, a corticosteroid, is often given to children with asthma, but it is not a quick-relief medication. The prednisone will take time to relieve the child's symptoms.
    2. Montelukast (Singulair) is an allergy medication that should be taken daily by asthmatics with significant allergies. Allergens are often triggers for asthmatics, so treating the child for allergies can help avoid an asthma attack. Montelukast (Singulair), however, does not help a child immediately with the symptoms of a particular asthma attack.
    3. **Albuterol is the quick-relief bronchodilator of choice for treating an asthma attack.**
    4. Fluticasone (Flovent) is a long-term therapy medication for asthmatics and is used daily to help prevent asthma attacks.

TEST-TAKING HINT: The test taker must know the medications used to treat asthma and which ones are used in which situations.

21. 1. **This child is exhibiting signs of severe asthma. This child should be seen first. The child no longer has wheezes and now has diminished breath sounds.**
    2. This child is exhibiting symptoms of mild asthma and should not be seen before the other children.
    3. This child is exhibiting signs of moderate asthma and should be watched but is not the patient of highest priority.
    4. This child is exhibiting signs of moderate asthma and is not the patient of highest priority.

TEST-TAKING HINT: The test taker can eliminate answers 2, 3, and 4 by knowing that diminished breath sounds are a sign the patient has a worsening condition. The other bit of information that is essential in this problem is the child's age. The younger the child, the faster the respiratory status can diminish.

22. 1. A child of 3 years old is too young to comply with incentive spirometry, and this activity won't increase the expiratory phase anyway.
    2. Breathing into a paper bag results in a prolonged inspiratory and expiratory phase.
    3. **Blowing a pinwheel is an excellent means of increasing a child's expiratory phase. Play is an effective means of engaging a child in therapeutic activities. Blowing bubbles is another method to increase the child's expiratory phase.**
    4. Taking deep breaths results in a prolonged inspiratory phase.

    TEST-TAKING HINT: The test taker can eliminate answers 1 and 4 because they do not increase the expiratory phase. Play is one of the best ways to engage young children in therapeutic activities.

23. 1. It is better to maintain 30% to 50% humidity in homes of asthmatic children. However, humidifiers are not recommended because they can harbor mold if they are not cleaned properly.
    2. Chemical cleaning is not recommended because the chemicals used can be a trigger and actually cause the child to have an asthma attack. The best recommendation is to remove all carpet from the house, if possible.
    3. Household pets are not recommended for children with asthma.
    4. **Leather furniture is recommended rather than upholstered furniture. Upholstered furniture can harbor large amounts of dust, whereas leather furniture may be wiped off regularly with a damp cloth.**

    TEST-TAKING HINT: The test taker can eliminate answer 3 because there is no known way to make a pet allergy-free. Household pets are discouraged for all children with asthma or severe allergies. Answer 2 can be eliminated if the test taker understands that chemical agents are triggers to asthma for many children.

24. 1. A viral illness does not require antibiotics. The patient would need to complete a course of antibiotics for bacterial tonsillitis.
    2. Viral tonsillitis is usually a self-limiting disease and does not require a follow-up appointment unless the child's symptoms worsen.
    3. **Acetaminophen (Tylenol) is recommended PRN for pain relief.**
    4. Warm compresses to the neck are not recommended, as they may in fact increase the inflammation. Cold compresses or ice packs are recommended for comfort.

    TEST-TAKING HINT: The test taker can eliminate answer 1 by knowing that antibiotics are not given for viral illnesses. Answer 4 can be eliminated by knowing that swelling and inflammation increase with heat. Cold causes vasoconstriction of the vessels, aiding in decreasing the amount of inflammation.

25. 1. Shallow breathing is a late sign of respiratory distress.
    2. **Tachypnea is an early sign of distress and is often the first sign of respiratory illness in infants.**
    3. Tachycardia is a compensatory response by the body. When a child has respiratory distress and is not oxygenating well, the body increases the heart rate in an attempt to improve oxygenation.
    4. Bradycardia is a late sign of respiratory distress.

    TEST-TAKING HINT: The test taker must know the early and late signs and symptoms of respiratory distress and be able to recognize them.

26. 1. **Children with mononucleosis are more susceptible to secondary infections. Therefore, they should be limited to visitors within the family, especially during the acute phase of illness.**
    2. Children with mononucleosis do not need to be on bedrest. Children usually self-limit their activities.
    3. Children with mononucleosis do not need a restricted diet. Often, they are very tired and are not interested in eating. The nurse and family must ensure that the children are taking in adequate nutrition.
    4. Children with mononucleosis usually have decreased appetite, but it is essential that they remain hydrated. There is no reason to restrict fluid intake.

TEST-TAKING HINT: The test taker can eliminate answers 2 and 3 by understanding mononucleosis. Children with mononucleosis are usually very tired, are not interested in engaging in vigorous activity, and are rarely interested in eating.

27. **2, 3.**
    1. Children do not need to stay home unless they have a fever. However, the children should be taught to cough or sneeze into their elbow and to wash their hands after sneezing or coughing.
    2. **Children should always wash their hands after using the restroom. In order to decrease the spread of influenza, however, it is more important for the children to wash their hands after sneezing or coughing.**
    3. **It is essential that children wash their hands after any contact with nasopharyngeal secretions.**
    4. Children should have a flu shot annually, but that information is best included in an educational session for the parents. There is little that children can do directly to ensure they receive flu shots. Children of this age are often frightened of shots and would not likely pass that information on to their parents.
    5. Drinking lots of water will keep the child hydrated but not stop the spread of influenza.

TEST-TAKING HINT: Answers 1 and 4 can be eliminated because both situations are under parental control.

28. 1. **Children between the ages of 6 and 23 months are at the highest risk for having complications as a result of the flu. Their immune systems are not as developed, so they are at a higher risk for influenza-related hospitalizations.**
    2. The flu vaccine should not be given to anyone who is immunocompromised.
    3. The flu vaccine is recommended for all ages, but the 7-year-old is not the highest priority. A child this age will likely recover without any complications.
    4. The flu vaccine is recommended for all ages, but the 18-year-old is not the highest priority. A person this age will likely recover without any complications.

TEST-TAKING HINT: The test taker can eliminate answers 2 and 3 by knowing that infants and the elderly are at highest risk for complications related to the flu.

29. 1. **Influenza is most contagious 24 hours before and 24 hours after onset of symptoms.**
    2. Influenza is most contagious 24 hours before and 24 hours after onset of symptoms.
    3. Influenza is most contagious 24 hours before and 24 hours after onset of symptoms.
    4. Influenza is most contagious 24 hours before and 24 hours after onset of symptoms.

TEST-TAKING HINT: This question requires the test taker to have knowledge of the communicability of influenza.

30. 1. The child is receiving intravenous fluids, so he is being hydrated. However, this response does not explain to the father why his son cannot eat.
    2. **Infants are at higher risk of aspiration because their airways are shorter and narrower than those of adults. An infant with influenza has lots of nasal secretions and coughs up mucus. With all the secretions, the infant is at an even higher risk of aspiration.**
    3. Eating burns calories, but if the baby is upset and crying, he is also expending energy. Therefore, this is not the best answer choice.
    4. If the child has nasal congestion, that may make it difficult for him to feed. However, the recommendation to parents is to bulb-suction an infant with nasal congestion before feeding.

TEST-TAKING HINT: The test taker can eliminate answer 1 because it does not give the father an explanation of why his son cannot eat.

31. 1. Repeated exposure to smoke damages the cilia in the ear, making the child more prone to ear infections.
    2. Children experience fewer ear infections as they age because their immune system is maturing.
    3. **Removing children's tonsils may not have any effect on their ear infections. Children who have repeated bouts of tonsillitis can have ear infections secondary to the tonsillitis, but there is no indication in this question that the child has a problem with tonsillitis.**
    4. Children who have repeated ear infections are at a higher risk of having decreased hearing during and between infections. Hearing loss directly affects a child's speech development.

TEST-TAKING HINT: The test taker can eliminate answers 1, 2, and 4 because those options are true.

32. 1. **It is essential that parents ensure their children remain hydrated during a URI. The best way to accomplish this is by giving small amounts of fluid frequently.**
    2. Over-the-counter cough and cold medicine is not recommended for any child younger than 6 years.
    3. Aspirin is not given to children to treat a viral infection because of the risk of developing Reye syndrome.
    4. Over-the-counter cough and cold medicine is not recommended for any child younger than 6 years.

    TEST-TAKING HINT: The test taker can eliminate answers 2 and 4 because over-the-counter cold and cough medications are not recommended for infants.

33. 1. The parent should administer all of the medication. Stopping the medication when symptoms subside may not clear up the ear infection and may actually cause more severe symptoms.
    2. Antihistamines have not been shown to decrease the number of ear infections a child gets.
    3. **It is essential that all the medication be given.**
    4. The child is old enough to participate in the administration of medication but should do so only in the presence of the parents.

    TEST-TAKING HINT: Answer 1 can be eliminated because a course of antibiotics should always be completed as ordered, no matter what the age of the child. Answer 4 can be eliminated because children would not be expected to administer their own medications without supervision by an adult.

34. 1. Montelukast (Singulair) is an allergy medication, but it has not been proved to help reduce the number of ear infections in children.
    2. **Tobacco smoke has been proved to increase the incidence of ear infections. The tobacco smoke damages mucociliary function, prolonging the inflammatory process and impeding drainage through the eustachian tube.**
    3. Otitis media is not transmitted from one child to another. Otitis is often preceded by a URI, so children who are around other children with URIs may contract one, increasing their chances of developing an ear infection.
    4. Wearing a hat outside will have no impact on whether a child contracts an ear infection.

    TEST-TAKING HINT: The test taker can eliminate answer 3 by understanding that otitis media is not a contagious disease process. Answer 4 can be eliminated if the test taker understands that otitis media is not caused by exposing the child to cold air.

35. **2, 3.**
    1. Surgical intervention is not a first line of treatment. Surgery is usually reserved for children who have suffered from recurrent ear infections.
    2. **A child with recurrent ear infections is a candidate for ear tubes.**
    3. **A 2-year-old who has had multiple ear infections is a perfect candidate for ear tubes. The other issue is that a 2-year-old is at the height of language development, which can be adversely affected by recurrent ear infections because they can interfere with hearing.**
    4. Surgery is not a prophylactic treatment. Just because the sibling has had several ear infections does not suggest that the 3-year-old will also have frequent ear infections. The 3-year-old has not had an ear infection yet.
    5. A 7-year-old who has had two ear infections is not the appropriate candidate. Surgical intervention is usually reserved for children who have suffered from recurrent ear infections.

    TEST-TAKING HINT: The test taker must also consider the developmental level of the child in this question. The 13-month-old and 2-year-old have had multiple infections and are also at a stage when language development is essential. If these children are not hearing appropriately, speech will also be delayed. Surgical intervention is reserved for those who have had recurrent infections.

36. 1. Hearing loss is not an issue that would be discussed following one ear infection. Children with recurrent untreated ear infections are more likely to develop hearing loss.
    2. Speech delays are not an issue that would be discussed following one ear infection. Children with recurrent untreated ear infections are more likely to develop some hearing loss, which often results in delayed language development.
    3. **When children acquire an ear infection at such a young age, there is an increased risk of recurrent infections.**

4. Surgical intervention is not a first line of treatment. Surgery is usually reserved for children who have suffered from recurrent ear infections.

TEST-TAKING HINT: Answers 1, 2, and 4 can be eliminated if the test taker understands that these are all long-term effects of recurrent ear infections. The question is asking about a single incident of otitis.

37. 1. It is important to educate the family about the signs and symptoms of an ear infection, but that is not the priority at this time. The infant has already been diagnosed with the infection.
2. The parents may need emotional support because they are likely suffering from a lack of sleep because their infant is ill. However, this will not solve their current problems with their infant.
3. **Providing pain relief for the infant is essential. With pain relief, the child will likely stop crying and rest better, as will the parents.**
4. Promoting drainage flow from the ear is important, but providing pain relief is the highest priority.

TEST-TAKING HINT: The test taker needs to consider the needs of the child and the parent at this time. If the pain is controlled, the parents and child will both be in a better state. The other items are all essential in providing care for the child with otitis, but pain relief offers the best opportunity for the child and the parent to return to normal conditions.

38. 1. RSV is not diagnosed by a blood test.
2. Nasal secretions are tested to determine whether a child has RSV.
3. **The child is swabbed for nasal secretions. The secretions are tested to determine whether a child has RSV.**
4. Viral cultures are not done very often because it takes several days to receive results. The culture does not have to be sent to an outside laboratory for evaluation.

TEST-TAKING HINT: The test taker can eliminate answers 1, 2, and 4 because the child's nasal secretions will be swabbed.

39. 1. **Palivizumab (Synagis) will not help the child who has already contracted the illness. Palivizumab (Synagis) is an immunization and a method of primary prevention.**

2. RSV is spread through direct contact with respiratory secretions, so it is a good idea to keep the ill child away from the healthy one.
3. RSV is spread through direct contact with respiratory secretions, so it is a good idea to have all persons coming in contact with the child wash their hands.
4. RSV is spread through direct contact with respiratory secretions, so it is a good idea to have ill persons avoid any contact with the children until they are well.

TEST-TAKING HINT: This question requires the test taker to understand how RSV is transmitted and how to prevent the spread of the virus.

40. 1. **The younger the child, the greater the risk for developing complications related to RSV. This infant is at highest risk because of age and premature status.**
2. This child has a tracheostomy, but this is not an indication that the child cannot be managed at home.
3. Most children with RSV can be managed at home. Children 2 years and younger are at highest risk for developing complications related to RSV. Children who were born prematurely, have cardiac conditions, or have chronic lung disease are also at higher risk for needing hospitalization. The 3-year-old with a congenital heart disease is not the highest risk among this group of patients.
4. Children who were born prematurely, have cardiac conditions, or have chronic lung disease are at a higher risk for needing hospitalization. This child was a premature infant but is now 4 years of age.

TEST-TAKING HINT: The test taker must consider that all of these children have some amount of risk for requiring hospitalization. The 2-month-old has two of the noted risk factors of being premature and a very young infant.

41. 1. Tachypnea, an increase in respiratory rate, should be monitored but is a common symptom of respiratory distress.
2. Retractions should be monitored; they can occur with respiratory distress.
3. Wheezing should be monitored and can occur with respiratory distress.
4. **Grunting is a sign of impending respiratory failure and is a very concerning physical finding.**

TEST-TAKING HINT: The test taker can eliminate answers 1, 2, and 3 by knowing the signs of respiratory distress. They warrant frequent respiratory assessment, but they are not the most concerning physical signs.

42. 1. RSV is a viral illness and is not treated with antibiotics.
    2. Steroids are not used to treat RSV.
    3. **Racemic epinephrine promotes mucosal vasoconstriction.**
    4. Acetaminophen (Tylenol) and ibuprofen (Motrin) can be given to the child for comfort, but they do not improve the child's respiratory status.

TEST-TAKING HINT: This is a knowledge-level question that requires the test taker to know how RSV is treated.

43. 1. **The humid night air will help decrease subglottic edema, easing the child's respiratory effort. The coughing should diminish significantly, and the child should be able to rest comfortably. If the symptoms do not improve after taking the child outside, the parent should have the child seen by a health-care provider.**
    2. There is no immediate need to bring the child to the ED. The child's symptoms will likely improve on the drive to the hospital because of the child's exposure to the night air.
    3. Over-the-counter cough suppressants are not recommended for children because they reduce their ability to clear secretions.
    4. Warm liquids may increase subglottic edema and actually aggravate the child's symptoms. Cool liquid or a Popsicle is the best choice.

TEST-TAKING HINT: The test taker must accurately identify that the question is describing a child with croup and know how croup is treated.

44. 1. This child has signs and symptoms of acute laryngitis and is not in a significant amount of distress.
    2. **This child has signs and symptoms of epiglottitis and should receive immediate emergency medical treatment. The patient has no spontaneous cough and has a frog-like croaking because of a significant airway obstruction.**
    3. This child has signs and symptoms of LTB and is not in significant respiratory distress.

4. This child has signs and symptoms of bacterial tracheitis and should be treated with antibiotics but is not the patient in the most significant amount of distress.

TEST-TAKING HINT: The test taker must accurately identify that the question is describing a child with epiglottitis. The test taker must also understand that epiglottitis is a pediatric emergency and can cause the child to have complete airway obstruction.

45. 1. Nasopharyngitis is a viral illness and does not require antibiotic therapy.
    2. Children who attend day care are more prone to catching viral illnesses, but it is not the nurse's place to tell the parents not to send their child to day care. Often families do not have a choice about using day care.
    3. **Nursing care for nasopharyngitis is primarily supportive. Keeping the child comfortable during the course of the illness is all the parents can do. Nasal congestion can be relieved using normal saline drops and bulb suction. Acetaminophen (Tylenol) can also be given for discomfort or a mild fever.**
    4. There is no reason to restrict the child to clear liquids. Many children have a decreased appetite during a respiratory illness, so the most important thing is to keep them hydrated.

TEST-TAKING HINT: This question requires the test taker to understand the cause of and treatment for nasopharyngitis.

46. 1. Retractions indicate some degree of respiratory distress but more information needs to be obtained. Other common symptoms of a respiratory illness, including low-grade fever and nasal congestion, are not overly concerning.
    2. **When children are sitting in the tripod position, they are having difficulty breathing. The child is sitting and leaning forward in order to breathe more easily. Diminished breath sounds are indicative of a worsening condition. A muffled cough indicates that the child has some subglottic edema. This child has several signs and symptoms of a worsening respiratory condition.**
    3. Coarse breath sounds, cough, and fussiness are common signs and symptoms of a respiratory illness.
    4. Restlessness, wheezes, poor feeding, and crying are signs and symptoms of a respiratory illness.

TEST-TAKING HINT: The test taker can eliminate answers 1, 3, and 4 if familiar with common signs and symptoms of respiratory illness.

47. 1. A blood test does not provide a diagnosis of epiglottitis. A CBC may show an increased white blood cell count, indicating the child has some sort of infection.
    2. A throat culture is not done to diagnose epiglottitis. It is contraindicated to insert anything into the mouth or throat of any child who is suspected of having epiglottitis. Inserting anything into the throat could cause the child to have a complete airway obstruction.
    3. **A lateral neck x-ray is a definitive test to diagnose epiglottitis. The child is at risk for complete airway obstruction and should always be accompanied by a nurse to the x-ray department.**
    4. Epiglottitis is not diagnosed based on signs and symptoms. A lateral neck film makes the diagnosis.

    TEST-TAKING HINT: The test taker can eliminate answers 1, 2, and 4 because epiglottitis is diagnosed by lateral neck films.

48. 1. This child is exhibiting signs and symptoms of epiglottitis and should be kept as comfortable as possible. Agitating the child may cause increased airway swelling and may lead to complete obstruction.
    2. Respiratory treatments often frighten children. This child is exhibiting signs and symptoms of epiglottitis and should be kept as comfortable as possible. Agitating the child may cause increased airway swelling and may lead to complete obstruction.
    3. This child is exhibiting signs and symptoms of epiglottitis and should be kept as comfortable as possible. Agitating the child may cause increased airway swelling and may lead to complete obstruction. The child should be allowed to remain on the parent's lap and be kept as comfortable as possible until a lateral neck film is obtained.
    4. **This child is exhibiting signs and symptoms of epiglottitis and should be kept as comfortable as possible. The child should be allowed to remain in the parent's lap until a lateral neck film is obtained for a definitive diagnosis.**

TEST-TAKING HINT: The test taker must accurately identify that the question is describing a child with epiglottitis and understand that agitation in this child can result in complete airway obstruction.

49. 1. **Epiglottitis is bacterial in nature and requires intravenous antibiotics. A 7- to 10-day course of oral antibiotics is usually ordered following the intravenous course of antibiotics.**
    2. Surgery is not the course of treatment for epiglottitis. Epiglottal swelling usually diminishes after 24 hours of intravenous antibiotics.
    3. Ribavirin is an antiviral medication used to treat RSV.
    4. Epiglottitis is a bacterial infection; a course of intravenous antibiotics is indicated.

    TEST-TAKING HINT: Understanding that epiglottitis is bacterial in nature will lead the test taker to choose the correct answer.

50. 1. Epiglottitis is most common in children from 2 to 5 years of age. The onset is very rapid. Telling parents not to blame themselves is not effective. Parents tend to blame themselves for their child's illnesses even though they are not responsible.
    2. The nurse should not tell the parent to seek medical attention for any and all signs of illness.
    3. Epiglottitis is rapidly progressive and cannot be predicted.
    4. **Epiglottitis is rapidly progressive and cannot be predicted.**

    TEST-TAKING HINT: When something happens to a child, the parents always blame themselves. Telling them epiglottitis is rapidly progressive may be helpful.

51. 1. All children should be treated as individuals when they are being treated for a particular illness. However, most children exhibit similar symptoms when they have the same diagnosis. Younger children have worse symptoms than older children because their immune systems are less developed.
    2. Children have airways that are shorter and narrower than those of adults. As children age, their airways begin to grow in length and diameter.
    3. Children are more prone to ear infections because they have eustachian tubes that are short and wide and lie in a horizontal plane.
    4. **Younger children have less developed immune systems and usually exhibit worse symptoms than older children.**

TEST-TAKING HINT: Answer 1 can be eliminated because it does not directly address the mother's question. Answer 2 can be eliminated if the test taker has knowledge of the anatomical structure of a child's airway. Answer 3 can be eliminated because the eustachian tubes have no direct relationship to acquiring croup.

52. 1. The child is exhibiting signs and symptoms of croup and is in mild respiratory distress.
    2. **The child has stridor, indicating airway edema, which can be relieved by aerosolized racemic epinephrine.**
    3. A tracheostomy is not indicated for this child. A tracheostomy would be indicated for a child with a complete airway obstruction.
    4. This child is exhibiting signs and symptoms of croup and has no indication of tonsillitis. A tonsillectomy is usually reserved for children who have recurrent tonsillitis.

TEST-TAKING HINT: The test taker must accurately identify that the question is describing a child with croup and know the accepted treatments.

53. 1. Cough suppressants are not recommended for children. Coughing is a protective mechanism, so do not try to stop it.
    2. Expectorants are not recommended for children younger than 6 years of age. There is no research information that they are effective.
    3. Cold and flu medications are not indicated for children younger than 6 years of age as there is no indication they are effective.
    4. **Warm fluids, humidification, and honey are the best treatments for a URI. But honey is not used in children less than 1 year of age because of the association with botulism.**

TEST-TAKING HINT: The latest recommendations for treatment of URIs in children are to treat the symptoms because cough medications are not effective.

54. 1. Pneumonia is most frequently caused by viruses but can also be caused by bacteria such as *Streptococcus pneumoniae*.
    2. **Children with bacterial pneumonia are usually sicker than children with viral pneumonia. Children with bacterial pneumonia can be treated effectively, but they require a course of antibiotics.**
    3. Children with viral pneumonia are not usually as ill as those with bacterial pneumonia. Treatment for viral pneumonia includes maintaining adequate oxygenation and comfort measures.
    4. Treatment for viral pneumonia includes maintaining adequate oxygenation and comfort measures.

TEST-TAKING HINT: The test taker must have an understanding of the differences between viral and bacterial infections.

55. 1. These are all common symptoms of pneumonia and should be monitored but do not require hospitalization. Most people with pneumonia are treated at home, with a focus on treating the symptoms and keeping the patient comfortable. Comfort measures include cool mist, chest physiotherapy (CPT), antipyretics, fluid intake, and family support.
    2. These are all common symptoms of pneumonia and should be monitored but do not require hospitalization.
    3. **The teen who has been vomiting for several days and is unable to tolerate oral fluids and medication should be admitted for intravenous hydration.**
    4. These are all common symptoms of pneumonia and should be monitored but do not require hospitalization.

TEST-TAKING HINT: The test taker can eliminate answers 1, 2, and 4 if familiar with the common signs and symptoms of pneumonia.

56. 1. The Trendelenburg position is not effective for improving respiratory effort. Patients with pneumonia are usually most comfortable in a semi-erect position.
    2. **Lying on the left side may provide the patient with the most comfort. Lying on the left splints the chest and reduces the pleural rubbing.**
    3. It is most comfortable for the patient to lie on the affected side. Lying on the left splints the chest and reduces the pleural rubbing.
    4. Lying in the supine position does not provide comfort for the patient and does not improve the child's respiratory effort.

TEST-TAKING HINT: The test taker can eliminate answers 1 and 4 because neither of them would improve the child's respiratory effort. Both these positions may actually cause the patient increased respiratory distress.

57. 1. The nurse should teach the parents about the signs and symptoms of aspiration pneumonia. The most valuable information relates to preventing aspiration pneumonia from occurring in the future.

2. The nurse should instruct the parents on the treatment plan of aspiration pneumonia, but that is not the most beneficial piece of information the nurse can provide. The most valuable information relates to preventing aspiration pneumonia from occurring in the future.

3. The nurse should instruct the parents on the risks associated with recurrent aspiration pneumonia, but that is not the most beneficial piece of information the nurse can provide. The most valuable information relates to preventing aspiration pneumonia from occurring in the future.

4. **The most valuable information the nurse can give the parents is how to prevent aspiration pneumonia from occurring in the future.**

TEST-TAKING HINT: The test taker can eliminate answers 1, 2, and 3 because they are all forms of tertiary prevention. Primary prevention is key to maximizing this child's function.

58. 1. A chest x-ray will only show radiopaque items (items that x-rays cannot go through easily), so it is not helpful in determining whether the child aspirated a carrot.

    2. **A bronchoscopy will allow the physician to visualize the airway and will help determine whether the child aspirated the carrot.**

    3. A blood gas will identify whether the child has suffered any respiratory compromise, but the ABG cannot definitively determine the cause of the compromise.

    4. A sputum culture may be helpful several days later to determine whether the child has developed aspiration pneumonia. Aspiration pneumonia may take several days or a week to develop following aspiration.

TEST-TAKING HINT: Answer 1 can be eliminated because items that are not radiopaque (opaque to x-rays) cannot be seen on an x-ray. Answers 3 and 4 can be eliminated because they do not provide confirmation regarding whether the child aspirated.

59. 1. Abdominal thrusts are not recommended for children younger than 1 year.

    2. Inserting a finger in the child's mouth may cause the object to be pushed further down the airway, making it more difficult to remove.

    3. The Heimlich maneuver should be performed only on adults.

4. **The current recommendation for infants younger than 1 year is to administer five back blows followed by five chest thrusts.**

TEST-TAKING HINT: The test taker can eliminate answers 1, 2, and 3 if familiar with CPR/BLS in infants and children.

60. 1. Teaching the parents signs and symptoms of foreign body aspiration is important, but it is a tertiary means of prevention and will not help the parents prevent the aspiration.

    2. Teaching the parents the therapeutic management of foreign body aspiration is important, but it is a tertiary means of prevention and will not help the parents prevent the aspiration.

    3. **Teaching parents the most common objects aspirated by toddlers will help them the most. Parents can avoid having those items in the household or in locations where toddlers may have access to them.**

    4. Teaching the parents the risks associated with foreign body aspiration is important, but it is a tertiary means of prevention and will not help the parents prevent the aspiration.

TEST-TAKING HINT: The test taker can eliminate answers 1, 2, and 4 because they are all forms of tertiary prevention. Primary prevention is key to preventing foreign body aspiration.

61. 1, 3, 4, 5.

    1. **Children with CF have difficulty absorbing nutrients because of the blockage of the pancreatic duct. Pancreatic enzymes cannot reach the duodenum to aid in digestion of food. These children often require up to 150% of the caloric intake of their peers. The nutritional recommendation for CF patients is high-calorie and high-protein.**

    2. A high-fat, high-carbohydrate diet is not recommended for adequate nutrition.

    3. **Exercise is effective in helping CF patients clear secretions.**

    4. **Minimizing pulmonary complications is essential to a better outcome for CF patients. Compliance with CPT, nebulizer treatments, and medications are all components of minimizing pulmonary complications.**

    5. **Medication compliance is a necessary part of maintaining pulmonary and gastrointestinal function.**

TEST-TAKING HINT: The test taker can eliminate answer 2 because patients are not placed on high-fat diets.

62. 60 mEq/L.
The definitive diagnosis of CF is made when a child has a sweat chloride level >60 mEq/L. A normal chloride level is <40 mEq/L.

TEST-TAKING HINT: The test taker must have knowledge of tests and normal values used to identify a diagnosis of CF.

Cardiovascular Disorders

6

KEYWORDS

The following words include English vocabulary, nursing/medical terminology, concepts, principles, or information relevant to content specifically addressed in the chapter or associated with topics presented in it. English dictionaries, your nursing textbooks, and medical dictionaries such as *Taber's Cyclopedic Medical Dictionary* are resources that can be used to expand your knowledge and understanding of these words and related information.

Bacterial endocarditis

Cardiac demand

Defects with decreased pulmonary flow

Defects with increased pulmonary flow

Obstructive defects

ABBREVIATIONS

Angiotensin receptor blockers (ARB)

Aortic stenosis (AS)

Aspirin (ASA)

Atrial septal defect (ASD)

Atrioventricular canal (AVC)

Bacterial endocarditis (BE)

Blood pressure (BP)

Cardiac output (CO)

Cerebrovascular accident (CVA)

Coarctation of the aorta (COA)

Congenital heart defect (CHD)

Congestive heart failure (CHF)

Heart rate (HR)

Kawasaki disease (KD)

Left sternal border (LSB)

Patent ductus arteriosus (PDA)

Pulmonic stenosis (PS)

Rheumatic fever (RF)

Supraventricular tachycardia (SVT)

Systemic vascular resistance (SVR)

Tetralogy of Fallot (TOF)

Ventricular septal defect (VSD)

QUESTIONS

1. What can an electrocardiogram (ECG) detect? **Select all that apply.**
   1. Ischemia.
   2. Injury.
   3. Cardiac output (CO).
   4. Dysrhythmias.
   5. Systemic vascular resistance (SVR).
   6. Occlusion pressure.
   7. Conduction delay.

2. A newborn is diagnosed with a congenital heart defect (CHD). The test results reveal that the lumen of the duct between the aorta and pulmonary artery remains open. This defect is known as _____.

3. Tetralogy of Fallot (TOF) involves which defects? **Select all that apply.**
   1. Ventricular septal defect (VSD).
   2. Right ventricular hypertrophy.
   3. Left ventricular hypertrophy.
   4. Pulmonic stenosis (PS).
   5. Pulmonic atresia.
   6. Overriding aorta.
   7. Patent ductus arteriosus (PDA).

4. A 10-year-old child is recovering from a severe sore throat. The parent states that the child complains of chest pain. The nurse observes that the child has swollen joints, nodules on the fingers, and a rash on the chest. The likely cause is _____.

5. What should the nurse assess prior to administering digoxin (Lanoxin)?
   1. Sclera.
   2. Apical pulse rate.
   3. Cough.
   4. Liver function test.

6. Which statement by a parent of an infant with congestive heart failure (CHF) who is being sent home on digoxin (Lanoxin) indicates the need for further education?
   1. "I will give the medication at regular 12-hour intervals."
   2. "If he vomits, I will not give a make-up dose."
   3. "If I miss a dose, I will not give an extra dose."
   4. "I will mix the digoxin in some formula to make it taste better."

7. Which finding might delay a cardiac catheterization procedure on a 1-year-old?
   1. 30th percentile for weight.
   2. Severe diaper rash.
   3. Allergy to soy.
   4. Oxygen saturation of 91% on room air.

8. The nurse is caring for a child who has undergone a cardiac catheterization. During recovery, the nurse notices the dressing is saturated with bright red blood. The nurse's first action is to:
   1. Call the interventional cardiologist.
   2. Notify the cardiac catheterization laboratory that the child will be returning.
   3. Apply a bulky pressure dressing over the present dressing.
   4. Apply direct pressure 1 inch above the puncture site.

9. Which interventions decrease cardiac demands in an infant with congestive heart failure (CHF)? **Select all that apply.**
   1. Allow parents to hold and rock their child.
   2. Feed only when the infant is crying.
   3. Keep the child uncovered to promote low body temperature.
   4. Make frequent position changes.
   5. Feed the child when sucking the fists.
   6. Change bed linens only when necessary.
   7. Organize nursing activities.

10. Indomethacin (Indocin) may be given to close which congenital heart defect (CHD) in newborns? _____

11. For the child with hypoplastic left heart syndrome, which drug may be given to allow the patent ductus arteriosus (PDA) to remain open until surgery? _____

12. On examination, a nurse hears a murmur at the left sternal border (LSB) in a child with diarrhea and fever. The parent asks why the health-care provider never said anything about the murmur. The nurse explains:
    1. "The health-care provider is not a cardiologist."
    2. "Murmurs are difficult to detect, especially in children."
    3. "The fever increased the intensity of the murmur."
    4. "We need to refer the child to an interventional cardiologist."

13. While assessing a newborn with respiratory distress, the nurse auscultates a machine-like heart murmur. Other findings are a wide pulse pressure, periods of apnea, increased $PaCO_2$, and decreased PO_2. The nurse suspects that the newborn has:
    1. Pulmonary hypertension.
    2. Patent ductus arteriosus (PDA).
    3. Ventricular septal defect (VSD).
    4. Bronchopulmonary dysplasia.

14. Which are the most serious complications for a child with Kawasaki disease (KD)? **Select all that apply.**
    1. Coronary thrombosis.
    2. Coronary stenosis.
    3. Coronary artery aneurysm.
    4. Hypocoagulability.
    5. Decreased sedimentation rate.
    6. Hypoplastic left heart syndrome.

15. A child who has reddened eyes with no discharge; red, swollen, and peeling palms and soles of the feet; dry, cracked lips; and a "strawberry tongue" most likely has
    _____.

16. The nurse is caring for a child with Kawasaki disease (KD). A student nurse who is on the unit asks if there are medications to treat this disease. The nurse's response to the student nurse is:
    1. Immunoglobulin G and aspirin.
    2. Immunoglobulin G and ACE inhibitors.
    3. Immunoglobulin E and heparin.
    4. Immunoglobulin E and ibuprofen (Motrin).

17. Congenital heart defects (CHDs) are classified by which of the following? **Select all that apply.**
    1. Cyanotic defect.
    2. Acyanotic defect.
    3. Defects with increased pulmonary blood flow.
    4. Defects with decreased pulmonary blood flow.
    5. Mixed defects.
    6. Obstructive defects.
    7. Pansystolic murmurs.

18. During a well-child checkup for an infant with tetralogy of Fallot (TOF), the child develops severe respiratory distress and becomes cyanotic. The nurse's first action should be to:
    1. Lay the child flat to promote hemostasis.
    2. Lay the child flat with legs elevated to increase blood flow to the heart.
    3. Sit the child on the parent's lap, with legs dangling, to promote venous pooling.
    4. Hold the child in knee-chest position to decrease venous blood return.

19. Hypoxic spells in the infant with a congenital heart defect (CHD) can cause which of the following? **Select all that apply.**
1. Polycythemia.
2. Blood clots.
3. Cerebrovascular accident (CVA).
4. Developmental delays.
5. Viral pericarditis.
6. Brain damage.
7. Alkalosis.

20. A 6-month-old who has episodes of cyanosis after crying could have the congenital heart defect (CHD) of decreased pulmonary blood flow called

_____.

21. A toddler who has been hospitalized for vomiting because of gastroenteritis is sleeping and difficult to wake up. Assessment reveals vital signs of a regular HR of 220 beats per minute, respiratory rate of 30 per minute, BP of 84/52, and capillary refill of 3 seconds. Which dysrhythmia does the nurse suspect in this child?
1. Rapid pulmonary flutter.
2. Sinus bradycardia.
3. Rapid atrial fibrillation.
4. Supraventricular tachycardia.

22. BP screenings to detect end-organ damage should be done routinely beginning at what age?
1. Birth.
2. 3 years.
3. 8 years.
4. 13 years.

23. What associated manifestation might the nurse occasionally find in a child diagnosed with Wilms tumor?
1. Atrial fibrillation.
2. Hypertension.
3. Endocarditis.
4. Hyperlipidemia.

24. Which drug should not be used to control secondary hypertension in a sexually active adolescent female who uses intermittent birth control?
1. Beta blockers.
2. Calcium channel blockers.
3. ACE inhibitors.
4. Diuretics.

25. A 16-year-old being treated for hypertension has a history of asthma. Which drug class should be avoided in treating this client's hypertension?
1. Beta blockers.
2. Calcium channel blockers.
3. ACE inhibitors.
4. Diuretics.

26. The _____ serves as the septal opening between the atria of the fetal heart.

27. While looking through the chart of an infant with a congenital heart defect (CHD) of decreased pulmonary blood flow, the nurse would expect which laboratory finding?
1. Decreased platelet count.
2. Polycythemia.
3. Decreased ferritin level.
4. Shift to the left.

28. The nurse is caring for a 9-month-old who was born with a congenital heart defect (CHD). Assessment reveals a HR of 160, capillary refill of 4 seconds, bilateral crackles, and sweat on the scalp. These are signs of _____.

29. Which of the following are examples of acquired heart disease? **Select all that apply.**
    1. Infective endocarditis.
    2. Hypoplastic left heart syndrome.
    3. Rheumatic fever (RF).
    4. Cardiomyopathy.
    5. Kawasaki disease (KD).
    6. Transposition of the great vessels.

30. A child diagnosed with congestive heart failure (CHF) is receiving maintenance doses of digoxin (Lanoxin) and furosemide (Lasix). She is rubbing her eyes when she is looking at the lights in the room, and her HR is 70 beats per minute. The nurse expects which laboratory finding?
    1. Hypokalemia.
    2. Hypomagnesemia.
    3. Hypocalcemia.
    4. Hypophosphatemia.

31. Which plan would be appropriate in helping to control congestive heart failure (CHF) in an infant?
    1. Promoting fluid restriction.
    2. Feeding a low-salt formula.
    3. Feeding in semi-Fowler position.
    4. Encouraging breast milk.

32. In which congenital heart defect (CHD) would the nurse need to take upper and lower extremity BPs?
    1. Transposition of the great vessels.
    2. Aortic stenosis (AS).
    3. Coarctation of the aorta (COA).
    4. Tetralogy of Fallot (TOF).

33. A 10-year-old has undergone a cardiac catheterization. At the end of the procedure, the nurse should first assess:
    1. Pain.
    2. Pulses.
    3. Hemoglobin and hematocrit levels.
    4. Catheterization report.

34. Which statement by the mother of a child with rheumatic fever (RF) shows she has good understanding of the care of her child? **Select all that apply.**
    1. "I will apply heat to his swollen joints to promote circulation."
    2. "I will have him do gentle stretching exercises to prevent contractures."
    3. "I will give him his ordered anti-inflammatory medication for pain and inflammation."
    4. "I will apply cold packs to his swollen joints to reduce pain."
    5. "I will take my child every month to the health-care provider's office for his penicillin shot."

35. A child has been diagnosed with valvular disease following rheumatic fever (RF). During patient teaching, the nurse discusses the child's long-term prophylactic therapy with antibiotics for dental procedures, surgery, and childbirth. The parents indicate they understand when they say:
    1. "She will need to take the antibiotics until she is 18 years old."
    2. "She will need to take the antibiotics for 5 years after the last attack."
    3. "She will need to take the antibiotics for 10 years after the last attack."
    4. "She will need to take the antibiotics for the rest of her life."

36. A child born with Down syndrome should be evaluated for which associated cardiac manifestation?
    1. Congenital heart defect (CHD).
    2. Systemic hypertension.
    3. Hyperlipidemia.
    4. Cardiomyopathy.

37. The Norwood procedure is used to correct:
    1. Transposition of the great vessels.
    2. Hypoplastic left heart syndrome.
    3. Tetralogy of Fallot (TOF).
    4. Patent ductus arteriosus (PDA).

38. A child has a Glasgow Coma Scale of 3, HR of 88 beats per minute and regular, respiratory rate of 22, BP of 78/52, and blood sugar of 35 mg/dL. The nurse asks the caregiver about accidental ingestion of which drug?
    1. Calcium channel blocker.
    2. Beta blocker.
    3. ACE inhibiter.
    4. ARB.

39. Exposure to which illness should be a cause to discontinue therapy and substitute dipyridamole (Persantine) in a child receiving aspirin therapy for Kawasaki disease (KD)?
    1. Chickenpox or influenza.
    2. *E. coli* or *Staphylococcus*.
    3. *Candida* or *Streptococcus* A.
    4. *Streptococcus* A or staphylococcus.

40. The nurse is caring for an 8-year-old girl whose parents indicate she has developed spastic movements of her extremities and trunk, facial grimace, and speech disturbances. They state it seems worse when she is anxious and does not occur while sleeping. The nurse questions the parents about which recent illness?
    1. Kawasaki disease (KD).
    2. Rheumatic fever (RF).
    3. Malignant hypertension.
    4. Atrial fibrillation.

41. The most common cardiac dysrhythmia in the pediatric population is:
    1. Ventricular tachycardia.
    2. Sinus bradycardia.
    3. Supraventricular tachycardia.
    4. First-degree heart block.

42. A nursing action that promotes ideal nutrition in an infant with congestive heart failure (CHF) is:
    1. Feeding formula that is supplemented with additional calories.
    2. Allowing the infant to nurse at each breast for 20 minutes.
    3. Providing large feedings every 5 hours.
    4. Using firm nipples with small openings to slow feedings.

43. An 18-month-old with a myelomeningocele is undergoing a cardiac catheterization. The mother expresses concern about the use of dye in the procedure. The child does not have any allergies. In addition to the concern for an iodine allergy, what other allergy should the nurse bring to the attention of the catheterization staff?
    1. Soy.
    2. Latex.
    3. Penicillin.
    4. Dairy.

44. Treatment for congestive heart failure (CHF) in an infant began 3 days ago and has included digoxin (Lanoxin) and furosemide (Lasix). The child no longer has retractions, lungs are clear, and HR is 96 beats per minute while the child sleeps. The nurse is confident that the child has diuresed successfully and has good renal perfusion when the nurse notes the child's urine output is:
    1. 0.5 cc/kg/hr.
    2. 1 cc/kg/hr.
    3. 30 cc/hr.
    4. 1 oz/hr.

45. A 3-month-old has been diagnosed with a ventricular septal defect (VSD). The flow of blood through the heart is _____.

46. The parents of a 3-month-old ask why their baby will not have an operation to correct a ventricular septal defect (VSD). The nurse's best response is:
    1. "It is always helpful to get a second opinion about any serious condition like this."
    2. "Your baby's defect is small and will likely close on its own by 1 year of age."
    3. "It is common for health-care providers to wait until an infant develops respiratory distress before they do the surgery."
    4. "With a small defect like this, they wait until the child is 10 years old to do the surgery."

47. The flow of blood through the heart with an atrial septal defect (ASD) is

    _____.

48. Patent ductus arteriosus causes what type of shunt? _____

49. A child has been seen by the school nurse for dizziness since the start of the school term. It happens when standing in line for recess and homeroom. The child now reports that she would rather sit and watch her friends play hopscotch because she cannot count out loud and jump at the same time. When the nurse asks her if her chest ever hurts, she says yes. Based on this history, the nurse suspects that she has:
    1. Ventricular septal defect (VSD).
    2. Aortic stenosis (AS).
    3. Mitral valve prolapse.
    4. Tricuspid atresia.

50. The school nurse has been following a child who comes to the office frequently for vague complaints of dizziness and headache. Today, she is brought in after fainting in the cafeteria following a nosebleed. Her BP is 122/85, and her radial pulses are bounding. The nurse suspects she has:
    1. Transposition of the great vessels.
    2. Coarctation of the aorta (COA).
    3. Aortic stenosis (AS).
    4. Pulmonic stenosis (PS).

51. Which medication should the nurse give to an infant diagnosed with transposition of the great vessels?
    1. Ibuprofen (Motrin).
    2. Betamethasone.
    3. Prostaglandin E.
    4. Indomethacin (Indocin).

52. Which statement by the mother of a child with rheumatic fever (RF) shows an understanding of prevention for her other children?
    1. "Whenever one of them gets a sore throat, I will give that child an antibiotic."
    2. "There is no treatment. It must run its course."
    3. "If their culture is positive for group A *Streptococcus*, I will give them their antibiotic."
    4. "If their culture is positive for *Staphylococcus* A, I will give them their antibiotic."

53. Which client could require feeding by gavage? **Select all that apply.**
    1. Infant with congestive heart failure (CHF).
    2. Infant with significant pulmonary stenosis.
    3. Toddler with repair of transposition of the great vessels.
    4. Toddler with Kawasaki disease (KD) in the acute phase.
    5. School-age child with rheumatic fever (RF) and chorea.

54. Which physiological changes occur as a result of hypoxemia in congestive heart failure (CHF)?
    1. Polycythemia and clubbing.
    2. Anemia and barrel chest.
    3. Increased white blood cells and low platelets.
    4. Elevated erythrocyte sedimentation rate and peripheral edema.

55. Aspirin has been ordered for the child with rheumatic fever (RF) in order to:
    1. Keep the patent ductus arteriosus (PDA) open.
    2. Reduce joint inflammation.
    3. Decrease swelling of strawberry tongue.
    4. Treat ventricular hypertrophy of endocarditis.

56. Which vaccines must be delayed for 11 months after the administration of gamma globulin? **Select all that apply.**
    1. Diphtheria, tetanus, and pertussis.
    2. Hepatitis B.
    3. Inactivated polio virus.
    4. Measles, mumps, and rubella.
    5. Varicella.

57. The mother of a toddler reports that the child's father has just had a myocardial infarction (MI). Because of this information, the nurse recommends the child have a(n):
    1. Electrocardiogram.
    2. Lipid profile.
    3. Echocardiogram.
    4. Cardiac catheterization.

58. During play, a toddler with a history of tetralogy of Fallot (TOF) might assume which position?
    1. Sitting.
    2. Supine.
    3. Squatting.
    4. Standing.

59. A heart transplant may be indicated for a child with severe heart failure and:
1. Patent ductus arteriosus (PDA).
2. Ventricular septal defect (VSD).
3. Hypoplastic left heart syndrome.
4. Pulmonic stenosis (PS).

60. Family discharge teaching has been effective when the parent of a toddler diagnosed with Kawasaki disease (KD) states:
1. "The arthritis in her knees is permanent. She will need knee replacements."
2. "I will give her diphenhydramine (Benadryl) for her peeling palms and soles of her feet."
3. "I know she will be irritable for 2 months after her symptoms started."
4. "I will continue with high doses of Tylenol for her inflammation."

61. Which assessments indicate that the parent of a 7-year-old is following the prescribed treatment for congestive heart failure (CHF)? **Select all that apply.**
1. HR of 56 beats per minute.
2. Elevated red blood cell count.
3. 50th percentile height and weight for age.
4. Urine output of 0.5 cc/kg/hr.
5. Playing basketball with other children his age.

ANSWERS AND RATIONALES

The correct answer number and rationale for why it is the correct answer are given in **boldface blue type.** Rationales for why the other possible answer options are incorrect also are given, but they are not in boldface type.

1. **1, 2, 4, 7.**
   1. **An electrocardiogram can indicate ischemia of the heart muscle.**
   2. **An electrocardiogram can indicate injury to the heart muscle.**
   3. An electrocardiogram does not indicate CO.
   4. **An electrocardiogram can show dysrhythmias.**
   5. An electrocardiogram does not show SVR.
   6. An electrocardiogram does not show occlusion pressures.
   7. **An electrocardiogram does show conduction delays.**

   TEST-TAKING HINT: The electrocardiogram checks the electrical system of the heart, not the mechanical system. CO is mechanical; occlusion pressure does not have to do with the electrocardiogram; and SVR measures pressures in the peripheral system.

2. **Patent ductus arteriosus (PDA).**

   TEST-TAKING HINT: This is a defect with increased pulmonary flow. It should close in the first few weeks of life.

3. **1, 2, 4, 6.**
   1. **TOF is a congenital defect with a ventricular septal defect, right ventricular hypertrophy, pulmonary valve stenosis, and overriding aorta.**
   2. **TOF is a congenital defect with ventricular septal defect, right ventricular hypertrophy, pulmonary valve stenosis, and overriding aorta.**
   3. TOF is a congenital defect with ventricular septal defect, right ventricular hypertrophy, pulmonary valve stenosis, and overriding aorta.
   4. **TOF is a congenital defect with ventricular septal defect, right ventricular hypertrophy, pulmonary valve stenosis, and overriding aorta.**
   5. TOF is a congenital defect with ventricular septal defect, right ventricular hypertrophy, pulmonary valve stenosis, and overriding aorta.

   6. **TOF is a congenital defect with ventricular septal defect, right ventricular hypertrophy, pulmonary valve stenosis, and overriding aorta.**
   7. PDA is not one of the defects in tetralogy of Fallot.

   TEST-TAKING HINT: Tetralogy of Fallot has four defects. Pulmonary stenosis causes decreased pulmonary flow.

4. **Rheumatic fever (RF).**
   To make the diagnosis of RF, major and minor criteria are used. Major criteria include carditis, subcutaneous nodules, erythema marginatum, chorea, and arthritis. Minor criteria include fever and previous history of RF.

   TEST-TAKING HINT: RF is an inflammatory disease caused by group A beta-hemolytic streptococcus.

5. 1. The sclera has nothing to do with CHF.
   2. **The apical pulse rate is assessed because digoxin (Lanoxin) decreases the HR; if the HR is <60, digoxin should not be administered.**
   3. Cough would not be assessed before administration. It is more commonly seen in patients who have been prescribed ACE inhibitors.
   4. Liver function tests are not assessed before digoxin (Lanoxin) is administered. Digoxin can lower HR and cause dysrhythmias.

   TEST-TAKING HINT: The test taker should know that the sclera and liver function tests have nothing to do with digoxin (Lanoxin). Cough could be associated with ACE inhibitors.

6. 1. This is appropriate for digoxin (Lanoxin) administration.
   2. This is appropriate for digoxin administration.
   3. This is appropriate for digoxin administration.
   4. **If the medication is mixed in his formula, and he refuses to drink the entire amount, the dose will be inadequate.**

   TEST-TAKING HINT: What if the child does not drink all the formula?

7. 1. This may be a reason the child needs the catheterization.
   2. **A child with severe diaper rash has potential for infection if the interventionist makes the standard groin approach.**
   3. Shellfish, not soy, is an allergy concern.
   4. This may be a reason the child needs the catheterization.

TEST-TAKING HINT: Consider the risk for infection as a delaying factor.

8. 1. This is not an appropriate action.
   2. This is not an appropriate action.
   3. This can be done after applying direct pressure 1 inch above the puncture site.
   4. **Applying direct pressure 1 inch above the puncture site will localize pressure over the vessel site.**

TEST-TAKING HINT: Consider the risk for volume depletion.

9. 1, 4, 5, 6, 7.
   1. **Rocking by the parents will comfort the infant and decrease demands.**
   2. The infant would not be fed when crying because crying increases cardiac demands. The infant might choke if the nipple is placed in the mouth and the child inhales when trying to swallow.
   3. Keep the child normothermic to reduce metabolic demands.
   4. **Frequent position changes will decrease the risk for infection by avoiding immobility with its potential for skin breakdown.**
   5. **An infant sucking the fists could indicate hunger.**
   6. **Change bed linens only when necessary to avoid disturbing the child.**
   7. **Organize nursing activities to avoid disturbing the child.**

TEST-TAKING HINT: Do all that can be done to decrease demands on the child.

10. Patent ductus arteriosus (PDA).

TEST-TAKING HINT: Prostaglandins allow the duct to remain open; thus, a prostaglandin inhibitor, such as indomethacin (Indocin) or ibuprofen (Motrin), can help close the duct.

11. Prostaglandin E.

TEST-TAKING HINT: Prostaglandin E maintains ductal patency to promote blood flow until the Norwood procedure is begun. Consider the opposite of wanting to close the PDA.

12. 1. This is not a collegial response.
   2. The increased CO of the fever increases the intensity of the murmur, making it easier to hear.
   3. **The increased CO of the fever increases the intensity of the murmur, making it easier to hear.**
   4. This child does not need to see an interventional cardiologist. The murmur needs to be diagnosed first, and then a treatment plan would be developed.

TEST-TAKING HINT: Consider the pathophysiology of fever.

13. 1. Pulmonary hypertension is a pulmonary condition, which does not create a heart murmur.
   2. **The main identifier in the stem is the machine-like murmur, which is the hallmark of a PDA.**
   3. A VSD does not produce a machine-like murmur.
   4. Bronchopulmonary dysplasia is a pulmonary condition, which does not create a heart murmur.

TEST-TAKING HINT: The test taker needs to know common murmur sounds.

14. 1, 2, 3.
   1. **Thrombosis, stenosis, and aneurysm affect blood vessels. The child with KD has hypercoagulability and an increased sedimentation rate due to inflammation.**
   2. **Thrombosis, stenosis, and aneurysm affect blood vessels. The child with KD has hypercoagulability and an increased sedimentation rate due to inflammation.**
   3. **Thrombosis, stenosis, and aneurysm affect blood vessels. The child with KD has hypercoagulability and an increased sedimentation rate due to inflammation.**
   4. The child with KD has hypercoagulability and an increased sedimentation rate due to inflammation.
   5. The child with KD has hypercoagulability and an increased sedimentation rate due to inflammation.
   6. Hypoplastic left heart syndrome is a CHD and has no relation to KD.

TEST-TAKING HINT: KD is an inflammation of small- and medium-sized blood vessels.

15. **Kawasaki disease (KD).**

    TEST-TAKING HINT: Classic signs of KD include red eyes with no discharge; dry, cracked lips; strawberry tongue; and red, swollen, and peeling palms and soles of the feet. Incidence of KD is higher in males. The strongest indicator for this disease is the hallmark strawberry tongue.

16. 1. **High-dose immunoglobulin G and salicylate (aspirin) therapy for inflammation are the current treatment for KD.**
    2. Immunoglobulin G is correct, but ACE inhibitors are incorrect for treatment.
    3. Heparin may be used for the child with an aneurysm, but not immunoglobulin E.
    4. Immunoglobulin E and ibuprofen (Motrin) are not correct.

    TEST-TAKING HINT: Consider anti-inflammatory medications for treatment of KD.

17. **3, 4, 5, 6.**
    1. Heart defects are no longer classified as cyanotic or acyanotic.
    2. Heart defects are no longer classified as cyanotic or acyanotic.
    3. **Heart defects are now classified as defects with increased or decreased pulmonary blood flow, mixed, obstructive, or acquired.**
    4. **Heart defects are now classified as defects with increased or decreased pulmonary blood flow, mixed, obstructive or acquired.**
    5. **Heart defects are now classified as defects with increased or decreased pulmonary blood flow mixed, obstructive, or acquired.**
    6. **Heart defects are now classified as defects with increased or decreased pulmonary blood flow, mixed, obstructive, or acquired.**
    7. A murmur may be heard with a CHD, but a murmur does not classify the defect.

    TEST-TAKING HINT: Know the new classifications, not the older ones.

18. 1. Laying the child flat would increase preload, increasing blood to the heart, therefore making respiratory distress worse.
    2. Laying the child flat with legs elevated would increase preload, increasing blood to the heart, therefore making respiratory distress worse.

    3. Sitting the child on the parent's lap with legs dangling might possibly help, but it would not be as effective as the knee-chest position in occluding the venous return.
    4. **The increase in the SVR would increase afterload and increase blood return to the pulmonary artery.**

    TEST-TAKING HINT: The test taker should choose the response that decreases the preload in this patient.

19. **1, 2, 3, 4, 6.**
    1. **Hypoxia causes polycythemia, which can lead to increased blood viscosity, which can lead to blood clots and a stroke (CVA).**
    2. **Hypoxia causes polycythemia, which can lead to increased blood viscosity, which can lead to blood clots and a stroke (CVA).**
    3. **Hypoxia causes polycythemia, which can lead to increased blood viscosity, which can lead to blood clots and a stroke (CVA).**
    4. **Developmental delays can be caused by multiple hospitalizations and surgeries. The child usually catches up to the appropriate level.**
    5. Hypoxia can increase the risk for bacterial endocarditis, not viral pericarditis.
    6. **Brain damage can be caused by hypoxia, blood clots, and stroke (CVA).**
    7. Hypoxic episodes cause acidosis, not alkalosis.

    TEST-TAKING HINT: Hypoxic episodes in a child with CHD ("tet spells") can cause polycythemia and strokes (CVAs).

20. **Tetralogy of Fallot (TOF).**
    "Tet" spells are characteristic of TOF.

    TEST-TAKING HINT: Know the congenital heart defect classifications.

21. 1. This is not a real dysrhythmia.
    2. Sinus bradycardia is a slow rate for the child's age.
    3. Rapid atrial fibrillation is an irregular rhythm.
    4. **SVT is often above 200 and a result of dehydration, which a vomiting child could have. The rapid rate causes a low CO, resulting in low BP and prolonged capillary refill.**

    TEST-TAKING HINT: The HR is regular and very rapid for a child of any age. The child has been vomiting, which can result in dehydration.

22. 1. Birth is too early, and readings are often not reliable because of patient movement.
    2. **Age 3 years is the recommended age to establish a baseline BP in a normal, healthy child.**
    3. Age 8 years is too late to detect early damage.
    4. Age 13 years is too late to detect early damage.

    TEST-TAKING HINT: The test taker needs to know that 3 years of age is the recommended age to begin BP measurements in healthy children.

23. 1. Wilms tumor does not affect or cause this condition.
    2. **Because Wilms tumor sits on the kidney, it can be associated with secondary hypertension. It does not affect or cause the other conditions.**
    3. Wilms tumor does not affect or cause this condition.
    4. Wilms tumor does not affect or cause this condition.

    TEST-TAKING HINT: Knowing that Wilms tumor is on top of the kidney should suggest that secondary hypertension is a possibility.

24. 1. ACE inhibitors and angiotensin II receptor blockers can cause birth defects. The others are not teratogenic.
    2. ACE inhibitors and angiotensin II receptor blockers can cause birth defects. The others are not teratogenic.
    3. **ACE inhibitors and angiotensin II receptor blockers can cause birth defects. The others are not teratogenic.**
    4. ACE inhibitors and angiotensin II receptors can cause birth defects. The others are not teratogenic.

    TEST-TAKING HINT: The test taker needs to know which of these drugs are teratogenic.

25. 1. **Beta blockers are not generally used in clients with asthma and hypertension because of concern the beta agonist will cause severe asthma attacks.**
    2. Calcium channel blockers do not have the effect of causing asthma attacks.
    3. ACE inhibitors do not have the effect of causing asthma attacks.
    4. Diuretics do not have the effect of causing asthma attacks.

    TEST-TAKING HINT: The test taker needs to know side effects of drugs.

26. **Foramen ovale.**

    TEST-TAKING HINT: The foramen ovale is the septal opening between the atria of the fetal heart. The test taker needs to know basic fetal circulation.

27. 1. The nurse should expect a normal platelet count in an infant with a CHD of decreased pulmonary blood flow.
    2. **Polycythemia is the result of the body attempting to increase the oxygen supply in the presence of hypoxia by increasing the total number of red blood cells to carry the oxygen.**
    3. Ferritin measures the amount of iron stored in the body and is not affected by decreased pulmonary blood flow.
    4. "Shift to the left" refers to an increase in the number of immature white blood cells.

    TEST-TAKING HINT: The test taker needs to know what laboratory values hypoxia can affect.

28. **Congestive heart failure (CHF).**

    TEST-TAKING HINT: All of these are signs of pump failure. The infant is likely to have diaphoresis only on the scalp. The signs are not unlike those of an adult with this condition.

29. 1, 3, 4, 5.
    1. **Infective endocarditis is an example of an acquired heart problem.**
    2. Hypoplastic left heart syndrome is a CHD.
    3. **RF is an acquired heart problem.**
    4. **Cardiomyopathy is an acquired heart problem.**
    5. **KD is an acquired heart problem.**
    6. Transposition of the great vessels is a CHD.

    TEST-TAKING HINT: "Acquired" means occurring after birth and seen in an otherwise normal and healthy heart.

30. 1. **The rubbing of the child's eyes may mean that she is seeing halos around the lights, indicating digoxin (Lanoxin) toxicity. The HR is slow for her age and also indicates digoxin toxicity. A decrease in serum potassium because of the furosemide (Lasix) can increase the risk for digoxin toxicity.**
    2. Hypomagnesemia does not affect digoxin and is not related to the child rubbing her eyes.
    3. Hypocalcemia does not affect digoxin and is not related to the child rubbing her eyes.
    4. Hypophosphatemia does not affect digoxin and is not related to the child rubbing her eyes.

TEST-TAKING HINT: The test taker knows that furosemide (Lasix) causes the loss of potassium and can cause digoxin (Lanoxin) toxicity.

31. 1. The nurse would not need to restrict fluids, as the child likely would not be getting overloaded with oral fluids.
    2. The infant likely will have sodium depletion because of the chronic diuretic use; the infant needs a normal source of sodium, so low-sodium formula would not be used.
    3. **The infant has a great deal of difficulty feeding with CHF, so even getting the maintenance fluids is a challenge. The infant is fed in the more upright position so that fluid in the lungs can go to the base of the lungs, allowing better expansion.**
    4. Breast milk has slightly less sodium than does formula, and the child needs a normal source of sodium because of the diuretic.

TEST-TAKING HINT: Infants are not able to concentrate urine well and may have sodium depletion, so they need a normal source of sodium.

32. 1. BPs would not need to be taken in both the upper and lower extremities in transposition of the great vessels. The aorta and pulmonary arteries are in opposite positions, which does not change the BP readings.
    2. AS is a narrowing of the aortic valve, which does not affect the BP in the extremities.
    3. **With COA there is narrowing of the aorta, which increases pressure proximal to the defect (upper extremities) and decreases pressure distal to the defect (lower extremities). There will be high BP and strong pulses in the upper extremities and lower-than-expected BP and weak pulses in the lower extremities.**
    4. TOF is a congenital cardiac problem with four defects that do not affect the BP in the extremities.

TEST-TAKING HINT: The test taker must know the anatomy of the cardiac defects and what assessments are to be made in each one.

33. 1. Pain needs to be assessed post procedure but is not the priority.
    2. **Checking for pulses, especially in the canulated extremity, would assure perfusion to that extremity and is the priority post procedure.**

3. Hemoglobin and hematocrit levels would be checked post procedure if the child had bled very much during or after the procedure.
    4. The catheterization report would be of interest to know what was determined from the procedure. This would also be good to check on the patient post procedure.

TEST-TAKING HINT: The test taker would know that the priority is assessing the cannulated extremity, checking for adequate perfusion.

34. 3, 5.
    1. During the acute phase, limit any manipulation of the joint and avoid heat or cold.
    2. During the acute phase, limit any manipulation of the joint and avoid heat or cold.
    3. **Anti-inflammatory medications are the drugs of choice for treatment of RF because RF is a systemic inflammatory disease that can follow strep infections.**
    4. During the acute phase, limit any manipulation of the joint and avoid heat or cold.
    5. **The parent will take the child to the clinic monthly for a penicillin injection to prevent recurrent strep infections.**

TEST-TAKING HINT: The test taker should know that aspirin is the drug of choice and that manipulation of the joint should be limited during the acute phase. Follow up care after the diagnosis includes monthly penicillin injections to prevent recurrent strep infections and cardiac damage.

35. 1. This could be true for a patient with a less severe form of RF.
    2. This could be true for a patient with a less severe form of RF.
    3. This could be true for a patient with a less severe form of RF.
    4. **Valvular involvement indicates significant damage, so antibiotics would be taken for the rest of her life.**

TEST-TAKING HINT: The test taker should know that the severity of the damage to the heart valves determines how long prophylactic antibiotics will be administered.

36. 1. **CHD is found often in children with Down syndrome.**
    2. This is not associated with Down syndrome.
    3. This is not associated with Down syndrome.
    4. This is not associated with Down syndrome.

TEST-TAKING HINT: A child with a genetic syndrome, such as Down, is likely to have other abnormalities.

37. 1. Transposition of the great vessels requires different surgical procedures.
    2. The Norwood procedure is specific to hypoplastic left heart syndrome.
    3. TOF requires different surgical procedures.
    4. PDA requires different surgical procedures.

    TEST-TAKING HINT: Review surgical treatment of CHD.

38. 1. Calcium channel blockers decrease the force of cardiac contraction and slow the electrical conduction of the heart, resulting in slowing of the HR. The HR is normal in this child.
    2. The beta blocker not only affects the heart and lungs but also blocks the beta sites in the liver, reducing the amount of glycogen available for use, causing hypoglycemia. The lower HR and BP also suggest ingestion of a cardiac medication.
    3. ACE inhibiters block the conversion of a protein from its inactive to its active form. The protein causes constriction of small blood vessels, which raises BP. By blocking this protein, BP is lowered.
    4. Angiotensin receptor blockers relax blood vessels, which lowers BP and makes it easier for the heart to pump blood.

    TEST-TAKING HINT: Know drug side effects. In this case, glycogen is blocked.

39. **1. Both chickenpox and influenza are viral in nature, so consider stopping the aspirin because of the danger of Reye syndrome.**
    2. *E. coli* and *Staphylococcus* are not viral, so Reye syndrome is not a factor.
    3. *Candida* is a strain of fungus, so aspirin could be used to treat fever, but is not recommended in children. *Streptococcus* A is a bacterium; Reye syndrome is not a factor.
    4. *Streptococcus* A and *Staphylococcus* are not viral, so Reye syndrome is not a factor.

    TEST-TAKING HINT: Consider Reye syndrome when the patient is taking aspirin and has a viral infection.

40. 1. KD does not result in this condition, called chorea or St. Vitus' dance.
    2. Chorea can be a manifestation of RF, with a higher incidence in females.
    3. Malignant hypertension does not result in this condition, called chorea or St. Vitus' dance.
    4. Atrial fibrillation is not an illness.

TEST-TAKING HINT: The test taker can eliminate answer 1 because KD can cause damage to coronary arteries.

41. 1. Ventricular tachycardia is uncommon in children.
    2. Sinus bradycardia is uncommon in children.
    3. Supraventricular tachycardia is most common in children.
    4. First-degree heart block is uncommon in children.

    TEST-TAKING HINT: Consider a tachycardiac rhythm in a pediatric patient.

42. **1. Formula can be supplemented with extra calories, either from a commercial supplement, such as Polycose, or from corn syrup. Calories in formula could increase from 20 kcal/oz to 30 kcal/oz or more.**
    2. The infant would get too tired while feeding, which increases cardiac demand. Limit breastfeeding to a half hour, or 15 minutes per side.
    3. Smaller feedings more often, such as every 2 to 3 hours, would decrease cardiac demand.
    4. Soft nipples that are easy for the infant to suck would make for less work getting nutrition.

    TEST-TAKING HINT: Allow the child to get the most nutrition most effectively.

43. 1. Children with spina bifida (myelomeningocele) often have a latex allergy. The catheter balloon is often made of latex, and all personnel caring for the patient should be made aware of the allergy.
    2. Children with spina bifida (myelomeningocele) often have a latex allergy. The catheter balloon is often made of latex, and all personnel caring for the patient should be made aware of the allergy.
    3. Children with spina bifida (myelomeningocele) often have a latex allergy. The catheter balloon is often made of latex, and all personnel caring for the patient should be made aware of the allergy.
    4. Children with spina bifida (myelomeningocele) often have a latex allergy. The catheter balloon is often made of latex, and all personnel caring for the patient should be made aware of the allergy.

    TEST-TAKING HINT: Material that composes the balloon catheter is made of latex, which is a common allergy in a child with a myelomeningocele.

44. 1. This is incorrect because 0.5 cc/kg/hr is below the normal pediatric urine output.
   2. **Normal pediatric urine output is 1 cc/kg/hr.**
   3. This is incorrect because 30 cc/hr is above the normal pediatric urine output.
   4. This is incorrect because 1 oz/hr is above the normal pediatric urine output.

   TEST-TAKING HINT: The test taker needs to know that normal urine output for a child is 1 cc/kg/hr.

45. **Left to right.**
   The pressures in the left side of the heart are greater, causing the flow of blood to be from an area of higher pressure to lower pressure, or left to right, increasing the pulmonary blood flow with the extra blood.

   TEST-TAKING HINT: The test taker should know that the classification for this defect is left to right.

46. 1. This is not a collegial response, and the nurse should explain to the parents why an operation is not necessary now.
   2. **Usually a VSD will close on its own within the first year of life.**
   3. It is not common for health-care providers to wait until respiratory distress develops because that puts the infant at greater risk for complications. The defect is small and will likely close on its own.
   4. Small defects usually close on their own within the first year.

   TEST-TAKING HINT: Know the various treatments depending on size of the defect. VSD is the most common CHD.

47. **Left to right.**
   The pressures in the left side of the heart are greater, causing the flow of blood to be from an area of higher pressure to lower pressure, or left to right, increasing the pulmonary blood flow with the extra blood.

   TEST-TAKING HINT: What is the CHD classification of ASD?

48. **Left to right.**
   Blood flows from the higher-pressure aorta to the lower-pressure pulmonary artery, resulting in a left to right shunt.

   TEST-TAKING HINT: What is the CHD classification of PDA?

49. 1. Murmur and CHF are often found in infancy.
   2. **AS can progress, and the child can develop exercise intolerance that can be better when resting.**
   3. Mitral valve prolapse causes a murmur and palpitations, usually in adulthood.
   4. Tricuspid atresia causes hypoxemia in infancy.

   TEST-TAKING HINT: What do "stenosis," "prolapse," and "atresia" mean, and what do those conditions cause?

50. 1. Transposition of the great vessels does not cause these symptoms.
   2. **In the older child, COA causes dizziness, headache, fainting, elevated blood pressure, and bounding radial pulses.**
   3. AS does not cause these symptoms.
   4. PS does not cause these symptoms.

   TEST-TAKING HINT: The test taker should recognize that the child's BP is elevated and her pulses are bounding, which are symptoms of COA.

51. 1. Ibuprofen (Motrin) blocks prostaglandins, which would speed up the closing of the PDA.
   2. Betamethasone blocks prostaglandins, which would speed up the closing of the PDA.
   3. **Prostaglandin E inhibits closing of the PDA, which connects the aorta and pulmonary artery.**
   4. Indomethacin (Indocin) is used to treat osteoarthritis and gout.

   TEST-TAKING HINT: The test taker should know that children who have transposition of the great vessels also have another cardiac defect, and the common one is PDA.

52. 1. Do not use an antibiotic if the disease is not bacterial in origin. Most sore throats are viral.
   2. RF is a bacterial infection caused by group A beta-hemolytic *Streptococcus*, and the drug of choice is penicillin.
   3. **RF is caused by a streptococcal infection, not by *Staphylococcus*.**
   4. RF is cause by a streptococcal infection, not by *Staphylococcus*.

   TEST-TAKING HINT: The test taker needs to know the cause of RF and how it is treated.

53. 1, 2.

 1. **The child may experience increased cardiac demand while feeding. Feedings by gavage eliminate that work and still provide high-calorie intake for growth.**
 2. **The child with significant pulmonary stenosis will tire easily, especially during a feeding, and may need to be gavage-fed.**
 3. Transposition of the great vessels should be repaired before the toddler years, so that child would not need to be gavage-fed.
 4. A toddler with KD in the acute phase does not need to be gavage-fed.
 5. An RF patient with St. Vitus' dance (chorea) does not need to be gavage-fed. Most of these children do not have CHF.

TEST-TAKING HINT: The test taker should consider how gavage feedings would affect the work of the heart.

54. 1. **The hypoxemia stimulates erythropoiesis, which causes polycythemia, in an attempt to increase oxygen by having more red blood cells carry oxygen. Clubbing of the fingers is a result of the polycythemia and hypoxemia.**
 2. Anemia and barrel chest do not occur as a result of hypoxemia. Hypoxemia stimulates the production of erythropoietin to increase the number of red blood cells to carry more oxygen. The barrel chest is the result of air trapping.
 3. Increased white blood cells occur as the result of an infection, not hypoxemia. Hypoxemia does not cause a decreased number of platelets.
 4. An elevated erythrocyte sedimentation rate is the result of inflammation in the body. Peripheral edema can be caused by CHF.

TEST-TAKING HINT: The test taker could eliminate answers 2, 3, and 4 by knowing that they do not cause hypoxemia in CHF.

55. 1. Aspirin is not used to treat this condition. A PDA does not occur with RF.
 2. **Joint inflammation is experienced in RF; aspirin therapy helps with inflammation and pain.**
 3. Strawberry tongue is manifested in strep throat; aspirin is not used to treat this disease.
 4. Aspirin is not used to treat this condition.

TEST-TAKING HINT: Know the manifestations of RF.

56. 4, 5.

 1. Diphtheria, tetanus, and pertussis vaccines can be given following administration of gamma globulin. These are killed vaccines, and the only vaccines not administered would be live vaccines such as measles, mumps, and rubella.
 2. Hepatitis B vaccine can be administered following gamma globulin. Live vaccines are held for at least 11 months.
 3. Inactivated polio virus vaccine can be given following gamma globulin administration. Live vaccines are held for 11 months.
 4. **The body might not produce the appropriate number of antibodies following gamma globulin infusion, so live virus vaccines should be delayed for 11 months.**
 5. **The body might not produce the appropriate number of antibodies following gamma globulin infusion, so live virus vaccines should be delayed for 11 months.**

TEST-TAKING HINT: The test taker needs to know which vaccines are killed and which are live.

57. 1. Current recommendations are for a lipid profile in children over 2 years with a first- or second-degree relative with stroke (CVA), myocardial infarction, angina, or sudden cardiac death. Also screen if parent, sibling, or grandparent has cholesterol of 240 mg/dL or greater.
 2. **Current recommendations are for a lipid profile in children over 2 years with a first- or second-degree relative with stroke (CVA), myocardial infarction, angina, or sudden cardiac death. Also screen if parent, sibling, or grandparent has cholesterol of 240 mg/dL or greater.**
 3. Current recommendations are for a lipid profile in children over 2 years with a first- or second-degree relative with stroke (CVA), myocardial infarction, angina, or sudden cardiac death. Also screen if parent, sibling, or grandparent has cholesterol of 240 mg/dL or greater.
 4. Current recommendations are for a lipid profile in children over 2 years with a first- or second-degree relative with stroke (CVA), myocardial infarction, angina, or sudden cardiac death. Also screen if parent, sibling, or grandparent has cholesterol of 240 mg/dL or greater.

TEST-TAKING HINT: Risk factors for the father's MI include elevated lipids, family history of heart disease, diabetes, and smoking.

58. 1. The toddler will naturally assume a squatting position to decrease preload by occluding venous flow from the lower extremities and increasing afterload. Increasing SVR in this position increases pulmonary blood flow.
   2. The toddler will naturally assume a squatting position to decrease preload by occluding venous flow from the lower extremities and increasing afterload. Increasing SVR in this position increases pulmonary blood flow.
   3. **The toddler will naturally assume this position to decrease preload by occluding venous flow from the lower extremities and increasing afterload. Increasing SVR in this position increases pulmonary blood flow.**
   4. The toddler will naturally assume a squatting position to decrease preload by occluding venous flow from the lower extremities and increasing afterload. Increasing SVR in this position increases pulmonary blood flow.

TEST-TAKING HINT: The child self-assumes this position during the "tet" spell which increases vascular return.

59. 1. Severe heart failure can be an indication for heart transplant if quality of life is decreased. PDAs usually close on their own or can be closed surgically.
   2. Severe heart failure can be an indication for heart transplant if quality of life is decreased. If small, VSDs can close on their own or be surgically closed.
   3. **Hypoplastic left heart syndrome is treated by the Norwood procedure, or heart transplant.**
   4. Severe heart failure can be an indication for heart transplant if quality of life is decreased. PS can be very constrictive to only slightly stenotic. Surgery is usually indicated for children with severe stenosis.

TEST-TAKING HINT: Consider severe heart failure and which complex of CHD would indicate a need for a heart transplant.

60. 1. Arthritis in KD is always temporary.
   2. Peeling palms and feet are painless and usually not itchy, so this medication would not be needed. Diphenhydramine (Benadryl) is an antihistamine used for itching and allergy symptoms.
   3. **Children can be irritable for 2 months after the symptoms of the disease start.**
   4. Acetaminophen (Tylenol) is never given in high doses due to liver failure, and it is not an anti-inflammatory. Aspirin is given in high doses for KD.

TEST-TAKING HINT: The test taker must know about KD to choose the best response.

61. 3, 5.
   1. HR of 56 beats per minute is likely the result of digoxin (Lanoxin) toxicity.
   2. Elevated count of red blood cells indicates polycythemia secondary to hypoxemia.
   3. **The 50th percentile height and weight for age shows good growth, indicating good nutrition and perfusion.**
   4. Urine output of 0.5 cc/kg/hr indicates that furosemide (Lasix) is not being given as ordered; the output is too low.
   5. **Playing basketball with children his age indicates he is following the prescribed treatment and responding well to it.**

TEST-TAKING HINT: The test taker should know the expected responses of medications used to treat CHF and indications of doing well.

Gastrointestinal Disorders

KEYWORDS

The following words include English vocabulary, nursing/medical terminology, concepts, principles, or information relevant to content specifically addressed in the chapter or associated with topics presented in it. English dictionaries, your nursing textbooks, and medical dictionaries such as *Taber's Cyclopedic Medical Dictionary* are resources that can be used to expand your knowledge and understanding of these words and related information.

Anorectal malformation
Anterior fontanel
Appendectomy
Bile
Biliary atresia
Bowel obstruction
Celiac disease
Cholestyramine
Cleft lip
Cleft palate
Congenital aganglionic megacolon
  (Hirschsprung disease)
Constipation
Dehydration
Electrolytes
Encopresis
Enterocolitis
Esophageal atresia
Esophagus
Fistula
Fluid maintenance
Fundus
Gastroenteritis
Gastroesophageal reflux
Gastrostomy tube
Gluten
Hepatitis
Imperforate anus
Intestinal villi

Intussusception
Jaundice
Jejunal biopsy
Kasai procedure
Malabsorption
Malaise
Metoclopramide (Reglan)
Necrotizing enterocolitis
Nissen fundoplication
Occult blood
Omeprazole (Prilosec)
Ondansetron (Zofran)
Patient-controlled analgesia
Peristalsis
Peritonitis
Polyhydramnios
Pyloric stenosis
Rotavirus
Rovsing sign
Short bowel syndrome
Stimulant laxative
Stoma
Stool softener
Sudden infant death syndrome
Tracheoesophageal fistula
Umbilical hernia
Vomiting
Yankauer suction
Zofran (ondansetron)

ABBREVIATIONS

Gastroesophageal reflux (GER)
Gastrostomy tube (GT)
Nasogastric tube (NGT)
Necrotizing enterocolitis (NEC)
Nothing by mouth (NPO)

Patient-controlled analgesia (PCA)
Parenteral nutrition (PN)
Short bowel syndrome (SBS)
Sudden infant death syndrome (SIDS)

QUESTIONS

1. The parent of a newborn asks, "Will my baby spit out the formula if it is too hot or too cold?" Which is the nurse's best response?
   1. "Babies have a tendency to reject hot fluids but not cold fluids, which could result in abdominal discomfort."
   2. "Babies have a tendency to reject cold fluids but not hot fluids, which could result in esophageal burns."
   3. "Your baby would most likely spit out formula that was too hot, but your baby could swallow some of it, which could result in a burn."
   4. "Your baby is too young to be physically capable of spitting out fluids and will automatically swallow anything."

2. The mother of a newborn asks the nurse why the infant has to nurse so frequently. Which is the best response?
   1. Formula tends to be more calorically dense, and formula-fed babies require fewer feedings than breastfed babies.
   2. The newborn's stomach capacity is small, and peristalsis is slow.
   3. The newborn's stomach capacity is small, and peristalsis is more rapid than in older children.
   4. Breastfed babies tend to take longer to complete a feeding than formula-fed babies.

3. A 4-month-old has had vomiting and diarrhea for 24 hours. The infant is fussy, and the anterior fontanel is sunken. The nurse notes the infant does not produce tears when crying. Which task will help confirm the diagnosis of dehydration?
   1. Urinalysis obtained by bagged specimen.
   2. Urinalysis obtained by sterile catheterization.
   3. Analysis of serum electrolytes.
   4. Analysis of cerebrospinal fluid.

4. A 4-month-old is brought to the emergency department with severe dehydration. The heart rate is 198, and her blood pressure is 68/38. The infant's anterior fontanel is sunken. The nurse notes that the infant does not cry when the intravenous line is inserted. The child's parents state that she has not "held anything down" in 18 hours. The nurse obtains a finger-stick blood sugar of 94. Which would the nurse expect to do immediately?
   1. Administer a bolus of normal saline.
   2. Administer a bolus of $D^{10}W$.
   3. Administer a bolus of normal saline with 5% dextrose added to the solution.
   4. Offer the child an oral rehydrating solution such as Pedialyte.

5. The nurse is caring for a 2-year-old child who was admitted to the pediatric unit for moderate dehydration due to vomiting and diarrhea. The child is restless with periods of irritability. The child is afebrile with a heart rate of 148 and a blood pressure of 90/42. Baseline laboratory tests reveal the following: Na 152, Cl 119, and glucose 115. The parents state that the child has not urinated in 12 hours. After establishing a saline lock, the nurse reviews the physician's orders. Which order should the nurse question?
   1. Administer a saline bolus of 10 mL/kg, which may be repeated if the child does not urinate.
   2. Recheck serum electrolytes in 12 hours.
   3. After the saline bolus, begin maintenance fluids of D5 ¼ NS with 10 mEq KCl/L.
   4. Give clear liquid diet as tolerated.

6. The parent of a 5-year-old states that the child has been having diarrhea for 24 hours, vomited twice 2 hours ago, and now claims to be thirsty. The parent asks what to offer the child because the child is refusing Pedialyte. Which is the nurse's most appropriate response?
   1. "You can offer clear diet soda such as Sprite and ginger ale."
   2. "Pedialyte is really the best thing for your child, who, if thirsty enough, will eventually drink it."
   3. "Pedialyte is really the best thing for your child. Allow your child some choice in the way to take it by offering small amounts in a spoon, medicine cup, or syringe."
   4. "It really does not matter what your child drinks as long as it is kept down. Try offering small amounts of fluids in medicine cups."

7. The nurse is caring for a 9-month-old with diarrhea secondary to rotavirus. The child has not vomited and is mildly dehydrated. Which is likely to be included in the discharge teaching?
   1. Administer loperamide (Imodium) as needed.
   2. Administer bismuth subsalicylate (Kaopectate) as needed.
   3. Continue breastfeeding per routine.
   4. The infant may return to day care 24 hours after antibiotics have been started.

8. Which child can be discharged without further evaluation?
   1. A 2-year-old who has had 24 hours of watery diarrhea that has changed to bloody diarrhea in the past 12 hours.
   2. A 3-year-old who had a relapse of one diarrhea episode after restarting a normal diet.
   3. A 6-year-old who has been having vomiting and diarrhea for 2 days and has decreased urine output.
   4. A 10-year-old who has just returned from a Scout camping trip and has had several episodes of diarrhea.

9. The nurse receives a call from the parent of a 10-month-old who has vomited three times in the past 8 hours. The parent describes the baby as playful and wanting to drink. The parent asks the nurse what to give the child. Select the nurse's best response.
   1. "Replace the next feeding with regular water, and see if that is better tolerated."
   2. "Do not allow your baby to eat any solids; give half the normal formula feeding, and see if that is better tolerated."
   3. "Do not let your baby eat or drink anything for 24 hours to give the stomach a chance to rest."
   4. "Give your child ½ ounce of Pedialyte every 10 minutes. If vomiting continues, wait an hour, and then repeat what you previously gave."

10. The parents of a 4-year-old ask the nurse how to manage their child's constipation. Select the nurse's best response.
1. "Add 2 ounces of apple or pear juice to the child's diet."
2. "Be sure your child eats a lot of fresh fruit such as apples and bananas."
3. "Encourage your child to drink more fluids."
4. "Decrease bulky foods such as whole-grain breads and brown rice."

11. A child is diagnosed with chronic constipation that has been unresponsive to dietary and activity changes. Which pharmacological measure is most appropriate?
1. Natural supplements and herbs.
2. Stimulant laxative.
3. Osmotic agent.
4. Pharmacological measures are not used in pediatric constipation.

12. Which instructions for a child diagnosed with encopresis should the nurse question? **Select all that apply.**
1. Limit the intake of milk.
2. Offer a diet high in protein.
3. Obtain a complete dietary log.
4. Follow up with a child psychologist.
5. After dinner, have the child sit on the toilet for 10 minutes.

13. The nurse is caring for an infant diagnosed with Hirschsprung disease. The mother states she is pregnant with a boy and wants to know if her new baby will likely have the disorder. Which is the nurse's best response?
1. "Genetics play a small role in Hirschsprung disease, so there is a chance the baby will develop it as well."
2. "There is no evidence to support a genetic link, so it is very unlikely the baby will also have it."
3. "It is rarely seen in boys, so it is not likely your new baby will have Hirschsprung disease."
4. "Hirschsprung disease is seen only in girls, so your new baby will not be at risk."

14. The nurse is caring for an infant newly diagnosed with Hirschsprung disease. What does the nurse understand about this infant's condition? **Select all that apply.**
1. There is a lack of peristalsis in the large intestine and an accumulation of bowel contents, leading to abdominal distention.
2. There is excessive peristalsis throughout the intestine, resulting in abdominal distention.
3. There is a small-bowel obstruction, leading to ribbon-like stools.
4. There is inflammation throughout the large intestine, leading to accumulation of intestinal contents and abdominal distention.
5. There is an accumulation of bowel contents, leading to non-passage of stools.

15. The nurse is caring for a 3-month-old being evaluated for possible Hirschsprung disease. His parents call the nurse and show her his diaper containing a large amount of mucus and bloody diarrhea. The nurse notes that the infant is irritable and his abdomen appears very distended. Which should be the nurse's next action?
1. Reassure the parents that this is an expected finding and not uncommon.
2. Call a code for a potential cardiac arrest and stay with the infant.
3. Immediately obtain all vital signs with a quick head-to-toe assessment.
4. Obtain a stool sample for occult blood.

16. The nurse is caring for an 8-week-old male who has just been diagnosed with Hirschsprung disease. The parents ask what they should expect. Which is the nurse's best response?
    1. "It is really an easy disease to manage. Most children are placed on stool softeners to help with constipation until it resolves."
    2. "A permanent stool diversion, called a colostomy, will be placed by the surgeon to bypass the narrowed area."
    3. "Daily bowel irrigations will help your child maintain regular bowel habits."
    4. "Although your child will require surgery, there are different ways to manage the disease, depending on how much bowel is involved."

17. Which should the nurse include in the plan of care to decrease symptoms of gastroesophageal reflux (GER) in a 2-month-old? **Select all that apply.**
    1. Place the infant in an infant seat immediately after feedings.
    2. Place the infant in the prone position immediately after feeding to decrease the risk of aspiration.
    3. Encourage the parents not to worry because most infants outgrow GER within the first year of life.
    4. Encourage the parents to hold the infant in an upright position for 30 minutes following a feeding.
    5. Suggest that the parents burp the infant after every 1–2 ounces consumed.

18. The nurse knows that Nissen fundoplication involves which of the following?
    1. The fundus of the stomach is wrapped around the inferior stomach, mimicking a lower esophageal sphincter.
    2. The fundus of the stomach is wrapped around the inferior esophagus, mimicking a cardiac sphincter.
    3. The fundus of the stomach is wrapped around the middle portion of the stomach, decreasing the capacity of the stomach.
    4. The fundus of the stomach is dilated, decreasing the likelihood of reflux.

19. The nurse is caring for a 4-month-old with gastroesophageal reflux (GER). The infant is due to receive rantadine (Zantac). Based on the medication's mechanism of action, when should this medication be administered?
    1. Immediately before a feeding.
    2. 30 minutes after the feeding.
    3. 30 minutes before the feeding.
    4. At bedtime.

20. The nurse is administering omeprazole (Prilosec) to a 3-month-old with gastroesophageal reflux (GER). The child's parents ask the nurse how the medication works. Which is the nurse's best response?
    1. "Prilosec is a proton pump inhibitor that is commonly used for reflux in infants."
    2. "Prilosec decreases stomach acid, so it will not be as irritating when your child spits up."
    3. "Prilosec helps food move through the stomach quicker, so there will be less chance for reflux."
    4. "Prilosec relaxes the pressure of the lower esophageal sphincter."

21. A 10-year-old is being evaluated for possible appendicitis and complains of nausea and sharp abdominal pain in the right lower quadrant. An abdominal ultrasound is scheduled, and a blood count has been obtained. The child vomits, finds the pain relieved, and calls the nurse. Which should be the nurse's next action?
    1. Cancel the ultrasound and obtain an order for oral ondansetron (Zofran).
    2. Cancel the ultrasound and prepare to administer an intravenous bolus.
    3. Prepare for the probable discharge of the patient.
    4. Immediately notify the health-care provider of the child's status.

22. The parents of a child being evaluated for appendicitis tell the nurse the health-care provider said their child has a positive Rovsing sign. They ask the nurse what this means. Which is the nurse's best response?
    1. "Your child's health-care provider should answer that question."
    2. "A positive Rovsing sign means the child feels pain in the right side of the abdomen when the left side is palpated."
    3. "A positive Rovsing sign means pain is felt when the physician removes the hand from the abdomen."
    4. "A positive Rovsing sign means pain is felt in the right lower quadrant when the child coughs."

23. Which is the best position for an 8-year-old who has just returned to the pediatric unit after an appendectomy for a ruptured appendix?
    1. Semi-Fowler.
    2. Prone.
    3. Right side-lying.
    4. Left side-lying.

24. The nurse is to receive a 4-year-old from the recovery room after an appendectomy. The parents have not seen the child since surgery and ask what to expect. Which is the nurse's best response?
    1. "Your child will be very sleepy, have an intravenous line in the hand, and have a nasal tube to help drain the stomach. If your child needs pain medication, it will be given intravenously."
    2. "Your child will be very sleepy, have an intravenous line in the hand, and have white stockings to help prevent blood clots. If your child needs pain medication, we will give it intravenously or provide a liquid to swallow."
    3. "Your child will be wide awake and will have an intravenous line in the hand. If your child needs pain medication, we will give it intravenously or provide a liquid to swallow."
    4. "Your child will be very sleepy and have an intravenous line in the hand. If your child needs pain medication, we will give it intravenously."

25. The nurse is caring for a 5-year-old who has just returned from having an appendectomy. Which is the optimal way to manage pain?
    1. Intravenous morphine as needed.
    2. Liquid acetaminophen (Tylenol) with codeine as needed.
    3. Morphine administered through a PCA pump.
    4. Intramuscular morphine as needed.

26. The nurse is caring for a 3-year-old who had an appendectomy 2 days ago. The child has a fever of 101.8°F (38.8°C) and breath sounds are slightly diminished in the right lower lobe. Which action is most appropriate?
    1. Teach the child how to use an incentive spirometer.
    2. Encourage the child to blow bubbles.
    3. Obtain an order for intravenous antibiotics.
    4. Obtain an order for acetaminophen (Tylenol).

27. The nurse is providing discharge instructions to the parents of a child who had an appendectomy for a ruptured appendix 5 days ago. The nurse knows that further education is required when the parent states which of the following? **Select all that apply.**
    1. "We will wait a few days before allowing our child to return to school."
    2. "We will wait 2 weeks before allowing our child to return to sports."
    3. "We will call the health-care provider's office if we notice any drainage around the wound."
    4. "We will encourage our child to go for walks every day."
    5. "We will encourage our child to eat at every meal and offer snacks."

28. Which manifestations should the nurse expect to find in a child in the early stages of acute hepatitis?
    1. Nausea, vomiting, and generalized malaise.
    2. Nausea, vomiting, and pain in the left upper quadrant.
    3. Generalized malaise and yellowing of the skin and sclera.
    4. Yellowing of the skin and sclera without any other generalized complaints.

29. Which foods should be offered to a child with hepatitis?
    1. A tuna sandwich on whole wheat bread and a cup of skim milk.
    2. Clear liquids, such as broth, and Jell-O.
    3. A hamburger, French fries, and a diet soda.
    4. A peanut butter sandwich and a milkshake.

30. Which would be an appropriate activity for the nurse to recommend to the parent of a preschooler just diagnosed with acute hepatitis?
    1. Climbing in a "playscape."
    2. Kicking a ball.
    3. Playing video games in bed.
    4. Playing with puzzles in bed.

31. Which manifestation would the nurse expect to see in a 4-week-old infant with biliary atresia?
    1. Abdominal distention, enlarged liver, enlarged spleen, clay-colored stool, and tea-colored urine.
    2. Abdominal distention, multiple bruises, bloody stools, and hematuria.
    3. Yellow sclera and skin tones, excessively oily skin, and prolonged bleeding times.
    4. No manifestations until the disease has progressed to the advanced stage.

32. The nurse is caring for an infant with biliary atresia. The parents ask why the child is receiving cholestyramine. Which is the nurse's best response?
    1. To lower the infant's cholesterol.
    2. To relieve the infant's itching.
    3. To help the infant gain weight.
    4. To help feedings be absorbed in a more efficient manner.

33. Which is an accurate description of a Kasai procedure?
    1. A palliative procedure in which the bile duct is attached to a loop of bowel to assist with bile drainage.
    2. A curative procedure in which a connection is made between the bile duct and a loop of bowel to assist with bile drainage.
    3. A curative procedure in which the bile duct is banded to prevent bile leakage.
    4. A palliative procedure in which the bile duct is banded to prevent bile leakage.

34. The parents of a newborn diagnosed with a cleft lip and palate ask the nurse when their child's lip and palate will most likely be repaired. Which is the nurse's best response?
    1. "The palate and the lip are usually repaired in the first few weeks of life so that the baby can grow and gain weight."
    2. "The palate and the lip are usually not repaired until the baby is approximately 6 months old so that the mouth has had enough time to grow."
    3. "The lip is repaired in the first few months of life, but the palate is not usually repaired until the child is 3 years old."
    4. "The lip is repaired in the first few weeks of life, but the palate is not usually repaired until the child is 18 months old."

35. The nurse is caring for a newborn with a cleft lip and palate. The mother states, "I will not be able to breastfeed my baby." Which is the nurse's best response?
    1. "It sounds like you are feeling discouraged. Would you like to talk about it?"
    2. "Sometimes breastfeeding is still an option for babies with a cleft lip and palate. Would you like more information?"
    3. "Although breastfeeding is not an option, you can pump your milk and then feed it to your baby with a special nipple."
    4. "We usually discourage breastfeeding babies with cleft lip and palate as it puts them at an increased risk for aspiration."

36. The nurse is caring for a 4-month-old who has just had an isolated cleft lip repaired. Select the best position for the child in the immediate post-operative period.
    1. Right side-lying.
    2. Left side-lying.
    3. Supine.
    4. Prone.

37. Which should be included in the plan of care for a 14-month-old whose cleft palate was repaired 12 hours ago? **Select all that apply.**
    1. Allow the infant to have familiar items of comfort such as a favorite stuffed animal and a "sippy" cup.
    2. Once liquids have been tolerated, encourage a bland diet such as soup, Jell-O, and saltine crackers.
    3. Administer pain medication on a regular schedule, as opposed to an as-needed schedule.
    4. Use a Yankauer suction catheter on the infant's mouth to decrease the risk of aspiration of oral secretions.
    5. When discharged, remove elbow restraints.

38. The nurse is caring for a newborn with esophageal atresia. When reviewing the mother's history, which would the nurse expect to find?
    1. Maternal polyhydramnios.
    2. Pregnancy lasting more than 38 weeks.
    3. Poor nutrition during pregnancy.
    4. Alcohol consumption during pregnancy.

39. Which should be the nurse's immediate action when a newborn begins to cough and choke and becomes cyanotic while feeding?
    1. Inform the health-care provider of the situation.
    2. Have the mother stop feeding the infant, and observe to see if the choking episode resolves on its own.
    3. Immediately determine the infant's oxygen saturation and have the mother stop feeding the infant.
    4. Take the infant from the mother and administer blow-by oxygen while obtaining the infant's oxygen saturation.

40. The nurse is caring for a newborn who has just been diagnosed with tracheoesophageal fistula and is scheduled for surgery. Which should the nurse expect to do in the preoperative period?
    1. Keep the child in a monitored crib, obtain frequent vital signs, and allow the parents to visit but not hold their infant.
    2. Administer intravenous fluids and antibiotics.
    3. Place the infant on 100% oxygen via a non-rebreather mask.
    4. Have the mother feed the infant slowly in a monitored area, stopping all feedings 4 to 6 hours before surgery.

41. The nurse is giving discharge instructions to the parent of a 1-month-old infant with tracheoesophageal fistula and a gastrostomy tube (GT). The nurse knows the mother understands the discharge teaching when she states:
    1. "I will give my baby feedings through the GT but place liquid medications in the corner of the mouth to be absorbed."
    2. "I will flush the GT with 2 ounces of water after each feeding to prevent the GT from clogging."
    3. "I will clean the area around the GT every day."
    4. "I will place petroleum jelly around the GT if any redness develops."

42. An expectant mother asks the nurse if her new baby will have an umbilical hernia. The nurse bases the response on the fact that it occurs:
    1. More often in large infants.
    2. In white infants more often than in African American infants.
    3. Twice as often in male infants.
    4. More often in premature infants.

43. The nurse is providing discharge teaching to the parents of an infant with an umbilical hernia. Which should be included in the plan of care?
    1. If the hernia has not resolved on its own by the age of 12 months, surgery is generally recommended.
    2. If the hernia appears to be more swollen or tender, seek medical care immediately.
    3. To help the hernia resolve, place a pressure dressing over the area gently.
    4. If the hernia is repaired surgically, there is a strong likelihood that it will return.

44. The nurse is caring for an infant with pyloric stenosis. The parent asks if any future children will likely have pyloric stenosis. Which is the nurse's best response?
    1. "You seem worried; would you like to discuss your concerns?"
    2. "It is very rare for a family to have more than one child with pyloric stenosis."
    3. "Pyloric stenosis can run in families. It is more common among males."
    4. "Although there can be a genetic link, it is very unusual for girls to have pyloric stenosis."

45. The nurse is caring for an 8-week-old infant being evaluated for pyloric stenosis. Which statement by the parent would be typical for a child with this diagnosis?
    1. "The baby is a very fussy eater and just does not want to eat."
    2. "The baby tends to have a very forceful vomiting episode about 30 minutes after most feedings."
    3. "The baby is always hungry after vomiting, so I feed her again."
    4. "The baby is happy in spite of getting really upset after spitting up."

46. The nurse is caring for a 7-week-old scheduled for a pyloromyotomy in 24 hours. Which would the nurse expect to find in the plan of care?
    1. Keep infant NPO; begin intravenous fluids at maintenance.
    2. Keep infant NPO; begin intravenous fluids at maintenance; place nasogastric tube (NGT) to low wall suction.
    3. Obtain serum electrolytes; keep infant NPO; do not attempt to pass NGT due to obstruction.
    4. Offer infant small frequent feedings; keep NPO 6 to 8 hours before surgery.

47. The nurse receives a call from the mother of a 6-month-old who describes her child as alternately sleepy and fussy. She states that her infant vomited once this morning and had two episodes of diarrhea. The last episode contained mucus and a small amount of blood. She asks the nurse what she should do. Which is the nurse's best response?
1. "Your infant will need to have some tests in the emergency department to determine whether anything serious is going on."
2. "Try feeding your infant in about 30 minutes; in the event of repeat vomiting, bring the infant to the emergency department for some tests and intravenous rehydration."
3. "Many infants display these symptoms when they develop an allergy to the formula they are receiving; try switching to a soy-based formula."
4. "Do not worry about the blood and mucus in the stool; it is not unusual for infants to have blood in their stools because their intestines are more sensitive."

48. The nurse is caring for a 5-month-old infant with a diagnosis of intussusception. The infant has periods of irritability during which the knees are brought to the chest and the infant cries, alternating with periods of lethargy. Vital signs are stable and within age-appropriate limits. The health-care provider elects to give an enema. The parents ask the purpose of the enema. Which is the nurse's most appropriate response?
1. "The enema will confirm the diagnosis. If the test result is positive, your child will need to have surgery to correct the intussusception."
2. "The enema will confirm the diagnosis. Although very unlikely, the enema may also help fix the intussusception so that your child will not immediately need surgery."
3. "The enema will help confirm the diagnosis and has a good chance of fixing the intussusception."
4. "The enema will help confirm the diagnosis and may temporarily fix the intussusception. If the bowel returns to normal, there is a strong likelihood that the intussusception will recur."

49. The nurse will soon receive a 4-month-old who has been diagnosed with intussusception. The infant is described as very lethargic with the following vital signs: T 101.8°F (38.7°C), HR 181, BP 68/38. The reporting nurse states the infant's abdomen is very rigid. Which is the most appropriate action for the receiving nurse?
1. Prepare to accompany the infant to a computed tomography scan to confirm the diagnosis.
2. Prepare to accompany the infant to the radiology department for a reducing enema.
3. Prepare to start a second intravenous line to administer fluids and antibiotics.
4. Prepare to get the infant ready for immediate surgical correction.

50. The nurse is providing discharge instructions to the parents of an infant who has had surgery to open a low imperforate anus. The nurse knows that the discharge instructions have been understood when the child's parents say:
1. "We will use an oral thermometer because we cannot use a rectal one."
2. "We will call the health-care provider if the stools change in consistency."
3. "Our infant will never be toilet-trained."
4. "We understand that it is not unusual for our infant's urine to contain stool."

51. The nurse caring for a neonate with an anorectal malformation notes that the infant has not passed any stool per rectum but that the infant's urine contains meconium. The nurse can make which assumption?
1. The child likely has a low anorectal malformation.
2. The child likely has a high anorectal malformation.
3. The child will not need a colostomy.
4. This malformation will be corrected with a nonoperative rectal pull-through.

52. The nurse is caring for a newborn with an anorectal malformation and a colostomy. The nurse knows that more education is needed when the infant's parent states which of the following?
    1. "I will make sure the stoma is red."
    2. "There should not be any discharge or irritation around the outside of the stoma."
    3. "I will keep a bag attached to avoid the contents of the small intestine coming in contact with the baby's skin."
    4. "As my baby grows, a pattern will develop over time, and there should be predictable bowel movements."

53. The parent of a child being evaluated for celiac disease asks the nurse why it is important to make dietary changes. Which is the nurse's best response?
    1. "The body's response to gluten causes damage to the mucosal cells in the intestine, leading to absorption problems."
    2. "The body's response to consumption of anything containing gluten is to create special cells called villi, which leads to more diarrhea."
    3. "The body's response to gluten causes the intestine to become more porous and hang on to more of the fat-soluble vitamins, leading to vitamin toxicity."
    4. "The body's response to gluten causes damage to the mucosal cells, leading to malabsorption of water and hard, constipated stools."

54. The nurse is caring for a 14-year-old with celiac disease. The nurse knows that the patient understands the diet instructions by ordering which of the following meals?
    1. Eggs, bacon, rye toast, and lactose-free milk.
    2. Pancakes, orange juice, and sausage links.
    3. Oat cereal, breakfast pastry, and nonfat skim milk.
    4. Cheese, banana slices, rice cakes, and whole milk.

55. Which would the nurse expect to be included to make the diagnosis of celiac disease in a child?
    1. Obtain complete blood count and serum electrolytes.
    2. Obtain complete blood count and stool sample; keep child NPO.
    3. Obtain stool sample and prepare child for jejunal biopsy.
    4. Obtain complete blood count and serum electrolytes; monitor child's response to gluten-containing diet.

56. Which manifestation suggests that an infant is developing necrotizing enterocolitis (NEC)?
    1. Absorption of bolus orogastric feedings at a faster rate than previous feedings.
    2. Bloody diarrhea.
    3. Increased bowel sounds.
    4. Appears hungry right before a scheduled feeding.

57. The nurse is caring for a 1-month-old term infant who experienced an anoxic episode at birth. The health-care team suspects that the infant is developing necrotizing enterocolitis (NEC). Which would the nurse expect to be included in the plan of care?
    1. Immediately remove the feeding nasogastric tube (NGT) from the infant.
    2. Obtain vital signs every 4 hours.
    3. Prepare to administer antibiotics intravenously.
    4. Change feedings to half-strength, administer slowly via a feeding pump.

58. More education about necrotizing enterocolitis (NEC) is needed in a nursing in-service when one of the participants states:
    1. "Encouraging the mother to pump her milk for the feedings helps prevent NEC."
    2. "Some sources state that the occurrence of NEC has increased because so many preterm infants are surviving."
    3. "When signs of sepsis appear, the infant will likely deteriorate quickly."
    4. "NEC occurs only in preemies and low-birth-weight infants."

59. The nurse is caring for an infant who has been diagnosed with short bowel syndrome (SBS). The parent asks how the disease will affect the child. Which is the nurse's best response?
    1. "Because your child has a shorter intestine than most, your child will likely experience constipation and will need to be placed on a bowel regimen."
    2. "Because your child has a shorter intestine than most, he will not be able to absorb all the nutrients and vitamins in food and will need to get nutrients in other ways."
    3. "Unfortunately, most children with this diagnosis do not do very well."
    4. "The prognosis and course of the disease have changed because hyperalimentation is available."

60. The nurse is caring for a 3-month-old infant who has short bowel syndrome (SBS) and has been receiving parenteral nutrition (PN). The parents ask if their child will ever be able to eat. Which is the nurse's best response?
    1. "Children with SBS are never able to eat and must receive all of their nutrition in intravenous form."
    2. "You will have to start feeding your child because children cannot be on PN longer than 6 months."
    3. "We will start feeding your child soon so that the bowel continues to receive stimulation."
    4. "Your child will start receiving tube feedings soon but will never be able to eat by mouth."

61. Which child may need extra fluids to prevent dehydration? **Select all that apply.**
    1. A 7-day-old receiving phototherapy.
    2. A 6-month-old with newly diagnosed pyloric stenosis.
    3. A 2-year-old with pneumonia.
    4. A 2-year-old with full-thickness burns to the chest, back, and abdomen.
    5. A 13-year-old who has just started her menses.

62. The nurse is interviewing the parents of a 6-year-old who has been experiencing constipation. Which could be a causative factor? **Select all that apply.**
    1. Hypothyroidism.
    2. Muscular dystrophy.
    3. Myelomeningocele.
    4. Drinks a lot of milk.
    5. Active in sports.

The correct answer number and rationale for why it is the correct answer are given in **boldface blue type.** Rationales for why the other possible answer options are incorrect also are given, but they are not in boldface type.

1. 1. Swallowing is a reflex in neonates; infants younger than 6 weeks cannot voluntarily control swallowing.
   2. Swallowing is a reflex in neonates; infants younger than 6 weeks cannot voluntarily control swallowing.
   3. The infant is not capable of selectively rejecting fluid because swallowing is a reflex until 6 weeks.
   4. **Swallowing is a reflex in infants younger than 6 weeks.**

   TEST-TAKING HINT: Swallowing is a reflex that is present until the age of 6 weeks. The test taker should eliminate answers 1, 2, and 3 because they suggest that the infant is capable of selectively rejecting fluids.

2. 1. The caloric content of breast milk and formula tends to be similar.
   2. Peristalsis in infants is greater than in older children.
   3. **The small-stomach capacity and rapid movement of fluid through the digestive system account for the need for small, frequent feedings.**
   4. Breastfed babies and formula-fed babies do not necessarily have a difference in feeding time.

   TEST-TAKING HINT: The test taker should eliminate answers 1 and 4 because they both form generalizations that are not supported by current literature.

3. 1. The information obtained from a urinalysis of an infant is not as helpful as serum electrolytes. The infant has limited ability to concentrate urine, so the specific gravity is not usually affected.
   2. The information obtained from a urinalysis of an infant is not as helpful as serum electrolytes. The infant has limited ability to concentrate urine, so the specific gravity is not usually affected. A urinalysis does not need to be obtained by catheterization.
   3. **The analysis of serum electrolytes offers the most information and assists with the diagnosis of dehydration.**
   4. Although critical in diagnosing meningitis, a lumber puncture and analysis of cerebrospinal fluid are not done to confirm dehydration.

   TEST-TAKING HINT: Infants have limited ability to concentrate urine, so answers 1 and 2 can be eliminated immediately.

4. 1. **Dehydration is corrected with the administration of an isotonic solution, such as normal saline or lactated Ringer solution.**
   2. Solutions containing dextrose should never be administered in bolus form because they may result in cerebral edema.
   3. Solutions containing dextrose should never be administered in bolus form because they may result in cerebral edema.
   4. Severe dehydration is not usually corrected with oral solutions; children with altered levels of consciousness should be kept NPO.

   TEST-TAKING HINT: The test taker should immediately eliminate answers 2 and 3 because they both suggest administering glucose in bolus form, which is always contraindicated in pediatric clients. Answer 4 should be eliminated because the infant is severely dehydrated and not responding to painful stimulation, which is suggested by the lack of a cry on intravenous insertion.

5. 1. Fluid boluses of normal saline are administered according to the child's body weight. It is not unusual to have to repeat the bolus multiple times in order to see an improvement in the child's condition.
   2. It is important to monitor serum electrolytes frequently in the dehydrated child.
   3. **Potassium is contraindicated because the child has not yet urinated. Potassium is not added to the maintenance fluid until kidney function has been verified.**
   4. The child with dehydration secondary to vomiting and diarrhea is placed on a clear liquid diet.

   TEST-TAKING HINT: Be aware of the usual ways in which dehydration is treated. Answer 3 should be selected because the description states that the child has not urinated.

6. 1. When Pedialyte is not tolerated, it is usually recommended that clear sodas and juices be diluted. Diet beverages are not recommended because the sugar is needed to help the sodium be reabsorbed.
2. Pedialyte is the best choice. If the child is not encouraged to drink Pedialyte, the child may become severely dehydrated. Other ways to encourage oral rehydration need to be considered.
3. **Pedialyte is the first choice, as recommended by the American Academy of Pediatrics. Offering the child appropriate choices may allow the child to feel empowered and less likely to refuse the Pedialyte. Small, frequent amounts are usually better tolerated.**
4. Offering small amounts of liquids is important. The type of beverage does matter because many fluids may increase vomiting and diarrhea.

TEST-TAKING HINT: The test taker should eliminate answer 2 because it offers an ultimatum to a child. The child is likely to refuse the Pedialyte, worsening the state of dehydration.

7. 1. Loperamide (Imodium) slows intestinal motility and allows overgrowth of organisms and should therefore be avoided.
2. Bismuth subsalicylate (Kaopectate) slows intestinal motility and allows overgrowth of organisms and should therefore be avoided.
3. **Breastfeeding is usually well tolerated and helps prevent death of intestinal villi and malabsorption.**
4. Antibiotics are not effective in viruses. Children should not return to day care while they are still having diarrhea.

TEST-TAKING HINT: The test taker can eliminate answer 4 because antibiotics are not effective with viruses such as rotavirus. Answers 1 and 2 can be eliminated because antidiarrheal agents are not recommended in the pediatric population.

8. 1. Diarrhea containing blood needs further evaluation to determine the source of the blood, and the child's blood counts and electrolyte balance need to be tested.
2. **It is common for children to have a relapse of diarrhea after resuming a regular diet.**

3. Children who have had vomiting and diarrhea for more than 2 days require evaluation to determine whether IV rehydration and hospital admission are necessary.
4. Diarrhea following a camping trip needs further evaluation because it may be caused by bacteria or parasites.

TEST-TAKING HINT: The test taker should eliminate answers 1 and 3 because they describe children who may have altered electrolytes and blood counts due to prolonged diarrhea.

9. 1. Free water should not be given because it does not contain any electrolytes and can lead to critical electrolyte imbalances.
2. Formula should be avoided, and clear liquids such as Pedialyte should be offered.
3. Twenty-four hours is too long for the infant to remain NPO. The infant needs to drink a rehydration solution such as Pedialyte in order to avoid severe dehydration.
4. **Offering small amounts of clear liquids is usually well tolerated. If the child vomits, make NPO for an hour to allow the stomach to rest and then restart fluids. The child in this scenario is described as playful and therefore does not appear to be at risk for dehydration.**

TEST-TAKING HINT: The test taker should eliminate answers 1 and 3 because they could cause harm to the infant.

10. 1. Two ounces of apple juice is most likely not a sufficient quantity to alter a 4-year-old child's bowel movements.
2. Although fresh fruits help decrease constipation, bananas tend to increase constipation.
3. **Increasing fluid consumption helps to decrease the hardness of the stool.**
4. Whole-grain bread and brown rice are high in fiber and help decrease constipation.

TEST-TAKING HINT: Answer 1 decreases constipation in an infant but not in a preschooler.

11. 1. Natural supplements and herbs are not recommended because the safety and efficacy are not standardized.
2. A stimulant laxative is not the drug of choice because it may increase abdominal discomfort and may lead to dependency.
3. **A stool softener (osmotic agent) is the drug of choice because it will lead to easier evacuation.**

4. Although diet and activity modification are tried first, medications are sometimes needed.

TEST-TAKING HINT: The test taker should eliminate answer 4 because it implies that medications are never given to the constipated child. In health care, there are very few cases of "never" and "always."

12. **2, 4.**
    1. Dairy products are limited because they can lead to constipation.
    2. **A diet high in protein will cause more constipation.**
    3. A complete dietary log should be kept to correlate the foods that lead to constipation.
    4. **The child and family would not be encouraged initially to seek counseling unless a psychological component to the encopresis had been identified.**
    5. Children with constipation/encopresis are advised to sit on the toilet for 10 minutes after dinner to take advantage of the gastrocolic reflex.

    TEST-TAKING HINT: Recall foods and behaviors that cause constipation in children and successful approaches to meet their needs.

13. 1. **There is a genetic component to Hirschsprung disease, so any future siblings are also at risk.**
    2. There is a genetic component to Hirschsprung disease.
    3. Hirschsprung disease is seen more commonly in males than females.
    4. Hirschsprung disease is seen in both males and females, but is more common in males.

    TEST-TAKING HINT: The test taker can eliminate answers 3 and 4 because they are similar and therefore would not likely be the correct answer.

14. **1, 5.**
    1. **In Hirschsprung disease, a portion of the large intestine has an area lacking in ganglion cells. This results in a lack of peristalsis as well as an accumulation of bowel contents and abdominal distention.**
    2. There is a lack of peristalsis at the aganglionic section of the bowel.
    3. Hirschsprung disease does not include a small-bowel obstruction.
    4. Hirschsprung disease does not present with inflammation throughout the large intestine.
    5. **There is accumulation of stool above the aganglionic bowel, which does not allow stool to pass through.**

TEST-TAKING HINT: The test taker should be familiar with the pathophysiology of Hirschsprung disease in order to select answers 1 and 5.

15. 1. All cases of bloody diarrhea need to be evaluated because this may be a sign of enterocolitis, which is a potentially fatal complication of Hirschsprung disease.
    2. Although this is a potentially critical complication, calling a code is not necessary at this time because the infant is irritable and not unconscious.
    3. **All vital signs need to be evaluated because the child with enterocolitis can quickly progress to a state of shock. A quick head-to-toe assessment will allow the nurse to evaluate the child's circulatory system.**
    4. It is not a priority to test the stool for occult blood, because there is obvious blood in the sample.

    TEST-TAKING HINT: The test taker should select answer 3 because there is not enough information to determine the status of the child. Obtaining vital signs will help the nurse to assess the situation.

16. 1. The constipation will not resolve with stool softeners. The affected bowel needs to be removed.
    2. Most colostomies are not permanent. The large intestine is usually reattached, and the colostomy is taken down.
    3. The child with Hirschsprung disease requires surgery to remove the aganglionic portion of the large intestine.
    4. **The aganglionic portion needs to be removed. Although most children have a temporary colostomy placed, many infants are able to bypass the colostomy and have the bowel immediately reattached.**

    TEST-TAKING HINT: The test taker should be led to answer 4 because it is the least restrictive of all answers and is the only one that states that the child will require surgery. Children with Hirschsprung disease are managed surgically.

17. **4, 5.**
    1. Placing the infant in an infant seat increases intra-abdominal pressure, putting the infant at increased risk for GER.
    2. The prone position is not recommended because it may lead to sudden infant death syndrome (SIDS).

3. Although most infants outgrow GER, providing the parents with this education will not help decrease the symptoms.

4. **Keeping the infant in an upright position is the best way to decrease the symptoms of GER. The infant can also be placed in the supine position with the head of the crib elevated. A harness can be used to keep the child from sliding down.**

5. **Burping the infant frequently may help decrease spitting up by expelling air from the stomach more often.**

TEST-TAKING HINT: The test taker may be led to answer 3. However, the question is looking for ways to decrease reflux. Although decreasing parental anxiety may help decrease reflux, the better answers are 4 and 5 because they are more likely to be part of an effective management plan.

18. 1. The fundus is wrapped around the inferior esophagus, not the inferior stomach.

2. **The Nissen fundoplication involves wrapping the fundus of the stomach around the inferior esophagus, creating a lower esophageal, or cardiac, sphincter.**

3. The fundus is not wrapped around the middle portion of the stomach. There is no benefit to decreasing the stomach's capacity.

4. The fundus of the stomach is not dilated.

TEST-TAKING HINT: The test taker needs to be familiar with surgical options for GER disease.

19. 1. If rantadine (Zantac) is administered immediately before a feeding, the medication will not have enough time to take effect.

2. This medication should be administered prior to a feeding to be effective.

3. **Rantadine (Zantac) decreases gastric acid secretion and should be administered 30 minutes before a feeding.**

4. This medication should be administered prior to a feeding to be effective.

TEST-TAKING HINT: The test taker needs to be familiar with the administration of rantadine (Zantac).

20. 1. Although this is an accurate description of the mechanism of action, it does not tell the parents how the medication functions.

2. **This accurate description gives the parents information that is clear and concise.**

3. Omeprazole (Prilosec) does not increase the rate of gastric emptying.

4. Omeprazole (Prilosec) does not relax the pressure of the lower esophageal sphincter.

TEST-TAKING HINT: The test taker should eliminate answers 1 and 4 because they do not communicate information in a manner that will be clear to many parents.

21. 1. The ultrasound should not be canceled but obtained emergently because the child probably has a perforated appendix. The child should be NPO because surgery is imminent.

2. The ultrasound should not be canceled but obtained emergently because the child probably has a perforated appendix.

3. The child will not be discharged because he most likely has a perforated appendix.

4. **The health-care provider should be notified immediately, because a sudden change or loss of pain often indicates a perforated appendix.**

TEST-TAKING HINT: The test taker should eliminate answers 1 and 2 because there is no reason to cancel the ultrasound. The health-care provider should always be notified of any changes in a patient's condition.

22. 1. This response is not helpful and dismisses the parents' concern.

2. **A positive Rovsing sign occurs when the left lower quadrant is palpated and pain is felt in the right lower quadrant.**

3. Pain that is felt when the hand is removed during palpation is called rebound tenderness.

4. Pain that is felt when the child coughs is called a positive cough sign.

TEST-TAKING HINT: The test taker should immediately eliminate answer 1 because it is not therapeutic and is dismissive.

23. 1. The semi-Fowler position does not provide the most comfort to the postoperative appendectomy child.

2. The prone position does not allow the nurse to visualize the incision easily and would probably be uncomfortable for the child.

3. **The right side-lying position promotes comfort and allows the peritoneal cavity to drain.**

4. The left side-lying position may not provide as much comfort and will not allow the peritoneal cavity to drain as freely as will the right side-lying position.

TEST-TAKING HINT: The test taker should be led to answer 3 because lying on the same side as the abdominal incision is usually the most comfortable for the child.

24. 1. An NGT is not needed when an appendix has not ruptured.
2. Antiembolic stockings are not used in children this young, who will likely be moving the lower extremities and ambulating.
3. The child in the immediate postoperative period is usually not wide awake.
4. **In the immediate postoperative period, the child is usually sleepy but can be roused. The child usually has an intravenous line for hydration and pain medication.**

TEST-TAKING HINT: The test taker should eliminate answer 1 because NGTs are not used unless the appendix has ruptured. Answer 2 can also be eliminated because a 4-year-old who is post appendectomy is not at risk for blood clots.

25. 1. Intravenous morphine given as needed may cause the child to have periods of pain when the medication has worn off. The child may also be hesitant to ask for pain medication, fearing an invasive procedure.
2. Liquid acetaminophen (Tylenol) with codeine may not offer sufficient pain control in the immediate postoperative period.
3. **Morphine administered through a PCA pump offers the child control over managing pain. The PCA pump also has the benefit of offering a basal rate as well as an as-needed rate for optimal pain management.**
4. The intramuscular route should be avoided if less invasive routes are available. A 5-year-old fears invasive procedures and may deny pain to avoid receiving an injection.

TEST-TAKING HINT: The test taker should recall that PCA pumps are very effective, even in young children.

26. 1. Many 3-year-olds have difficulty understanding how to use an incentive spirometer.
2. **Blowing bubbles is a developmentally appropriate way to help the preschooler take deep breaths and cough.**
3. In the early postoperative period, a fever is likely a respiratory issue and not a result of infection of the incision.
4. Although acetaminophen (Tylenol) may be administered, encouraging the child to breathe deeply and cough will help prevent the fever from returning.

TEST-TAKING HINT: The test taker should be aware that a fever in the first few days after surgery is generally due to pulmonary complications, so answer 3 can be eliminated. Remembering the developmental needs of the child, the test taker should select answer 2.

27. 2, 3.
1. The child should wait a few days before returning to school to avoid being easily fatigued.
2. **The child should wait 6 weeks before returning to any strenuous activity.**
3. **Any signs of infection should be reported to the surgeon.**
4. The child should be encouraged to walk every day because it will help the bowels return to normal and help the child regain stamina.
5. Encouraging the child to eat three meals per day and snacks in between is important following surgery to restore stamina and help with healing.

TEST-TAKING HINT: The test taker should note that the question is asking which of the answers indicate that more education is needed. Answer 2 should be selected because 2 weeks is too early to return to strenuous sports. Answer 3 should be selected because the surgeon, not the general health-care provider, should be contacted.

28. 1. **The early stage of acute hepatitis is referred to as the anicteric phase, during which the child usually complains of nausea, vomiting, and generalized malaise.**
2. A tender enlarged liver is noted in the right upper quadrant.
3. The child does not appear jaundiced until the icteric phase.
4. The child does not appear jaundiced until the icteric phase. The child usually does not feel well during the early stages of acute hepatitis.

TEST-TAKING HINT: The test taker needs to be familiar with the manifestations of acute hepatitis. Knowing that the early stage is referred to as the anicteric phase, answers 3 and 4 can be eliminated.

29. 1. **A diet that is high in protein and carbohydrates helps maintain caloric intake and protein stores while preventing muscle wasting. A low-fat diet prevents abdominal distention.**

2. The child should be encouraged to consume a diet higher in protein.
3. The child should be encouraged to consume a low-fat diet.
4. The child should be encouraged to consume a low-fat diet.

TEST-TAKING HINT: The child with hepatitis is usually placed on a diet that is high in both protein and carbohydrates but low in fat.

30. 1. The child with acute hepatitis usually does not feel well, and activities should be limited to quiet, restful ones.
    2. The child with acute hepatitis usually does not feel well, and activities should be limited to quiet, restful ones.
    3. Video games can be played by preschoolers but are not the most appropriate choice.
    4. **Playing with puzzles is a developmentally appropriate activity for a preschooler on bedrest.**

TEST-TAKING HINT: The test taker should incorporate developmentally appropriate activities for the child in the early stages of acute hepatitis. Answers 1 and 2 can be eliminated because they are not activities that can be done while resting. Answer 4 should be selected because it is a better activity for a preschooler.

31. 1. **The infant with biliary atresia usually has an enlarged liver and spleen. The stools appear clay-colored because of the absence of bile pigments. The urine is tea-colored because of the excretion of bile salts.**
    2. The urine typically contains bile salts, not blood. There is usually no blood noted in the stool.
    3. The skin is usually dry and itchy, not oily.
    4. Manifestations of biliary atresia usually appear by 3 weeks of life.

TEST-TAKING HINT: The test taker needs to be familiar with the manifestations of biliary atresia and should be led to select answer 1.

32. 1. Although cholestyramine is used to lower cholesterol, its primary purpose in the child with biliary atresia is to relieve pruritus.
    2. **The primary reason cholestyramine is administered to the child with biliary atresia is to relieve pruritus.**
    3. Cholestyramine is not administered to help the child gain weight.
    4. Cholestyramine does not assist with the absorption of feedings.

TEST-TAKING HINT: The test taker needs to consider the manifestations of the disease process when considering why medications are administered. The liver is unable to eliminate bile, which leads to intense pruritus.

33. 1. **The Kasai procedure is a palliative procedure in which the bile duct is attached to a loop of bowel to assist with bile drainage.**
    2. The procedure is palliative, not curative because most children require a liver transplant after a few years.
    3. The Kasai procedure is not curative and does not band the bile duct.
    4. The Kasai procedure is palliative but does not band the bile duct.

TEST-TAKING HINT: The test taker can eliminate answers 2 and 3, because the majority of cases of biliary atresia require a liver transplant. The Kasai procedure is performed to give the child a few years to grow before requiring a transplant.

34. 1. The palate is not repaired until the child is approximately 18 months old to allow for facial growth. Waiting beyond 18 months may interfere with speech.
    2. The lip is usually repaired in the first few weeks of life, and the palate is usually repaired at approximately 18 months.
    3. The palate is repaired earlier than 3 years so that speech development is not impaired.
    4. **The lip is repaired in the first few weeks of life, but the palate is not usually repaired until the child is 18 months old.**

TEST-TAKING HINT: The test taker should consider the palate's involvement in the development of speech and therefore eliminate answer 3. The palate is usually given at least a year to grow sufficiently.

35. 1. Encouraging parents to express their feelings is important, but it is more appropriate to give the parents information on breastfeeding.
    2. **Some mothers are able to breastfeed their infants who have a cleft lip and palate. The breast can help fill in the cleft and help the infant create suction.**
    3. Breastfeeding is sometimes an option.
    4. Breastfeeding does not increase the risk of aspiration among infants with a cleft lip and palate.

TEST-TAKING HINT: The test taker should be led to select answer 2 because the breast can sometimes act to fill in the cleft.

36. 1. The infant may rub the face on the bedding if positioned on the side.
    2. The infant may rub the face on the bedding if positioned on the side.
    3. **The supine position is preferred because there is decreased risk of the infant rubbing the suture line.**
    4. The infant may rub the face on the bedding if positioned on the abdomen.

    TEST-TAKING HINT: The test taker should be led to answer 3 because it is the only option in which the suture line is not at increased risk for injury.

37. **1, 3.**
    1. **The child should not be allowed to use anything that creates suction in the mouth, such as pacifiers or straws. "Sippy" cups are acceptable.**
    2. The child should not have anything hard in the mouth, such as crackers, cookies, or a spoon.
    3. **Pain medication should be administered regularly to avoid crying, which places stress on the suture line.**
    4. A Yankauer suction should not be used in the mouth because it creates suction and is a hard instrument that could irritate the suture line. The child should be positioned to allow secretions to drain out of the child's mouth. Suction should be used only in the event of an emergency.
    5. Elbow restraints are used until the repaired palate has healed. When at home, the parents need to monitor the child closely if restraints are removed to move the arms or for bathing.

    TEST-TAKING HINT: The child who has had a cleft palate repair should have nothing in the mouth that could irritate the suture line. Answers 2 and 4 can be eliminated.

38. 1. **Maternal polyhydramnios is present because the infant cannot swallow and absorb the amniotic fluid in utero.**
    2. Many mothers of infants with esophageal atresia deliver early because of the pressure of the unabsorbed amniotic fluid.
    3. Although good nutrition is important in every pregnancy, there is not a direct relationship between diet and esophageal atresia.
    4. Although alcohol should not be consumed in any pregnancy, there is not a direct link between alcohol and esophageal atresia.

    TEST-TAKING HINT: The test taker should select answer 1 because esophageal atresia prevents the fetus from ingesting amniotic fluid, leading to increased amniotic fluid in utero.

39. 1. The infant's feeding should be stopped immediately and oxygen administered. The nurse should call for help but should not leave the infant while in distress.
    2. The mother should stop feeding the infant, but oxygen should be applied while the infant is cyanotic. The infant should be placed on a monitor, and vital signs should be obtained.
    3. Although obtaining oxygen saturations is extremely important, the infant is visually cyanotic, so the nurse should administer oxygen as a priority.
    4. **The infant should be taken from the mother and placed in the crib where the nurse can assess the baby. Oxygen should be administered immediately, and vital signs should be obtained.**

    TEST-TAKING HINT: The test taker should be led to answer 4 because the baby is cyanotic and needs oxygen.

40. 1. The infant should be monitored, and vital signs should be obtained frequently, but the parents should be encouraged to hold their baby.
    2. **Intravenous fluids are administered to prevent dehydration because the infant is NPO. Intravenous antibiotics are administered to prevent pneumonia because aspiration of secretions is likely.**
    3. The infant should receive only the amount of oxygen needed to keep saturations above 94%.
    4. As soon as the diagnosis is made, the infant is made NPO because the risk for aspiration is extremely high.

    TEST-TAKING HINT: Infants with tracheoesophageal fistula are at great risk for aspiration and subsequent pneumonia. With this knowledge, the test taker should eliminate answer 4 and select answer 2.

41. 1. Medications can also be placed in the GT.
    2. Two ounces of water is too much water for an infant and could cause electrolyte imbalances. The tube can be flushed with 3 to 5 mL of water to prevent clogging.
    3. **The area around the GT should be cleaned daily to prevent an infection.**

4. If redness develops, the parents should call the physician because an infection could be present.

TEST-TAKING HINT: The test taker should immediately eliminate answer 1 because medications and feedings can be placed in the GT. The test taker should know that 2 ounces of water after each feeding is a large amount (recalling that infants are typically fed at least every 4 hours).

42. 1. Umbilical hernias occur more often in low-birth-weight infants.
    2. Umbilical hernias occur more often in African American infants than in white infants.
    3. Umbilical hernias affect males and females equally.
    4. **Umbilical hernias occur more often in premature infants.**

TEST-TAKING HINT: The test taker needs to be familiar with the occurrence of umbilical hernias.

43. 1. Most umbilical hernias resolve spontaneously by age 2 to 3 years. Surgery is not usually recommended until the age of 3 because the hernia may resolve before that.
    2. **If the hernia appears larger, swollen, or tender, the intestine may be trapped, which is a surgical emergency.**
    3. A pressure dressing should never be placed over the hernia because it can cause irritation and does not help the hernia resolve.
    4. If the hernia is corrected surgically, the recurrence rate is low.

TEST-TAKING HINT: The test taker should be led to select answer 2 because a change in the hernia indicates an incarcerated hernia, which is an emergency.

44. 1. This approach sounds like the nurse is avoiding the parent's question. It would be better to offer the information and then ask about the parent's concerns.
    2. It is not at all uncommon for a family to have multiple children with pyloric stenosis.
    3. **Pyloric stenosis can run in families, and it is more common in males.**
    4. Although pyloric stenosis occurs more often in males, it can occur in females, especially in siblings of a child with pyloric stenosis.

TEST-TAKING HINT: The test taker needs to be familiar with pyloric stenosis.

45. 1. Infants with pyloric stenosis tend to be perpetually hungry because most of their feedings do not get absorbed.
    2. Infants with pyloric stenosis vomit immediately after a feeding, especially as the pylorus becomes more hypertrophied.
    3. **Infants with pyloric stenosis are always hungry and often appear malnourished.**
    4. Most infants with pyloric stenosis are irritable because they are hungry. Parents do not usually describe the vomiting episodes as "spitting up" because infants tend to have projectile vomiting.

TEST-TAKING HINT: Recall the dynamics of pyloric stenosis. Because feedings are not absorbed, the infant is irritable and hungry. The test taker can eliminate answers 1 and 4 and select answer 3.

46. 1. In addition to giving fluids intravenously and keeping the infant NPO, an NGT is placed to decompress the stomach.
    2. **In addition to giving fluids intravenously and keeping the infant NPO, an NGT is placed to decompress the stomach.**
    3. The pylorus is distal to the stomach, so an NGT is placed above the obstruction.
    4. The infant is made NPO as soon as diagnosis is confirmed. Allowing the infant to feed perpetuates the vomiting and continued hypertrophy of the pylorus.

TEST-TAKING HINT: The test taker should consider the pathophysiology of pyloric stenosis and eliminate answers 1, 3, and 4.

47. 1. **The infant is displaying signs of intussusception. This is an emergency that needs to be evaluated to prevent ischemia and perforation.**
    2. The mother should be told not to give the infant anything by mouth and bring the infant immediately to the emergency department.
    3. Although similar symptoms may be seen among infants with allergies, a more serious illness must first be ruled out. It is uncommon to see lethargy as a response to an allergy.
    4. All bloody stools should be evaluated.

TEST-TAKING HINT: The child is described as lethargic and is having diarrhea and vomiting. This child needs to be seen to rule out an intussusception. At the very least, the mother should be told to bring the child to the emergency department because the described signs could also be seen in severe dehydration. The test taker should be led to select answer 1.

48. 1. The enema is used for confirmation of diagnosis and reduction. In most cases of intussusception in young children, an enema is successful in reducing the intussusception.
   2. In most cases of intussusception in young children, an enema is successful in reducing the intussusception.
   3. **In most cases of intussusception in young children, an enema is successful in reducing the intussusception.**
   4. There is not a high likelihood that the intussusception will recur.

   TEST-TAKING HINT: The test taker needs to be aware that intussusceptions in young children respond well to reduction by enema.

49. 1. The child has already been diagnosed and appears to have developed peritonitis, which is a surgical emergency.
   2. Although reducing enemas have a high success rate among infants with intussusception, they are contraindicated in the presence of peritonitis.
   3. Although a second intravenous line may be needed, the nurse's first priority is getting the child to the operating room.
   4. **Intussusception with peritonitis is a surgical emergency, so preparing the infant for surgery is the nurse's top priority.**

   TEST-TAKING HINT: The child has already been diagnosed and is displaying signs of shock and peritonitis. The nurse must act quickly and get the child the surgical attention needed to avoid disastrous consequences.

50. 1. Although a rectal thermometer should never be used in a child with an anorectal malformation, an oral thermometer should not be used in an infant or young child.
   2. **A change in stool consistency is important to report because it could indicate stenosis of the rectum.**
   3. The child with a low anorectal malformation should be capable of achieving bowel continence.
   4. Any stool in the urine should be reported because it indicates a fistula is present.

   TEST-TAKING HINT: The test taker should eliminate answer 3 as it contains the word "never." There are very few circumstances in health care in which "never" is the case.

51. 1. The child who has stool in the urine has a fistula connecting the rectum to the urinary tract, and the anorectal malformation cannot be low.
   2. **The presence of stool in the urine indicates that the anorectal malformation is high.**
   3. This child probably needs a colostomy.
   4. This malformation requires surgical correction.

   TEST-TAKING HINT: The test taker needs to consider that stool is present in the urine, indicating a fistula is present and a more complex anorectal malformation exists, so answers 1 and 4 can be eliminated.

52. 1. The stoma should be red in color, indicating good perfusion.
   2. Discharge or irritation around the stoma could indicate the presence of an infection.
   3. **The colostomy contains stool from the large intestine; an ileostomy contains the very irritating stool from the small intestine.**
   4. Babies usually develop a pattern to their bowel habits as they grow.

   TEST-TAKING HINT: Although it is important to keep a bag attached to the colostomy, the contents are not the irritating effluent of an ileostomy.

53. 1. **The inability to digest protein leads to an accumulation of an amino acid that is toxic to the mucosal cells and villi, leading to absorption problems.**
   2. Extra villi cells are not created. Instead, villi become damaged, leading to absorption problems.
   3. The intestine does not become more porous. There is difficulty with absorbing vitamins, leading to deficiencies, not toxicity.
   4. The child experiences diarrhea, not constipation.

   TEST-TAKING HINT: The test taker needs to recall the pathophysiology of celiac disease in order to select answer 1. By recalling that the child with celiac usually appears malnourished and experiences diarrhea, the test taker can eliminate answers 3 and 4.

54. 1. Rye toast contains gluten.
   2. Unless otherwise indicated, pancakes are made of wheat flour, which contains gluten.
   3. Oat cereal and breakfast pastry contain gluten.
   4. **Cheese, banana slices, rice cakes, and whole milk do not contain gluten.**

TEST-TAKING HINT: The test taker needs to recall that children with celiac disease cannot tolerate gluten, which is found in wheat, barley, rye, and oats. Answers 1, 2, and 3 contain gluten.

55. 1. Although a blood count and serum electrolyte evaluation will likely be included in the child's evaluation, the diagnosis cannot be confirmed without a stool sample and jejunal biopsy.
    2. The child is not usually kept NPO but is monitored to assess the response to the gluten-free diet.
    3. **A stool sample for analysis of fat and a jejunal biopsy can confirm the diagnosis.**
    4. The child's response to a gluten-free diet is monitored.

TEST-TAKING HINT: The test taker should eliminate answers 1, 2, and 4 because they do not include preparing the child for a jejunal biopsy, which is the key to a definitive diagnosis of celiac disease.

56. 1. The feedings tend to take longer and often do not get absorbed before the next scheduled feeding.
    2. **Bloody diarrhea can indicate that the infant has NEC.**
    3. Bowel sounds tend to decrease, not increase.
    4. The infant does not appear hungry but irritable.

TEST-TAKING HINT: The test taker needs to be familiar with manifestations of NEC and be led to select answer 2.

57. 1. The feedings should immediately be stopped, but the NGT should be placed to allow decompression of the stomach.
    2. Vital signs should be obtained more frequently than every 4 hours because the infant is at high risk for peritonitis and sepsis.
    3. **Intravenous antibiotics are administered to prevent or treat sepsis.**
    4. Feedings are stopped immediately when a suspicion of NEC is present.

TEST-TAKING HINT: The test taker needs to consider the plan of care for an infant with NEC. This child is at risk for becoming critically ill, so feedings are stopped and vital signs are monitored very closely.

58. 1. It is thought that the breast milk contains macrophages that help fight infection, preventing NEC.

2. Because NEC is seen primarily in preterm and low-birth-weight infants, their increased survival rate has led to an increase in the occurrence of NEC.
3. The infant's condition deteriorates rapidly when sepsis occurs, so early recognition and treatment are essential.
4. **Although much more common in preterm and low-birth-weight infants, NEC is also seen in term infants as well.**

TEST-TAKING HINT: The test taker needs to be familiar with general concepts associated with NEC. Answer 4 contains the word "only," which is an absolute value that is rarely used in health care.

59. 1. Children with SBS experience diarrhea, not constipation.
    2. **Because the intestine is used for absorption, children with SBS usually need alternative forms of nutrition such as hyperalimentation.**
    3. Without knowing how much intestine is involved, the nurse cannot make this assumption about prognosis and should not share this information with the infant's parents.
    4. It is therapeutic to acknowledge the parents' concern. Without knowing the parents' knowledge base, this response may or may not be above the level of their comprehension.

TEST-TAKING HINT: The test taker should eliminate answer 1 because it is false. Answer 3 can also be eliminated because it makes a generalization that should not be made without knowing the details of the child's diagnosis.

60. 1. It is important for children with SBS to receive some feedings, either by tube or mouth, so that the intestine receives some stimulation.
    2. Although PN can cause long-term challenges, there is not an absolute time limit.
    3. **It is important to begin feedings as soon as the bowel is healed so that it receives stimulation and does not atrophy.**
    4. Feedings are provided by mouth or tube based on each child's needs.

TEST-TAKING HINT: The test taker could eliminate answers 1 and 4 because they contain the word "never," which is rarely used in health-care scenarios.

61. 1, 2, 3, 4.
    1. The lights in phototherapy increase insensible fluid loss, requiring the nurse to monitor fluid status closely.
    2. The infant with pyloric stenosis is likely to be dehydrated as a result of persistent vomiting.
    3. A 2-year-old with pneumonia may have increased insensible fluid loss as a result of tachypnea associated with respiratory illness. The nurse needs to monitor fluid status cautiously because fluid overload can result in increased respiratory distress.
    4. The child with a burn experiences extensive extracellular fluid loss and is at great risk for dehydration. The younger child is at greater risk because of greater proportionate body surface area.
    5. An adolescent starting her menses is not at risk for dehydration.

    TEST-TAKING HINT: The test taker needs to know that an infant needing phototherapy, an infant with persistent vomiting, a child with pneumonia, and a child with burns require more fluids because of the risk of dehydration.

62. 1, 2, 3, 4.
    1. Hypothyroidism can be a causative factor in constipation.
    2. Weakened abdominal muscles can be seen in muscular dystrophy and can lead to constipation.
    3. Myelomeningocele affects the innervation of the rectum and can lead to constipation.
    4. Excessive milk consumption can lead to constipation.
    5. Activity tends to decrease constipation and increase regularity.

    TEST-TAKING HINT: The test taker needs to know which of these conditions can cause constipation.

Genitourinary Disorders

KEYWORDS

The following words include English vocabulary, nursing/medical terminology, concepts, principles, or information relevant to content specifically addressed in the chapter or associated with topics presented in it. English dictionaries, your nursing textbooks, and medical dictionaries such as *Taber's Cyclopedic Medical Dictionary* are resources that can be used to expand your knowledge and understanding of these words and related information.

Albuminemia

Bladder exstrophy

Cryptorchidism

Dialysate

Disequilibrium syndrome

Enuresis

Epispadias

Glomerulonephritis

Hematuria

Hemodialysis

Hydronephrosis

Hypospadias

Inguinal hernia

Peritoneal dialysis

Proteinuria

Testicular torsion

ABBREVIATIONS

Acute kidney injury (AKI)

Blood urea nitrogen (BUN)

Chronic kidney disease (CKD)

Desmopressin acetate (DDAVP)

Hemolytic uremic syndrome (HUS)

Kilogram (kg)

Milliliter (mL)

Minimal change nephrotic syndrome (MCNS)

Magnetic resonance imaging (MRI) scan

Urinary tract infection (UTI)

Vesicoureteral reflux (VUR)

Voiding cystourethrogram (VCUG)

QUESTIONS

1. The bladder capacity of a 3-year-old is approximately how much?
   1. 1.5 fl. oz.
   2. 3 fl. oz.
   3. 4 fl. oz.
   4. 5 fl. oz.

2. The nurse is caring for a 4-year-old who weighs 15 kg. At the end of a 10-hour period, the nurse notes the urine output to be 150 mL. What action does the nurse take?
   1. Notifies the health-care provider because this urine output is too low.
   2. Encourages the child to increase oral intake to increase urine output.
   3. Records the child's urine output in the chart.
   4. Administers isotonic fluid intravenously to help with rehydration.

3. A child had a urinary tract infection (UTI) 3 months ago and was treated with an oral antibiotic. A follow-up urinalysis revealed normal results. The child has had no other problems until this visit when the child was diagnosed with another UTI. Which is the most appropriate plan?
   1. Obtain urinalysis and urine culture.
   2. Evaluate for renal failure.
   3. Admit to the pediatric unit.
   4. Send home on an antibiotic.
   5. Schedule a VCUG.

4. Which should the nurse teach a group of girls and parents about the importance of preventing urinary tract infections (UTIs)?
   1. Avoiding constipation has no effect on the occurrence of UTIs.
   2. After urinating, always wipe from back to front to prevent fecal contamination.
   3. Hygiene is an important preventive measure and can be accomplished with frequent tub baths.
   4. Increasing fluids will help prevent and treat UTIs.

5. Which child does not need a urinalysis to evaluate for a urinary tract infection (UTI)?
   1. A 4-month-old female presenting with a 2-day history of fussiness and poor appetite; current vital signs include axillary T 100.8°F (38.2°C), HR 120 beats per minute.
   2. A 4-year-old female who states, "It hurts when I pee"; she has been urinating every 30 minutes; vital signs are within normal range.
   3. An 8-year-old male presenting with a finger laceration; mother states he had surgical re-implantation of his ureters 2 years ago.
   4. A 12-year-old female complaining of pain to her lower right back; she denies any burning or frequency at this time; oral temperature of 101.5°F (38.6°C).

6. Which is the best way to obtain a urine sample in an 8-month-old being evaluated for a urinary tract infection (UTI)?
   1. Carefully cleanse the perineum from front to back and apply a self-adhesive urine collection bag to the perineum.
   2. Insert an indwelling Foley catheter, obtain the sample, and wait for results.
   3. Place a sterile cotton ball in the diaper and immediately obtain the sample with a syringe after the first void.
   4. Using a straight catheter, obtain the sample and immediately remove the catheter without waiting for the results of the urine sample.

7. Which child is at risk for developing glomerulonephritis?
   1. A 3-year-old who had impetigo 1 week ago.
   2. A 5-year-old with a history of five UTIs in the previous year.
   3. A 6-year-old with new-onset type 1 diabetes.
   4. A 10-year-old recovering from viral pneumonia.

8. Which combination of signs is commonly associated with glomerulonephritis?
   1. Massive proteinuria, hematuria, decreased urinary output, and lethargy.
   2. Mild proteinuria, increased urinary output, and lethargy.
   3. Mild proteinuria, hematuria, decreased urinary output, and lethargy.
   4. Massive proteinuria, decreased urinary output, and hypotension.

9. The parent of a child with glomerulonephritis asks the nurse why the urine is such a funny color. Which is the nurse's best response?
   1. "It is not uncommon for the urine to be discolored when children are receiving steroids and blood pressure medications."
   2. "There is blood in your child's urine that causes it to be tea-colored."
   3. "Your child's urine is very concentrated, so it appears to be discolored."
   4. "A ketogenic diet often causes the urine to be tea-colored."

10. Which finding requires immediate attention in a child with glomerulonephritis?
    1. Sleeping most of the day and being very "cranky" when awake; blood pressure is 170/90.
    2. Urine output is 190 mL in an 8-hour period and is the color of Coca-Cola.
    3. Complaining of a severe headache and photophobia.
    4. Refusing breakfast and lunch and stating he "just is not hungry."

11. The parents of a child with glomerulonephritis ask how they will know their child is improving after they go home. Which are the nurse's best responses? **Select all that apply.**
    1. "Your child's urine output will increase, and the urine will become less tea-colored."
    2. "Your child will have more energy as lab tests become more normal."
    3. "Your child's appetite will decrease as urine output increases."
    4. "Your child's laboratory values will become more normal."
    5. "Your child's weight will increase as the urine becomes less tea-colored."

12. Which statement by a parent is most consistent with minimal change nephrotic syndrome (MCNS)?
    1. "My child missed 2 days of school last week because of a really bad cold."
    2. "After camping last week, my child's legs were covered in bug bites."
    3. "My child came home from school a week ago because of vomiting and stomach cramps."
    4. "We have a pet turtle, but no one washes their hands after playing with the turtle."

13. The clinical manifestations of minimal change nephrotic syndrome (MCNS) are due to which of the following?
    1. Chemical changes in the composition of albumin.
    2. Increased permeability of the glomeruli.
    3. Obstruction of the capillaries of the glomeruli.
    4. Loss of the kidneys' ability to excrete waste and concentrate urine.

14. The parents of a child hospitalized with minimal change nephrotic syndrome (MCNS) ask why the last blood test revealed elevated lipids. Which is the nurse's best response?
    1. "If your child had just eaten a fatty meal, the lipids may have been falsely elevated."
    2. "It's not unusual to see elevated lipids in children because of the dietary habits of today."
    3. "Because your child is losing so much protein, the liver is stimulated and makes more lipids."
    4. "Your child's blood is very concentrated because of the edema, so the lipids are falsely elevated."

15. A child with minimal change nephrotic syndrome (MCNS) has generalized edema. The skin appears stretched, and areas of breakdown are noted over the bony prominences. The child has been receiving furosemide (Lasix) twice daily for several days. Which does the nurse expect to be included in the treatment plan to reduce edema?
    1. An increase in the amount and frequency of furosemide (Lasix).
    2. Addition of a second diuretic, such as mannitol.
    3. Administration of intravenous albumin.
    4. Elimination of all fluids and sodium from the child's diet.

16. A parent asks the nurse how to prevent the child from having minimal change nephrotic syndrome (MCNS) again. Which is the nurse's best response?
    1. "It is very rare for a child to have a relapse after having fully recovered."
    2. "Unfortunately, many children have cycles of relapse, and there is very little that can be done to prevent it."
    3. "Your child is much less likely to get sick again if sodium is decreased in the diet."
    4. "Try to keep your child away from sick children because relapses have been associated with infectious illnesses."

17. The nurse is caring for a newborn with hypospadias. His parents ask if circumcision is an option. Which is the nurse's best response?
    1. "Circumcision is a fading practice and is now contraindicated in most children."
    2. "Circumcision in children with hypospadias is recommended because it helps prevent infection."
    3. "Circumcision is an option, but it cannot be done at this time."
    4. "Circumcision can never be performed in a child with hypospadias."

18. An infant is scheduled for a hypospadias and chordee repair. The parent asks the nurse, "I understand why the hypospadias repair is necessary, but do they have to fix the chordee as well?" Which is the nurse's best response?
    1. "I understand your concern. Parents do not want their children to undergo extra surgery."
    2. "The chordee repair is done strictly for cosmetic reasons that may affect your son as he ages."
    3. "The repair is done to optimize sexual functioning when he is older."
    4. "This is the best time to repair the chordee because he will be having surgery anyway."

19. A 13-month-old is discharged following repair of his epispadias. Which statement made by the parents indicates they understand the discharge teaching?
    1. "If a mucous plug forms in the urinary drainage tube, we will irrigate it gently to prevent a blockage."
    2. "If a mucous plug forms in the urinary drainage tube, we will allow it to pass on its own because this is a sign of healing."
    3. "We will make sure the dressing is loosely applied to increase the toddler's comfort."
    4. "If we notice any yellow drainage, we will know that everything is healing well."

20. Which would the nurse most likely find in the history of a child with hemolytic uremic syndrome (HUS)? **Select all that apply.**
    1. Frequent UTIs and possible vesicoureteral reflux (VUR).
    2. Vomiting and diarrhea before admission.
    3. Bee sting and localized edema of the site for 3 days.
    4. Previously healthy with no signs of illness.
    5. Anorexia and bruising.

21. The manifestations of hemolytic uremic syndrome (HUS) are due primarily to which event?
    1. The swollen lining of the small blood vessels damages the red blood cells, which are then removed by the spleen, leading to anemia.
    2. There is a disturbance of the glomerular basement membrane, allowing large proteins to pass through.
    3. The red blood cell changes shape, causing it to obstruct microcirculation.
    4. There is a depression in the production of all formed elements of the blood.

22. Which laboratory results besides hematuria are most consistent with hemolytic uremic syndrome (HUS)?
    1. Massive proteinuria, elevated blood urea nitrogen and creatinine.
    2. Mild proteinuria, decreased blood urea nitrogen and creatinine.
    3. Mild proteinuria, increased blood urea nitrogen and creatinine.
    4. Massive proteinuria, decreased blood urea nitrogen and creatinine.

23. A child with hemolytic uremic syndrome (HUS) is very pale and lethargic. Stools have progressed from watery to bloody diarrhea. Blood work indicates low hemoglobin and hematocrit levels. The child has not had any urine output in 24 hours. The nurse expects administration of blood products and what else to be added to the plan of care?
    1. Initiation of dialysis.
    2. Close observation of the child's hemodynamic status.
    3. Diuretic therapy to force urinary output.
    4. Monitoring of urinary output.

24. Which needs to be present to diagnose hemolytic uremic syndrome (HUS)?
    1. Increased red blood cells with a low reticulocyte count, increased platelet count, and renal failure.
    2. Decreased red blood cells with a high reticulocyte count, decreased platelet count, and renal failure.
    3. Increased red blood cells with a high reticulocyte count, increased platelet count, and renal failure.
    4. Decreased red blood cells with a low reticulocyte count, decreased platelet count, and renal failure.

25. A 5-year-old is discharged from the hospital following the diagnosis of hemolytic uremic syndrome (HUS). The child has been free of diarrhea for 1 week, and renal function has returned. The parent asks the nurse when the child can return to school. Which is the nurse's best response?
    1. "Immediately, as your child is no longer contagious."
    2. "It would be best to keep your child home for a few more weeks because the immune system is weak, and there could be a relapse of HUS."
    3. "Your child will be contagious for approximately another 10 days, so it is best to not allow a return just yet."
    4. "It would be best to keep your child home to monitor urinary output."

26. Which is a care priority for a newborn diagnosed with bladder exstrophy and a malformed pelvis?
    1. Change the diaper frequently and assess for skin breakdown.
    2. Keep the exposed bladder open in a warm and dry environment to avoid any heat loss.
    3. Offer formula for infant growth and fluid management.
    4. Cluster all care to allow the child to sleep, grow, and gain strength for the upcoming surgical repair.

27. Which medication would most likely be included in the postoperative care of a child with repair of bladder exstrophy?
    1. Furosemide (Lasix).
    2. Mannitol.
    3. Meperidine (Demerol).
    4. Oxybutynin (Ditropan).

28. The nurse is providing discharge instructions to the parents of an infant born with bladder exstrophy who had a continent urinary reservoir placed. Which statement should be included?
1. "Allow your child to sleep on the abdomen to provide comfort during the immediate post-operative period."
2. "As your child grows, be cautious around playgrounds because the surface could be a health hazard."
3. "As your child grows, be sure to encourage many different foods because it is not likely that food allergies will develop."
4. "Encourage your child's development, by having brightly colored objects around, such as balloons."

29. Which causes the clinical manifestations of hydronephrosis?
1. A structural abnormality in the urinary system causes urine to back up and can cause pressure and cell death.
2. A structural abnormality causes urine to flow too freely through the urinary system, leading to fluid and electrolyte imbalances.
3. Decreased production of urine in one or both kidneys results in an electrolyte imbalance.
4. Urine with an abnormal electrolyte balance and concentration leads to increased blood pressure and subsequent increased glomerular filtration rate.

30. In addition to increased blood pressure, which findings would most likely be found in a child with hydronephrosis?
1. Metabolic alkalosis and positive renal ultrasound.
2. Metabolic acidosis and negative renal ultrasound.
3. Metabolic alkalosis and bacterial growth in the urine.
4. Metabolic acidosis, polydipsia, and polyuria.

31. Which should be included in the plan of care for a child diagnosed with hydronephrosis?
1. Intake and output as well as vital signs should be strictly monitored.
2. Fluids and sodium in the diet should be limited.
3. Steroids should be administered as ordered.
4. Limited contact with other people to avoid infection.

32. The nurse in a diabetic clinic sees a 10-year-old who is a new diabetic and has had trouble maintaining blood glucose levels within normal limits. The child's parent states the child has had several daytime "accidents." The nurse knows that this is referred to as which of the following?
1. Primary enuresis.
2. Secondary enuresis.
3. Diurnal enuresis.
4. Nocturnal enuresis.

33. The parent of a 7-year-old voices concern over the child's continued bed-wetting at night. The parent, on going to bed, has tried getting the child up at 11:30 p.m., but the child still wakes up wet. Which is the nurse's best response about what the parent should do next?
1. "There is a medication called DDAVP that decreases the volume of the urine. The physician thinks that will work for your child."
2. "When your child wakes up wet, be very firm and indicate how displeased you are. Have your child change the sheets to see how much work is involved."
3. "Limit fluids in the evening and start a reward system in which your child can choose a reward after a certain number of dry nights."
4. "Bed-wetting alarms are readily available, and most children do very well with them."

34. An adolescent woke up complaining of intense pain and swelling of the scrotal area and abdominal pain. He has vomited twice. Which should the nurse suggest?
   1. Encourage him to drink clear liquids until the vomiting subsides; if he gets worse, bring him to the emergency room.
   2. Bring him to the health-care provider's office for evaluation.
   3. Take him to the emergency department immediately.
   4. Encourage him to rest; apply ice to the scrotal area and go to the emergency department if the pain does not improve.

35. Which causes the symptoms in testicular torsion?
   1. Twisting of the spermatic cord interrupts the blood supply.
   2. Swelling of the scrotal sac leads to testicular displacement.
   3. Unmanaged undescended testes cause testicular displacement.
   4. Microthrombi formation in the vessels of the spermatic cord causes interruption of the blood supply.

36. The nurse evaluates postoperative teaching for repair of testicular torsion as successful when the parent of an adolescent says which the following?
   1. "I will encourage him to rest for a few days, but he can return to football practice in a week."
   2. "I will keep him in bed for 4 days and let him gradually increase his activity after that."
   3. "I will seek therapy as he ages because he is now infertile."
   4. "I will make sure he does testicular self-examination monthly."

37. Which protrusion into the groin of a female most likely causes inguinal hernias?
   1. Bowel.
   2. Fallopian tube.
   3. Large thrombus formation.
   4. Muscle tissue.

38. The parents of a 6-week-old male ask the nurse if there is a difference between an inguinal hernia and a hydrocele. Which is the nurse's best response?
   1. "The terms are used interchangeably and mean the same thing."
   2. "The symptoms are similar, but an inguinal hernia occurs when tissue protrudes into the groin, whereas a hydrocele is a fluid-filled mass in the scrotum."
   3. " 'Hydrocele' is the term used when an inguinal hernia occurs in females."
   4. "A hydrocele presents in a manner similar to that of an inguinal hernia but causes increased concern because it is often malignant."

39. The nurse evaluates the parents' understanding of the teaching about an inguinal hernia as successful when they say which of the following?
   1. "There are no risks associated with waiting to have the hernia reduced; surgery is done for cosmetic reasons."
   2. "It is normal to see the bulge in the baby's groin decrease with a bowel movement."
   3. "We will wait for surgery until the baby is older because narcotics for pain control will be required for several days."
   4. "It is normal for the bulge in the baby's groin to look smaller when the baby is asleep."

40. Which would the nurse expect to hear the parents of an infant with an incarcerated hernia report?
   1. Acute onset of pain, abdominal distention, and a mass that cannot be reduced.
   2. Gradual onset of pain, abdominal distention, and a mass that cannot be reduced.
   3. Acute onset of pain, abdominal distention, and a mass that is easily reduced.
   4. Gradual onset of pain, abdominal distention, and a mass that is easily reduced.

41. The parent of a 3-year-old is shocked to hear the diagnosis of Wilms tumor and says, "How could I have missed a lump this big?" Which is the nurse's best response?
    1. "Do not be hard on yourself. It's easy to overlook something that has probably been growing for months when we see our children on a regular basis."
    2. "I understand you must be very upset. Your child would have had a better prognosis had you caught it earlier."
    3. "It really takes a trained professional to recognize something like this."
    4. "Do not blame yourself. This mass grows so fast that it was probably not noticeable a few days ago."

42. Which would the nurse expect to find on assessment in a child with Wilms tumor?
    1. Decreased blood pressure, increased temperature, and a firm mass located in one flank area.
    2. Increased blood pressure, normal temperature, and a firm mass located in one flank area.
    3. Increased blood pressure, normal temperature, and a firm mass located on one side of the midline of the abdomen.
    4. Decreased blood pressure, normal temperature, and a firm mass located on one side or the other of the midline of the abdomen.

43. A child diagnosed with a Wilms tumor is scheduled for an MRI scan of the lungs. The parent asks the nurse the reason for this test as a Wilms tumor involves the kidney, not the lung. Which is the nurse's best response?
    1. "I'm not sure why your child is going for this test. I will check and get back to you."
    2. "It sounds like we made a mistake. I will check and get back to you."
    3. "The test is done to check to see if the disease has spread to the lungs."
    4. "We want to check the lungs to make sure your child is healthy enough to tolerate surgery."

44. The parents overhear the health-care team refer to their child's disease as in stage III. The parents ask the nurse what this means. Which is the nurse's best response?
    1. "The tumor is confined to the abdomen, but it has spread to the lymph nodes or peritoneal area; the prognosis is poor."
    2. "The tumor is confined to the abdomen, but it has spread to the lymph nodes or peritoneal area; the prognosis is very good."
    3. "The tumor has been found in three other organs beyond the peritoneal area; the prognosis is good."
    4. "The tumor has spread to other organs beyond the peritoneal area; the prognosis is poor."

45. The nurse is caring for a child due for surgery on a Wilms tumor. The child's procedure will consist of which of the following?
    1. Only the affected kidney will be removed.
    2. Both the affected kidney and the other kidney will be removed in case of recurrence.
    3. The mass will be removed from the affected kidney.
    4. The mass will be removed from the affected kidney, and a biopsy of the tissue of the unaffected kidney will be done.

46. The nurse anticipates that the child who has had a kidney removed will have a high level of pain and will require invasive and noninvasive measures for pain relief. The nurse anticipates that the child will have pain because of which of the following?
    1. The kidney is removed laparoscopically, and there will be residual pain from accumulated air in the abdomen.
    2. There is a postoperative shift of fluids and organs in the abdominal cavity, leading to increased discomfort.
    3. The chemotherapy makes the child more sensitive to pain.
    4. The radiation therapy makes the child less sensitive to pain.

47. The parents of a 7-year-old tell the nurse they do not understand the difference between CKD and AKI. Which is the nurse's best response?
    1. "There really is not much difference because the terms are used interchangeably."
    2. "Most children experience AKI. It is highly unusual for a child to experience CKD."
    3. "CKD tends to occur suddenly and is irreversible."
    4. "AKI is often reversible, whereas CKD results in permanent deterioration of kidney function."

48. A child had a tonsillectomy 6 days ago and was seen in the emergency room 4 hours ago because of postoperative hemorrhage. The parent noted that her child was "swallowing a lot and finally began vomiting large amounts of blood." The child's vital signs are as follows: T 99.5°F (37.5°C), HR 124, BP 84/48, and RR 26. The nurse knows that this child is at risk for which type of renal problem?
    1. CKD due to advanced disease process.
    2. Prerenal failure due to dehydration.
    3. Primary kidney damage due to a lack of urine flowing through the system.
    4. Postrenal failure due to a hypotensive state.

49. A child diagnosed with acute kidney injury (AKI) complains of "not feeling well," having "butterflies in the chest," and arms and legs "feeling like Jell-O." The cardiac monitor shows that the QRS complex is wider than it was and that an occasional premature ventricular contraction (PVC) is seen. Which would the nurse expect to administer?
    1. An isotonic saline solution with 20 mEq KCl/L.
    2. Sodium bicarbonate via slow intravenous push.
    3. Calcium gluconate via slow intravenous push.
    4. Oral potassium supplements.

50. A 10-kg toddler is diagnosed with AKI, is afebrile, and has a 24-hour urine output of 110 mL. After calculating daily fluid maintenance, which would the nurse expect the toddler's daily allotment of fluids to be?
    1. Sips of clear fluids and ice chips only.
    2. 350 mL of oral and intravenous fluids.
    3. 1000 mL of oral and intravenous fluids.
    4. 2000 mL of oral and intravenous fluids.

51. The nurse is caring for a 1-year-old diagnosed with AKI. Edema is noted throughout the child's body, and the liver is enlarged. The child's urine output is less than 0.5 mL/kg/hr, and vital signs are as follows: HR 146, BP 176/92, and RR 42. The child is noted to have nasal flaring and retractions with inspiration. The lung sounds are coarse throughout. Despite receiving oral sodium polystyrene sulfonate (Kayexalate), the child's serum potassium continues to rise. Which treatment will provide the most benefit to the child?
    1. Additional rectal sodium polystyrene sulfonate (Kayexalate).
    2. Intravenous furosemide (Lasix).
    3. Endotracheal intubation and ventilatory assistance.
    4. Placement of a Tenckhoff catheter for peritoneal dialysis.

52. The parent of a child diagnosed with AKI asks the nurse why peritoneal dialysis was selected instead of hemodialysis. Which is the nurse's best response?
    1. "Hemodialysis is not used in the pediatric population."
    2. "Peritoneal dialysis has no complications, so it is a treatment used without hesitation."
    3. "Peritoneal dialysis removes fluid at a slower rate than hemodialysis, so many complications are avoided."
    4. "Peritoneal dialysis is much more efficient than hemodialysis."

53. The nurse is caring for a 12-year-old receiving peritoneal dialysis. The nurse notes the return to be cloudy, and the child is complaining of abdominal pain. The child's parents ask what the next step will likely be. Which is the nurse's best response?
    1. "We will probably place antibiotics in the dialysis fluid before the next dwell time."
    2. "Many children experience cloudy returns. We do not usually worry about it."
    3. "We will probably give your child some oral antibiotics just to make sure nothing else develops."
    4. "The abdominal pain is likely due to the fluid going in too slowly. We will increase the rate of administration with the next fill."

54. A child receiving peritoneal dialysis has not been having adequate volume in the return. The child is currently edematous and hypertensive. Which would the nurse anticipate the health-care provider to do?
    1. Increase the glucose concentration of the dialysate.
    2. Decrease the glucose concentration of the dialysate.
    3. Administer antihypertensives and diuretics but not change the dialysate concentration.
    4. Decrease the dwell time of the dialysate.

55. During hemodialysis, the nurse notes that a 10-year-old becomes confused and restless. The child complains of a headache and nausea and has generalized muscle twitching. This can be prevented by which of the following?
    1. Slowing the rate of solute removal during dialysis.
    2. Ensuring the patient is warm during dialysis.
    3. Administering antibiotics before dialysis.
    4. Obtaining an accurate weight the night before dialysis.

56. Chronic hypertension in the child who has CKD is due to which of the following?
    1. Retention of sodium and water.
    2. Obstruction of the urinary system.
    3. Accumulation of waste products in the body.
    4. Generalized metabolic alkalosis.

57. Which best describes the electrolyte imbalance that occurs in CKD?
    1. Decreased serum phosphorus and calcium levels.
    2. Depletion of phosphorus and calcium stores from the bones.
    3. Change in the structure of the bones, causing calcium to remain in the bones.
    4. Nutritional needs are poorly met, leading to a decrease in many electrolytes such as calcium and phosphorus.

58. The diet for a child with CKD should be high in calories and include:
    1. Low protein and all minerals and electrolytes.
    2. Low protein and minerals.
    3. High protein and calcium and low potassium and phosphorus.
    4. High protein, phosphorus, and calcium and low potassium and sodium.

59. One week after kidney transplant, a child complains about abdominal pain, and the parents note that the child has been very fussy. The nurse notes a 10% weight gain as well as elevated BUN and creatinine levels. Which of the following medications would the child most likely be taking?
    1. Codeine tablets.
    2. Furosemide (Lasix).
    3. Polyethylene glycol 3350 (MiraLAX).
    4. Corticosteroids.

60. A renal transplantation is which of the following?
    1. A curative procedure that will free the child from any more treatment modalities.
    2. An ideal treatment option for families with a history of dialysis noncompliance.
    3. A treatment option that will free the child from dialysis.
    4. A treatment option that is very new to the pediatric population.

61. The parents of a 3-year-old are concerned that the child is having "more accidents" during the day. Which questions would be appropriate for the nurse to ask to obtain more information? **Select all that apply.**
    1. "Has there been a stressful event in the child's life, such as the birth of a sibling?"
    2. "Has anyone else in the family had problems with accidents?"
    3. "Does your child seem to be drinking more than usual?"
    4. "Is your child more fussy, and does your child seem to be in pain when urinating?"
    5. "Is your child having difficulties at preschool?"

62. Which is true of a Wilms tumor? **Select all that apply.**
    1. It is also referred to as neuroblastoma.
    2. It can occur at any age but is seen most often between the ages of 2 and 5 years.
    3. It can occur on its own or can be associated with many congenital anomalies.
    4. It is a slow-growing tumor.
    5. It is associated with a poor prognosis.

The correct answer number and rationale for why it is the correct answer are given in **boldface blue type**. Rationales for why the other possible answer options are incorrect also are given, but they are not in boldface type.

1. 1. The capacity of the bladder in fluid ounces can be estimated by adding 2 to the child's age in years.
   2. The capacity of the bladder in fluid ounces can be estimated by adding 2 to the child's age in years.
   3. The capacity of the bladder in fluid ounces can be estimated by adding 2 to the child's age in years.
   4. **The capacity of the bladder in fluid ounces can be estimated by adding 2 to the child's age in years.**

   TEST-TAKING HINT: The test taker can eliminate answer 1 because 1.5 fl oz represents a very small bladder capacity.

2. 1. The child weighs 15 kg, and the expected urine output is 0.5–1 mL/kg/hr. 0.5 × 15 kg = 7.5 mL; 1 mL × 15 kg = 15 mL. 7.5–15 mL/hour × 10 hours = 75–150 mL of urine for the 10-hour period. Therefore, the output is not too low.
   2. The child weighs 15 kg, and the expected urine output is 0.5–1 mL/kg/hr. 0.5 × 15 kg = 7.5 mL; 1 mL × 15 kg = 15 mL. 7.5–15 mL/hour × 10 hours = 75–150 mL of urine for the 10-hour period. The urine output is not too low, so the nurse does not need to encourage more fluids.
   3. **Recording the child's urine output in the chart is the appropriate action because the urine output is within the expected range of 0.5–1 mL/kg/hr, or 75–150 mL for the 10-hour period.**
   4. The child weighs 15 kg and the expected urine output is 0.5–1 mL/kg/hr. 0.5 × 15 kg = 7.5 mL; 1 mL × 15 kg = 15 mL. 7.5–15 mL/hour × 10 hours = 75–150 mL of urine for the 10-hour period. Therefore, it is not too low. The child is hydrated.

   TEST-TAKING HINT: The test taker can eliminate answers 1, 2, and 4 because they address strategies for caring for a dehydrated child.

3. 1. **Urinalysis and urine culture are routinely used to diagnose UTIs. VCUG is used to determine the extent of urinary tract involvement when a renal ultrasound shows scaring or possible reflux. If the child has a UTI related to bubble baths, constipation, or wiping back to front, a VCUG would not be ordered.**
   2. There are no data to suggest that renal failure should be evaluated.
   3. A UTI is usually treated with oral antibiotics at home and does not routinely require admission to the hospital.
   4. A second UTI requires more extensive evaluation and diagnostic testing.
   5. If the child has a UTI related to bubble baths, constipation, or wiping back to front, a VCUG would not be ordered.

   TEST-TAKING HINT: The test taker can eliminate answer 2 because it is the only answer that does not address the UTI. Answer 1 is the best choice because it will provide more data about the cause of the child's recurrent UTIs.

4. 1. The increased pressure associated with evacuating hardened stool can result in the backflow of urine into the bladder, leading to infection.
   2. To prevent infection, a female child should wipe from front to back.
   3. Tub baths are not recommended because they may cause irritation of the urethra, leading to infection.
   4. **Increasing fluids will help flush the bladder of any organisms, encourage urination, and prevent stasis of urine.**

   TEST-TAKING HINT: The test taker can eliminate answers 1, 2, and 3 because they do not provide accurate information.

5. 1. Fussiness and lack of appetite can indicate a UTI. Signs of infection, such as fever and increased heart rate, should be evaluated to determine whether an infection exists.
   2. Frequency and urgency are classic signs of a UTI.
   3. **Although this child has had a history of urinary infections, the child is currently not displaying any signs and therefore does not need a urinalysis at this time.**

4. Pain to the lower right back can indicate infection of the upper urinary tract. Although the child currently denies any burning or frequency, the child currently has a fever coupled with flank pain, which needs evaluation.

TEST-TAKING HINT: The test taker should be led to answer 3 because it states that the child is not currently having any manifestations of a UTI.

6. 1. A sample obtained from a urine bag would contain microorganisms from the skin, causing contamination of the sample.
2. There is no need to leave the catheter in because it serves as a portal for infection.
3. The cotton ball would not remain sterile and would therefore contaminate the urine sample.
4. **An in-and-out catheterization is the best way to obtain a urine culture in a child who is not yet toilet-trained.**

TEST-TAKING HINT: The test taker can eliminate answers 1 and 3 because they both lead to a contaminated sample.

7. 1. **Impetigo is a skin infection caused by the streptococcal organism that is commonly associated with glomerulonephritis.**
2. Frequent UTIs have not been associated with glomerulonephritis.
3. Type 1 diabetes is not a cause of glomerulonephritis.
4. Glomerulonephritis can be caused by a streptococcal organism, not a viral pneumonia.

TEST-TAKING HINT: The test taker may be distracted by answer 4, but that choice is a viral infection so that makes it an incorrect choice.

8. 1. Unlike nephrotic syndrome, protein is lost in mild-to-moderate amounts.
2. Urinary output is decreased in the child with glomerulonephritis.
3. **Mild-to-moderate proteinuria, hematuria, decreased urinary output, and lethargy are common findings in glomerulonephritis.**
4. Hypertension, not hypotension, is a common finding in glomerulonephritis.

TEST-TAKING HINT: The test taker should eliminate answers 1 and 4 because glomerulonephritis does not cause massive proteinuria. Answer 2 can be eliminated because increased urine output is not associated with glomerulonephritis.

9. 1. Steroids and antihypertensives do not cause urine to change color.
2. **Blood in the child's urine causes it to be tea-colored.**
3. The tea color of the urine is due to hematuria, not concentration.
4. The child with glomerulonephritis is not on a ketogenic diet. The ketogenic diet does not cause the urine to change color.

TEST-TAKING HINT: The test taker can immediately eliminate answer 4 because the child is not placed on a ketogenic diet.

10. 1. Children with glomerulonephritis usually have an elevated blood pressure and tend to rest most of the day.
2. The urine output is often decreased, and the urine is often tea-colored due to hematuria.
3. **A severe headache and photophobia can be signs of encephalopathy due to hypertension, and the child needs immediate attention.**
4. Anorexia is often seen with glomerulonephritis.

TEST-TAKING HINT: The test taker should eliminate answers 1, 2, and 4 because they are manifestations of glomerulonephritis.

11. 1, 5.
1. **When glomerulonephritis is improving, urine output increases, and the urine becomes less tea-colored. These are signs that can be monitored at home by the child's parents.**
2. As glomerulonephritis improves, the child should have more energy and require less rest, but lab test values are not something that will be readily apparent to the family at home.
3. The child's appetite should increase as the condition improves.
4. Although the laboratory test values will normalize, this is not something that will be readily apparent to the family at home.
5. **The child's weight will increase as the urine resumes a more normal color, indicating lab values are returning to normal and the child is better.**

TEST-TAKING HINT: The test taker should be led to answers 1 and 5 because the manifestations represent improvement in the disease process that can be easily recognized by the parents.

12. 1. **An upper respiratory infection often precedes MCNS by a few days.**
2. Bug bites are not typically associated with MCNS.

3. Vomiting and abdominal cramping are not typically associated with MCNS.
4. Pet turtles often carry salmonella, which can cause vomiting and diarrhea but not MCNS.

TEST-TAKING HINT: The test taker should be led to answer 1 because MCNS is most often associated with upper respiratory infections.

13. 1. Albumin does not undergo any chemical changes in MCNS.
    2. **Increased permeability of the glomeruli in MCNS allows large substances such as protein to pass through and be excreted in the urine.**
    3. Obstruction of the capillaries of the glomeruli due to the formation of antibody-antigen complexes occurs in glomerulonephritis.
    4. Loss of the kidneys' ability to excrete waste and concentrate urine occurs in renal failure.

TEST-TAKING HINT: The test taker should recognize the pathophysiology of MCNS.

14. 1. In MCNS, the lipids are truly elevated. Lipoprotein production is increased because of the increased stimulation of the liver caused by hypoalbuminemia.
    2. The elevated lipids are unrelated to the child's dietary habits.
    3. **In MCNS, the lipids are truly elevated. Lipoprotein production is increased because of the increased stimulation of the liver caused by hypoalbuminemia.**
    4. The lipids are not falsely elevated.

TEST-TAKING HINT: The test taker can eliminate answers 1 and 2 because they do not represent changes associated with a disease process.

15. 1. The dosage of the diuretic may be adjusted, but other medications such as albumin are likely to be used.
    2. Mannitol is not usually used in the treatment of MCNS.
    3. **In cases of severe edema, albumin is used to help return the fluid to the bloodstream from the subcutaneous tissue.**
    4. Although sodium and fluids are restricted in the severely edematous child, they are not eliminated completely.

TEST-TAKING HINT: The test taker can eliminate answer 2 because mannitol is used to treat cerebral edema.

16. 1. It is not unusual for a child to experience relapses.
    2. Many children do experience relapses, but exposure to infectious illnesses has been linked to relapses.
    3. There is no correlation between the consumption of sodium and minimal change nephrotic syndrome.
    4. **Exposure to infectious illness has been linked to the relapse of minimal change nephrotic syndrome.**

TEST-TAKING HINT: The test taker can eliminate answers 1 and 2 because relapses are common and can be prevented.

17. 1. Routine circumcision is recommended by the American Academy of Pediatrics; it is not contraindicated in most children.
    2. It is not recommended that circumcision of children with hypospadias be done immediately because the foreskin may be needed later for repair of the defect.
    3. **It is usually recommended that circumcision be delayed in the child with hypospadias because the foreskin may be needed for repair of the defect.**
    4. Circumcision can usually be performed in the child with hypospadias when the defect is corrected.

TEST-TAKING HINT: The test taker can eliminate answer 4 because "never" is infrequently the case in health care.

18. 1. This response is empathetic. It does not, however, answer the parent's concern, whereas a simple explanation would immediately do so.
    2. Although a cosmetic component exists, straightening the penis is important for future sexual function.
    3. **Releasing the chordee surgically is necessary for future sexual function.**
    4. Although the two surgeries are usually done simultaneously, each has its own importance and necessity.

TEST-TAKING HINT: The test taker should be led to answer 3 because it provides the parents with a simple, accurate explanation.

19. 1. **Any mucous plugs should be removed by irrigation to prevent blockage of the urinary drainage system.**
    2. The mucous plug should be removed by irrigation because it could cause a blockage of the urinary drainage system.
    3. The dressing is usually a compression type of dressing that helps decrease edema.

4. Foul-smelling yellow drainage is often a sign of infection that needs to be evaluated.

TEST-TAKING HINT: The test taker can eliminate answers 2 and 4 because they have potential to cause injury to the child.

20. **2, 5.**
    1. Frequent UTIs and VUR do not lead to HUS.
    2. **HUS is often preceded by diarrhea that may be caused by *E. coli* present in undercooked meat.**
    3. Insect stings are not associated with HUS.
    4. HUS is usually preceded by diarrhea.
    5. **Anorexia and bruising (purura and/or petechiae) are common clinical manifestations.**

    TEST-TAKING HINT: The test taker can eliminate answer 1 because there is no correlation between UTIs and HUS.

21. 1. **The swollen lining of the small blood vessels damages the red blood cells, which are then removed by the spleen.**
    2. The increased permeability of the basement membrane occurs in MCNS.
    3. The red blood cell changing shape is typical of sickle cell anemia.
    4. The depression of all formed elements of the blood occurs in aplastic anemia.

    TEST-TAKING HINT: The question requires familiarity with the pathophysiology of HUS.

22. 1. Protein is not lost in massive amounts in HUS.
    2. BUN and creatinine are usually increased in HUS.
    3. **Hematuria, mild proteinuria, and increased BUN and creatinine are all present in HUS.**
    4. Protein is not lost in massive amounts in HUS.

    TEST-TAKING HINT: The test taker can eliminate answer 4 because ketonuria is not associated with HUS.

23. 1. **Because the child is symptomatic, dialysis is the treatment of choice.**
    2. Because the child is symptomatic, dialysis is the treatment of choice.
    3. Diuretics are given to prevent fluid overload, but they cannot cause the child in renal failure to produce urine.
    4. The nurse would expect the plan to include dialysis because the child is no longer producing urine. Urinary output would still be monitored.

TEST-TAKING HINT: The test taker can eliminate answer 3 because diuretics will not cause a child in renal failure to produce urine. The nurse can expect urine output (or lack thereof) to be monitored and dialysis to be started.

24. 1. The triad in HUS includes decreased red blood cells (with a high reticulocyte count as the body attempts to produce more red blood cells), decreased platelet count, and renal failure.
    2. **The triad in HUS includes decreased red blood cells (with a high reticulocyte count as the body attempts to produce more red blood cells), decreased platelet count, and renal failure.**
    3. The triad in HUS includes decreased red blood cells (with a high reticulocyte count as the body attempts to produce more red blood cells), decreased platelet count, and renal failure.
    4. The triad in HUS includes decreased red blood cells (with a high reticulocyte count as the body attempts to produce more red blood cells), decreased platelet count, and renal failure.

    TEST-TAKING HINT: The test taker can eliminate answers 1 and 3 because platelets are not increased in HUS.

25. 1. Children with HUS are considered contagious for up to 17 days after the resolution of diarrhea and should be placed on contact isolation.
    2. Once the child recovers from HUS, there is usually no relapse.
    3. **Children with HUS are considered contagious for up to 17 days after the resolution of diarrhea and should be placed on contact isolation.**
    4. Once free of diarrhea for approximately 17 days, the child is considered not to be contagious and should be encouraged to return to developmentally appropriate activities as tolerated.

    TEST-TAKING HINT: The test taker can eliminate answer 1 because the child is still considered contagious.

26. 1. **Preventing infection from stool contamination and skin breakdown is the top priority of care.**
    2. Protect the bladder mucosa with a film wrap to keep the mucosa moist. Do not keep it open where it can be exposed to pathogens or subject to irritation from drying.

3. Infant formula would not provide enough fluid for this infant. An umbilical artery catheter would be inserted to provide fluids because of large insensible fluid losses from the exposed viscera.
4. Although the child should be encouraged to rest, it is important to change the diaper immediately to prevent fecal contamination and subsequent infection.

TEST-TAKING HINT: The test taker can eliminate answers 2 and 3 because they have potential to cause harm to the infant.

27. 1. Furosemide (Lasix) is a loop diuretic that is not routinely used in the care of the child with a repair of bladder exstrophy.
    2. Mannitol is an osmotic diuretic that is not routinely used in the care of the child with a repair of bladder exstrophy.
    3. Meperidine (Demerol) is a narcotic that is not a first-line drug for pain management after a bladder reconstruction.
    4. **Oxybutynin (Ditropan) is used to help control bladder spasms.**

TEST-TAKING HINT: The test taker can eliminate answer 2 because mannitol is a diuretic that is used for central nervous system edema.

28. 1. The infant should not be allowed to sleep on the abdomen because the prone position has been associated with sudden infant death syndrome.
    2. **Many children with urological malformations are prone to latex allergies. The surfaces of playgrounds are often made of rubber, which contains latex.**
    3. Many children with urological malformations are prone to latex allergies. Foods such as bananas can cause a latex allergy.
    4. Although children need a stimulating environment, balloons are dangerous because many contain latex and can also be a choking hazard.

TEST-TAKING HINT: The test taker can eliminate answer 1 because infants should be placed to sleep on their back to prevent sudden infant death syndrome.

29. 1. **Hydronephrosis is due to a structural abnormality in the urinary system, causing urine to back up, leading to pressure and potential cell death.**
    2. Hydronephrosis is due to pressure created by an obstruction, causing urine to back up. There is no free flow of urine.

3. A decreased production of urine does not lead to hydronephrosis.
4. Hydronephrosis is not caused by abnormalities in the urine.

TEST-TAKING HINT: This question requires familiarity with the pathophysiology of hydronephrosis.

30. 1. A positive renal ultrasound would indicate a blockage, causing hydronephrosis. Metabolic acidosis occurs, not alkalosis.
    2. Metabolic acidosis occurs because there is a reduction in hydrogen ion secretion from the distal nephron. A positive renal ultrasound would indicate a blockage, causing hydronephrosis.
    3. Metabolic acidosis, not alkalosis, occurs because there is a reduction in hydrogen ion secretion from the distal nephron. There is bacterial growth in the urine due to the urinary stasis caused by the obstruction.
    4. **Metabolic acidosis is caused by a reduction in hydrogen ion secretion from the distal nephron. Polydipsia and polyuria occur as the kidney's ability to concentrate urine decreases. There is bacterial growth in the urine due to the urinary stasis caused by the obstruction.**

TEST-TAKING HINT: The test taker can eliminate answers 1 and 3 because hydronephrosis does not lead to metabolic alkalosis.

31. 1. **Fluid status is monitored to ensure adequate urinary output. Assessing blood pressure monitors kidney function.**
    2. Fluid and sodium restriction are not required in hydronephrosis.
    3. Steroids are not routinely used in the treatment of hydronephrosis.
    4. Limiting the child's exposure to other people does not help prevent UTIs.

TEST-TAKING HINT: The test taker can eliminate answer 2 because fluids and sodium are not limited in the child's diet.

32. 1. Primary enuresis refers to urinary incontinence in a child who has never had voluntary bladder control.
    2. **Secondary enuresis refers to urinary incontinence in a child who previously had bladder control.**
    3. Diurnal enuresis refers to daytime urinary incontinence not caused by something else.
    4. Nocturnal enuresis refers to nighttime urinary incontinence.

TEST-TAKING HINT: The test taker should be led to answer 2 because the enuresis is secondary to something else, in this case a disease process.

33. 1. Although DDAVP is used for enuresis, it is not the first treatment chosen. Behavior modification and positive reinforcement are usually tried first.
2. Having the child help with changing the bed is a good idea. The child should be approached in a positive manner, however, not a punitive one, so as not to threaten self-esteem.
3. **Limiting the child's fluids in the evening will help decrease the nocturnal urge to void. Providing positive reinforcement and allowing the child to choose a reward will increase the child's sense of control.**
4. Enuresis alarms are readily available, but behavior modification and positive reinforcement are usually tried first.

TEST-TAKING HINT: The test taker can eliminate answer 2 because negative reinforcement is not recommended and is not helpful.

34. 1. The child is having symptoms of testicular torsion, which is a surgical emergency and needs immediate attention. The child should not wait to go to the emergency department and should be told not to drink anything in anticipation of surgery.
2. Testicular torsion is a surgical emergency, and time should not be wasted at the health-care provider's office when the child needs surgery.
3. **The child is having symptoms of testicular torsion, which is a surgical emergency and needs immediate attention.**
4. The child should be brought to the emergency department immediately because testicular torsion is a surgical emergency. Ice and scrotal support can be used for relief of discomfort, but bringing the child to the emergency room is the priority.

TEST-TAKING HINT: The test taker should be led to answer 3 because testicular torsion is a surgical emergency.

35. 1. **Testicular torsion is caused by an interruption of the blood supply due to twisting of the spermatic cord.**
2. Swelling of the scrotal sac occurs because of testicular torsion; it is not a cause of testicular torsion.

3. Unmanaged undescended testes may be a risk factor for but are not a cause of testicular torsion.
4. Microthrombi formation in the vessels of the spermatic cord does not occur in testicular torsion.

TEST-TAKING HINT: This question depends on familiarity with the pathophysiology of testicular torsion.

36. 1. Lifting and strenuous activity should be avoided for 2 to 4 weeks.
2. The child should not be placed on bedrest and should be encouraged to gradually increase activity while resting as necessary.
3. Most cases of testicular torsion involve only one testis, so most children do not become infertile.
4. **The child and family should be taught the importance of testicular self-examination.**

TEST-TAKING HINT: The test taker can eliminate answer 1 because this activity could place the postoperative teen at risk for injury.

37. 1. Bowel is the most common tissue to protrude into the groin in males.
2. **Fallopian tube or an ovary is the most common tissue to protrude into the groin in females.**
3. Large thrombus formation does not commonly protrude into the groin.
4. Muscle tissue does not commonly protrude into the groin.

TEST-TAKING HINT: The test taker should be led to answer 2 because the question specifically states that the child is a female.

38. 1. The terms are not used interchangeably. "Inguinal hernia" refers to protrusion of abdominal tissue into the groin, and "hydrocele" refers to a fluid-filled mass in the scrotum.
2. **The symptoms are similar, but an inguinal hernia occurs when tissue protrudes into the groin; a hydrocele is a fluid-filled mass in the scrotum.**
3. A hydrocele does not occur in females.
4. A hydrocele is not associated with an increased risk of malignancy.

TEST-TAKING HINT: This question depends on knowledge of the definitions of "inguinal hernia" and "hydrocele."

39. 1. Surgery is usually done at an early age to avoid incarceration, in which the hernia causes impaired circulation to the surrounding tissue.
2. The hernia tends to look larger when the child strains or has a bowel movement because of increased intra-abdominal pressure.
3. The surgery is usually done on an outpatient basis, and narcotics are not usually needed.
4. **The hernia often appears smaller when the child is asleep.**

TEST-TAKING HINT: **The test taker can eliminate answer 1 because there are risks associated with waiting for the repair, and surgery is not done solely for cosmetic reasons.**

40. 1. **Signs of an incarcerated hernia include an acute onset of pain, abdominal distention, and a mass that cannot be reduced. Other signs are bloody stools, edema of the scrotum, and a history of poor feeding.**
2. The pain is not gradual, but rather acute, in onset.
3. The mass is not easily reduced.
4. The mass is not easily reduced, and the child experiences acute, not gradual, onset of pain.

TEST-TAKING HINT: **The test taker can eliminate answers 2 and 4 because the onset of pain is not gradual.**

41. 1. Wilms tumor grows very rapidly and doubles in size in less than 2 weeks.
2. This response places blame on the parent. Wilms tumor has a very good prognosis, even when first diagnosed at a more advanced stage.
3. This response is condescending and does not acknowledge the parent as the person who knows the child best.
4. **The tumor is fast-growing and could very easily not have been evident a few days earlier.**

TEST-TAKING HINT: **The test taker can eliminate answer 2 because the nurse should never cause the parent to feel guilt and responsibility over any diagnosis.**

42. 1. The blood pressure may be increased, not decreased, if there is renal damage. The mass will be located on one side or the other of the midline of the abdomen. There is no reason for the child's temperature to be affected.

2. The blood pressure may be increased if there is renal damage. The mass will be located on one side or the other of the midline of the abdomen. There is no reason for the child's temperature to be affected.
3. **The blood pressure may be increased if there is renal damage. The mass will be located on one side or the other of the midline of the abdomen. There is no reason for the child's temperature to be affected.**
4. The blood pressure may be increased, not decreased, if there is renal damage. The mass is located on one side or the other of the midline of the abdomen. There is no reason for the child's temperature to be affected.

TEST-TAKING HINT: **The test taker can eliminate answers 1 and 2 because the mass is felt in the abdomen, not the back.**

43. 1. When the nurse is unsure of the answer, it is best to check and get back to the parents. The nurse should be aware that tests of other organs are often performed to evaluate for the presence of metastases.
2. The test is ordered to check for metastasis to the lungs.
3. **The test is done to see if the disease has spread to the lungs.**
4. A chest x-ray, not a magnetic resonance image, is ordered routinely to evaluate the health of the lungs prior to surgery.

TEST-TAKING HINT: **The test taker should be led to answer 3 because further testing evaluates metastasis to other organs.**

44. 1. The tumor is confined to the abdomen but has spread to the lymph nodes or peritoneal area. The prognosis is still very good.
2. **The tumor is confined to the abdomen but has spread to the lymph nodes or peritoneal area. The prognosis is still very good.**
3. Stage III does not indicate that the tumor has spread to three other organs.
4. The tumor has not spread to other organs beyond the peritoneal area. This would represent stage IV, but with aggressive treatment the child would still have a good prognosis.

TEST-TAKING HINT: **The test taker should be led to answer 2 because this represents stage III.**

45. 1. **The treatment of a Wilms tumor involves removal of the affected kidney.**
2. Removal of the unaffected kidney is not necessary and is not done.

3. The entire kidney is removed.
4. A biopsy of the tissue of the unaffected kidney is not necessary and is not obtained.

TEST-TAKING HINT: The test taker should eliminate answers 3 and 4 because the entire kidney is removed, not only the mass.

46. 1. A large incision is used because the kidney is not removed laparoscopically at this time.
    2. **There is a postoperative shift of fluids and organs in the abdominal cavity, leading to increased discomfort.**
    3. The increased pain is due to shifting of fluid and organs.
    4. The increased pain is due to shifting of fluid and organs.

TEST-TAKING HINT: The test taker should eliminate answer 1 because the kidney is not removed laparoscopically.

47. 1. Both disease processes are characterized by the kidney's inability to excrete waste. CKD occurs gradually and is irreversible, whereas AKI occurs suddenly and may be reversible.
    2. Children can experience CKD and AKI.
    3. CKD is irreversible, and it tends to occur gradually.
    4. **AKI is often reversible, whereas CKD results in permanent deterioration of kidney function.**

TEST-TAKING HINT: The test taker should eliminate answer 1 because the terms "acute" and "chronic" are not used interchangeably.

48. 1. CKD occurs gradually.
    2. **Examples of causes of prerenal failure include dehydration and hemorrhage.**
    3. Primary kidney failure occurs when the kidney experiences a direct injury. Examples include HUS and glomerulonephritis.
    4. Postrenal failure occurs when there is an obstruction to urinary flow. Hypotension does not cause postrenal failure.

TEST-TAKING HINT: The test taker should eliminate answer 1 because there is no evidence of a chronic disease process.

49. 1. The patient is demonstrating signs of hyperkalemia; therefore, intravenous potassium would be contraindicated.
    2. Sodium bicarbonate would be administered when metabolic acidosis is present.
    3. **Calcium gluconate is the drug of choice for cardiac irritability secondary to hyperkalemia.**

4. The patient is demonstrating signs of hyperkalemia; therefore, oral potassium supplements would be contraindicated.

TEST-TAKING HINT: The test taker should eliminate answers 1 and 4 because the patient is already showing signs of increased potassium levels.

50. 1. Sips of clear fluids and ice chips would not replace the insensible losses. All oral intake needs to be measured and accurately recorded because "sips" can be very subjective.
    2. **350 mL is approximately a third of the daily fluid requirement and is recommended for the child in the oliguric phase of AKI. If the child were febrile, the fluid intake would be increased.**
    3. 1000 mL represents the daily fluid requirement in a healthy child.
    4. 2000 mL is double the fluid requirement of a healthy child and is contraindicated in a child in the oliguric phase of AKI.

TEST-TAKING HINT: The question specifies that the child is afebrile; therefore, the test taker can eliminate answers 3 and 4 because extra fluid is not required.

51. 1. Although the child will likely receive additional sodium polystyrene sulfonate (Kayexalate), the child's condition will likely not improve without dialysis.
    2. Although the child will likely receive intravenous furosemide (Lasix), the child's condition will likely not improve without dialysis.
    3. Endotracheal intubation and ventilatory assistance may be required, but ultimately the child will need dialysis.
    4. **Placement of a Tenckhoff catheter for peritoneal dialysis is needed when the child's condition deteriorates despite medical treatment.**

TEST-TAKING HINT: The test taker should be led to answer 4 because dialysis is the treatment required to reverse the existing clinical manifestations.

52. 1. Hemodialysis is used in the pediatric population.
    2. Peritoneal dialysis has many complications, such as peritonitis.
    3. **Peritoneal dialysis removes fluid at a slower rate that is more easily controlled than that of hemodialysis.**
    4. Hemodialysis is much more efficient than peritoneal dialysis.

TEST-TAKING HINT: The test taker should eliminate answer 2 because very few treatments are without complications.

53. 1. **Cloudy returns and abdominal pain are signs of peritonitis and are usually treated with the administration of antibiotics in the dialysis fluid.**
    2. Cloudy returns and abdominal pain are signs of peritonitis and need to be treated.
    3. Cloudy returns and abdominal pain are signs of peritonitis and are usually treated with the administration of antibiotics in the dialysis fluid.
    4. Cloudy returns and abdominal pain are signs of peritonitis. In addition to peritonitis, abdominal pain can be caused by the rapid infusion of dialysis fluid.

TEST-TAKING HINT: The test taker can eliminate answer 4 because pain would be increased if the rate of administration were increased.

54. 1. **Increasing the concentration of glucose will pull more fluid into the return.**
    2. Decreasing the concentration of glucose will pull less fluid into the return.
    3. Antihypertensives and diuretics may be administered, but changing the concentration of glucose in the dialysate will help regulate the fluid balance.
    4. Increasing the dwell time would help pull more fluid into the return. Decreasing the dwell time would pull less fluid into the return.

TEST-TAKING HINT: The test taker should eliminate answers 2 and 4 because they decrease the amount of return.

55. 1. **The child is experiencing signs of disequilibrium syndrome, which is caused by free water shifting from intravascular spaces and can be prevented by slowing the rate of dialysis.**
    2. The patient's temperature is not a causative factor in disequilibrium syndrome.
    3. Antibiotics are used to prevent peritonitis, not disequilibrium syndrome.
    4. The child's weight should be obtained immediately prior to dialysis.

TEST-TAKING HINT: The test taker should eliminate answers 2 and 3 because they are not associated with disequilibrium syndrome.

56. 1. **The retention of sodium and water leads to hypertension.**
    2. Obstruction of the urinary system can lead to renal failure but is not a direct cause of hypertension.
    3. The accumulation of waste products leads to metabolic acidosis.
    4. In CKD, the body experiences a state of metabolic acidosis, not alkalosis.

TEST-TAKING HINT: The test taker should eliminate answer 4 because metabolic alkalosis is not associated with CKD.

57. 1. The kidneys are unable to excrete phosphorus, so phosphorus levels increase and calcium levels fall.
    2. **The calcium and phosphorus levels are drawn from the bones in response to low calcium levels.**
    3. The calcium is drawn from the bones in response to low serum calcium levels.
    4. Although the child may not be consuming enough calcium, dietary deficiency is not the primary cause of hypocalcemia.

TEST-TAKING HINT: The test taker should eliminate answer 4 because dietary imbalances are not the primary cause of hypocalcemia in renal problems.

58. 1. The child's diet should be high in calories and protein, but not all minerals and electrolytes should be high. Sodium, potassium, and phosphorus should be restricted.
    2. The child with CKD needs a diet high in protein.
    3. **The child with CKD needs a diet high in calories, protein, and calcium and low in potassium and phosphorus.**
    4. Phosphorus should be restricted because the kidneys are unable to excrete phosphorus.

TEST-TAKING HINT: The test taker should eliminate answer 2 because it is important for the child to have a diet high in protein.

59. 1. The child is demonstrating signs of rejection. Although pain control is always important, antirejection medications are of utmost importance.
    2. Furosemide (Lasix) may be given to reduce edema, but antirejection medications are the most important for this child.
    3. Polyethylene glycol 3350 (MiraLAX) will help with constipation, but it will not help prevent rejection.
    4. **Corticosteroids are considered part of the antirejection regimen that is essential after a kidney transplant.**

TEST-TAKING HINT: The test taker should be led to answer 4 because it is the only listed answer that is part of an antirejection regimen. Steroids can cause irritability and weight gain.

60. 1. There are extensive post-transplant care requirements.
2. This treatment option is not ideal for families with a history of noncompliance because there is extensive post-transplant care associated with the receipt of a kidney.
3. **Renal transplantation frees the patient from dialysis.**
4. Renal transplantation is not new to the pediatric population.

TEST-TAKING HINT: The test taker should eliminate answer 1 because transplantation is a treatment, not a cure.

61. 1, 2, 3, 4.
1. **Stressors such as the birth of a sibling can lead to incontinence in a child who previously had bladder control.**
2. **A pattern of enuresis can often be seen in families.**
3. **Increased thirst and incontinence can be associated with diabetes.**
4. **Fussiness and incontinence can be associated with UTIs.**
5. Preschool-age children may have difficulties at school, but the other information would be of more help to the nurse in gathering more information on enuresis.

TEST-TAKING HINT: The test taker should be able to eliminate answer 5 by knowing which are the most important questions to ask.

62. 2, 3.
1. It is referred to as a nephroblastoma, not a neuroblastoma.
2. **It can occur at any age but is seen most often between the ages of 2 and 5 years.**
3. **It can occur on its own or can be associated with many congenital anomalies.**
4. It is a tumor that grows very quickly.
5. It is associated with a very good prognosis.

TEST-TAKING HINT: The test taker would have to know about Wilms tumor to answer the question.

Endocrine Disorders 9

KEYWORDS

The following words include English vocabulary, nursing/medical terminology, concepts, principles, or information relevant to content specifically addressed in the chapter or associated with topics presented in it. English dictionaries, your nursing textbooks, and medical dictionaries such as *Taber's Cyclopedic Medical Dictionary* are resources that can be used to expand your knowledge and understanding of these words and related information.

Adrenal gland
Gonadotropin
Hyperthyroidism
Hypothyroidism
Pancreas

Pituitary gland
Type 1 diabetes (insulin-dependent diabetes)
Type 2 diabetes (noninsulin-dependent diabetes)

ABBREVIATIONS

Adrenocorticotropic hormone (ACTH)
Antidiuretic hormone (ADH)
Chronic kidney disease (CKD)
Diabetes insipidus (DI)
Diabetes mellitus (DM)
Emergency department (ED)
Health-care provider (HCP)
Insulin-dependent diabetes mellitus (IDDM)
Insulin-like growth factor-1 (IGF-1)

Insulin-like growth factor binding protein-3 (IGFBP-3)
Noninsulin-dependent diabetes mellitus (NIDDM)
Primary care provider (PCP)
Syndrome of inappropriate antidiuretic hormone (SIADH)
Thyrocalcitonin (TC)
Thyroid hormone (TH)
Thyroid-stimulating hormone (TSH)

QUESTIONS

1. At a follow-up visit for an 8-year-old who is being evaluated for short stature, the nurse measures and plots the child's height on the growth chart. Which explanation should the nurse give the child and family?
   1. "We want to make sure you were measured accurately the last two visits."
   2. "We need to calculate how tall you will be when you grow to adult height."
   3. "We need to see how much you have grown since your last visit."
   4. "We need to know your height so that a dosage of medication can be calculated for you."

2. What key information should be explained to the family of a 3-year-old who has short stature and abnormal laboratory test results?
   1. Because of the diurnal rhythm of the body, growth hormone levels are elevated following the onset of sleep.
   2. Exercise can stimulate growth hormone secretion.
   3. The initial screening tests need to be repeated for accuracy.
   4. Growth hormone levels in children are so low that stimulation testing must be done.

3. A 6-year-old white girl comes with her mother for evaluation of her acne, breast buds, axillary hair, and body odor. What information should the nurse explain to them?
   1. This is a typical age for girls to go into puberty.
   2. Encourage the girl to dress and act appropriately for her chronological age.
   3. She should be on birth control because she is fertile.
   4. She may be short if her epiphyses close early.

4. A nurse is caring for an infant who is very fussy and has a diagnosis of diabetes insipidus (DI). Which parameters should the nurse monitor while the infant is on fluid restrictions? **Select all that apply.**
   1. Oral intake.
   2. Urine output.
   3. Appearance of the mucous membranes.
   4. Change in pulse and temperature.
   5. Lethargy and pain.

5. A 12-year-old comes to the clinic with a diagnosis of Graves disease. What information should the nurse discuss with the child?
   1. Suggest weight loss.
   2. Encourage attending school.
   3. Emphasize that the disease will go into remission.
   4. Encourage the child to take responsibility for daily medications.

6. The school nurse notices that a 14-year-old who used to be an excellent student and very active in sports is losing weight and acting very nervous. The teen was recently checked by the primary care provider (PCP), who noted the teen had a very low level of TSH. The nurse recognizes that the teen has which condition?
   1. Hashimoto thyroid disease.
   2. Graves disease.
   3. Hypothyroidism.
   4. Juvenile autoimmune thyroiditis.

7. A newborn develops tetany and has a seizure prior to discharge from the nursery. The newborn is diagnosed with hypocalcemia secondary to hypoparathyroidism and is started on calcium and vitamin D. Which information would be most important for the nurse to teach the parents?
   1. They should observe the baby for signs of tetany and seizures.
   2. They should observe for weakness, nausea, vomiting, and diarrhea.
   3. They should administer the calcium and vitamin D daily as prescribed.
   4. They should call the clinic if they have any questions about care of the newborn.

8. A teen who was hospitalized for chronic kidney disease (CKD) develops symptoms of polyuria, polydipsia, and bone pain. Which body mineral might be causing these symptoms?
   1. Elevated calcium.
   2. Low phosphorus.
   3. Low magnesium.
   4. High aluminum hydroxide.

9. The family of a young child has been told the child has diabetes insipidus (DI). What information should the nurse emphasize to the family?
   1. One caregiver needs to learn to give the injections of vasopressin.
   2. Children should wear MedicAlert tags if they are over 5 years old.
   3. Diabetes insipidus is different from diabetes mellitus.
   4. Over time, the child may grow out of the need for medication.

10. A nurse is working with a child who has had a bone age evaluation. Which explanation of the test should the nurse give?
    1. "The bone age will give you a diagnosis of your child's short stature."
    2. "If the bone age is delayed, the child will continue to grow taller."
    3. "The x-ray of the bones is compared with that of the age-appropriate, standardized bone age."
    4. "If the bone age is not delayed, no further treatment is needed."

11. Which descriptive terms should be used to describe a school-age child with myxedematous skin/eyes/hair changes?
    1. The skin is oily and scaly.
    2. The skin has pale, thickened patches.
    3. The skin is moist.
    4. The eyes are puffy, the hair is sparse, and the skin is dry.

12. A child is brought to the ED with what is presumed to be acute adrenocortical insufficiency. Which of the following should the nurse do first?
    1. Insert an IV line to administer fluids and cortisol.
    2. Prepare for admission to the intensive care unit.
    3. Indicate the likelihood of a slow recovery.
    4. Discuss the likelihood of the child's imminent death.

13. A child with Addison disease takes oral cortisol supplements. What teaching should be done at each visit? **Select all that apply.**
    1. "Keep an extra month's supply of all medications on hand at all times."
    2. "Wear a MedicAlert bracelet at all times."
    3. "The child is less susceptible to infections."
    4. "Weight gain will occur."
    5. "Your child is more susceptible to infections."

14. The nurse is instructing a family on the side effects of oral cortisol. What aspects of administering the medication should the nurse emphasize?
    1. Weight gain and dietary management.
    2. Bitterness of the taste of the medication.
    3. Excitability that results from the medication.
    4. Taking the medication with food to decrease gastric irritation.

15. An infant is born with ambiguous genitalia. Genetic testing and an ultrasound are ordered. The infant has a large clitoris, but there is no vaginal orifice. The labia appear to be sac-like, darkened tissue. No testes are located. What suggestion should the nurse offer the family?
    1. Take the baby home, and wait until the gender is determined to name it.
    2. Because the parents wanted a boy, give the baby a boy's name.
    3. Give the baby a neutral name that fits either a boy or a girl.
    4. Call the infant "baby" until they know the gender.

16. A baby has hypertension as a result of partial 21-hydroxylase deficiency. The parents ask the nurse to clarify why the baby is being sent home on cortisone. Which is the nurse's best response about cortisone? It:
    1. Increases the utilization of fatty acids for energy.
    2. Depresses the secretion of ACTH.
    3. Stimulates the adrenal glands.
    4. Increases the response to inflammation.

17. A school-age child is diagnosed with bilateral pheochromocytomas. Which clinical manifestations should the nurse check for in this child?
   1. Hypertension headache and decreased gastrointestinal activity.
   2. Hypoglycemia, lethargy, and increased gastrointestinal activity.
   3. Bradycardia, diarrhea, and weight gain.
   4. Hypotension, constipation, and anuria.

18. A teen comes into the clinic with complaints of having been under a lot of stress recently. The teen is being treated for Addison disease and is taking cortisol and aldosterone orally. Today, the teen shows symptoms of muscle weakness, fatigue, salt craving, and dehydration. What should the nurse discuss with the teen regarding the medications?
   1. The dosages may need to be decreased in times of stress.
   2. The dosages may need to be increased in times of stress.
   3. The aldosterone should be stopped, and the cortisol should be increased.
   4. The cortisol may need to be given IV to raise its level.

19. A 6-year-old is diagnosed with growth hormone deficiency. A prescription is written for a dose of 0.025 mg/kg of somatotropin subcutaneously three times weekly. The child weighs 59.4 lb. Which dose of medication should the nurse administer three times weekly?
   1. 0.5 mg.
   2. 0.675 mg.
   3. 1 mg.
   4. 2 mg.

20. Somatotropin comes in a vial of 5 mg and is mixed with a diluent of 5 mL. There is 5 mL of solution in each vial. What amount of the solution should the nurse draw up to give a 1 mg dose?
   1. 0.5 mL.
   2. 0.675 mL.
   3. 1 mL.
   4. 2 mL.

21. A 7-year-old is diagnosed with central precocious puberty. The child is to receive a monthly intramuscular (IM) injection of leuprolide acetate (Lupron). The child has great fear of pain and needles and requires considerable stress reduction techniques each time an injection is due. What could the nurse suggest that might help manage the pain?
   1. Apply a eutectic mixture of local anesthetics (EMLA) of lidocaine and prilocaine to the site at least 60 minutes before the injection.
   2. Have extra help on hand to help hold the child down.
   3. Apply cold to the area prior to injection.
   4. Identify a reward to bribe the child to behave during the injection.

22. A child weighs 21 kg. The parent asks for the weight in pounds. Which is the correct equivalent?
   1. 9.5 lb.
   2. 46.2 lb oz.
   3. 50 lb.
   4. 60 lb.

23. Parents bring their teen to the clinic with a tender, enlarged right breast. The nurse explains that which hormone(s) secreted by the anterior pituitary influence(s) this process?
   1. Thyrotropin.
   2. Gonadotropin.
   3. Oxytocin.
   4. Somatotropin.

24. A toddler is admitted to the pediatric floor for hypopituitarism following removal of a craniopharyngioma. The toddler has polyuria, polydipsia, and dehydration. Which area of the brain was most affected by the surgery?
    1. Posterior pituitary.
    2. Anterior pituitary.
    3. Autonomic nervous system.
    4. Sympathetic nervous system.

25. Which hormone(s) does the anterior pituitary secrete? **Select all that apply.**
    1. Thyroxine.
    2. Luteinizing hormone.
    3. Prolactin (luteotropic hormone).
    4. ACTH.
    5. Epinephrine.
    6. Cortisol.

26. The adrenal cortex secretes sex hormones. Identify which hormones would result in feminization of a young male child. **Select all that apply.**
    1. Estrogen.
    2. Testosterone.
    3. Progesterone.
    4. Cortisol.
    5. Androgens.

27. Which test(s) could be utilized to determine cortisol levels in a child with suspected Cushing syndrome? **Select all that apply.**
    1. Fasting blood glucose.
    2. Thyroid panel (TSH, T3, T4).
    3. 24-hour urine for 17-hydroxycorticoids.
    4. Radiographic studies of the bones.
    5. Cortisone suppression test.
    6. Urine culture.
    7. Complete blood count.

28. A teen comes into the clinic with anxiety. Over the past 2 weeks, the teen has had some muscle twitching and has a positive Chvostek sign. Which explanation could the nurse provide to the parent about a Chvostek sign?
    1. It is a facial muscle spasm elicited by tapping the facial nerve.
    2. Muscle pain that occurs when touched.
    3. The sign occurs because of increased intracranial pressure.
    4. The sign is a result of a vitamin D overdose.

29. A child is working on a school project on glands and asks the clinic nurse to explain the function of the thymus gland. Which answer would the nurse provide?
    1. It produces hormones that help with digestion.
    2. It is a gland that disappears by the time a baby is born.
    3. A major function is to stimulate the pituitary to act as the master gland.
    4. The gland helps with immunity in fetal life and early childhood.

30. A parent with a toddler who has ambiguous genitalia asks the nurse how long it will be before the child identifies his or her gender. Which is the best answer?
    1. "A child does not know his or her gender until he or she is a teen."
    2. "A child knows his or her gender by the age of 18 to 30 months."
    3. "A child knows from the time of birth what his or her gender is."
    4. "A child of 4 to 6 years is beginning to learn his or her gender."

31. According to the growth chart below, an 8-kg boy who is 9 months old is in the _____ percentile of weight-for-age?

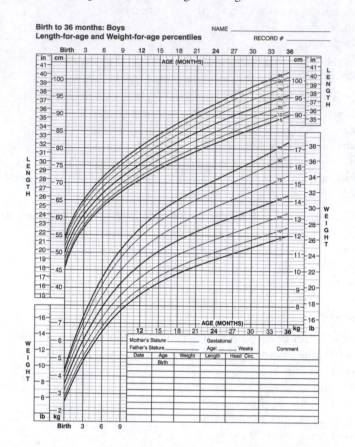

Birth to 36 months: Boys
Length-for-age and Weight-for-age percentiles

NAME _____

RECORD # _____

32. The parent brings the growth record along with the 21-month-old child to a new clinic for a well-child visit. The record shows a birth weight of 8 lb; the 6-month weight was 16 lb; the 12-month weight was 18 lb; and the 15-month weight was 19 lb. With the record showing that the toddler's weight-for-age has been decreasing, the nurse should do what initially?
1. Omit plotting the previous weight-for-age on the new growth chart.
2. Point out the growth chart to the new health-care provider (HCP).
3. Consider the toddler a child with failure to thrive.
4. Weigh the child and plot on a new growth chart.

33. The thyroid gland secretes two types of hormones, thyroid hormone (TH) and thyrocalcitonin (TC). Mark TH or TC in the correct spaces below.
1. _____ This hormone regulates the metabolic rate of all cells.
2. _____ This hormone regulates body heat production.
3. _____ This hormone affects milk production during lactation; it also affects menstrual flow.
4. _____ This hormone maintains calcium metabolism.
5. _____ This hormone affects appetite and the secretion of gastrointestinal substances.
6. _____ This hormone increases gluconeogenesis and utilization of glucose.

34. A child with adrenal insufficiency is sick with influenza. The parent calls the office and wants to know what to do. What is the first thing the nurse should advise this parent?
1. Withhold all medications and bring the child to the office.
2. Encourage the child to drink water and juices.
3. Give the child a dose of hydrocortisone and bring the child to the office.
4. Let the child rest; the child will be better in the morning.

35. A toddler is being evaluated for syndrome of inappropriate antidiuretic hormone (SIADH). The nurse should observe the child for which symptoms? **Select all that apply.**
    1. Dehydration.
    2. Fluid retention.
    3. Hyponatremia.
    4. Hypoglycemia.
    5. Myxedema.

36. What should the parent of a child with diabetes insipidus (DI) be taught about administering desmopressin acetate nasal spray? **Select all that apply.**
    1. The use of the flexible nasal tube.
    2. Nasal congestion causes this route to be ineffective.
    3. The medication should be administered every 48 hours.
    4. The medication should be administered every 8 to 12 hours.
    5. Overmedication results in signs of SIADH.
    6. Nasal sprays do not always work as well as injections.

37. A school-age child comes in with a sore throat and fever. The child was recently diagnosed with Graves disease and is taking propylthiouracil. What concerns should the nurse have about this child?
    1. The child must not be taking her medication.
    2. The child may have leukopenia.
    3. The child needs to start an antibiotic.
    4. The child is not getting enough sleep.

38. An 8-year-old with type 1 diabetes mellitus is complaining of a headache and dizziness and is visibly perspiring. Which of the following should the nurse do first?
    1. Administer glucagon intramuscularly.
    2. Offer the child 8 oz of milk.
    3. Administer rapid-acting insulin lispro (Humalog).
    4. Offer the child 8 oz of water or calorie-free liquid.

39. The nurse is caring for a 10-year-old post parathyroidectomy. Discharge teaching should include which of the following?
    1. How to administer injectable growth hormone.
    2. The importance of supplemental calcium in the diet.
    3. The importance of increasing iodine in the diet.
    4. How to administer subcutaneous insulin.

40. The nurse is teaching the family about caring for their 7-year-old, who has been diagnosed with type 1 diabetes mellitus. What information should the nurse provide about this condition?
    1. Best managed through diet, exercise, and oral medication.
    2. Can be prevented by proper nutrition and monitoring blood glucose levels.
    3. Characterized mainly by insulin resistance.
    4. Characterized mainly by insulin deficiency.

41. The most appropriate nursing diagnosis for a child with type 1 diabetes mellitus is which of the following?
    1. Risk for infection related to reduced body defenses.
    2. Impaired urinary elimination (enuresis).
    3. Risk for injury related to medical treatment.
    4. Anticipatory grieving.

42. The nurse caring for a client with type 1 diabetes mellitus is teaching how to self-administer insulin. Which is the proper injection technique?
    1. Position the needle with the bevel facing downward before injection.
    2. Spread the skin prior to intramuscular injection.
    3. Aspirate for blood return prior to injection.
    4. Elevate the subcutaneous tissue before injection.

43. The nurse is caring for a child who complains of constant hunger, constant thirst, frequent urination, and recent weight loss without dieting. Which can the nurse expect to be included in care for this child?
    1. Limiting daily fluid intake.
    2. Weight management consulting.
    3. Strict intake and output monitoring.
    4. Frequent blood glucose testing.

44. The nurse is obtaining the medical history of an 11-year-old diagnosed with hypopituitarism. An important question for the nurse to ask the parents is which of the following?
    1. "Is the child receiving vasopressin intramuscularly or subcutaneously?"
    2. "What time of day do you administer growth hormone?"
    3. "Does your child have any concerns about being taller than the peer group?"
    4. "How often is your child testing blood glucose?"

45. Which is an important nursing intervention for a child with a diagnosis of hyperthyroidism?
    1. Encourage an increase in physical activity.
    2. Do preoperative teaching for thyroidectomy.
    3. Promote opportunities for periods of rest.
    4. Do dietary planning to increase caloric intake.

46. A 13-year-old with type 2 diabetes mellitus asks the nurse, "Why do I need to have this hemoglobin A1c test?" The nurse's response is based on which of the following?
    1. To determine how balanced the child's diet has been.
    2. To make sure the child is not anemic.
    3. To determine how controlled the child's blood sugar has been.
    4. To make sure the child's blood ketone level is normal.

47. The nurse caring for a 14-year-old girl with diabetes insipidus (DI) understands which of the following about this disorder?
    1. DI is treated on a short-term basis with hormone replacement therapy.
    2. DI may cause anorexia if proper meal planning is not addressed.
    3. DI is treated with vasopressin on a lifelong basis.
    4. DI requires strict fluid limitation until it resolves.

48. A 7-year-old is tested for diabetes insipidus (DI). Twenty-four hours after his fluid restriction has begun, the nurse notes that his urine continues to be clear and pale, with a low specific gravity. Which is the most likely reason for this?
    1. Twenty-four hours is too early to evaluate effects of fluid restriction.
    2. The urine should be concentrated, and it is unlikely the child has DI.
    3. The child may have been sneaking fluids and needs closer observation.
    4. In DI, fluid restriction does not cause urine concentration.

49. The nurse has completed discharge teaching for the family of a 10-year-old diagnosed with diabetes insipidus (DI). Which statement best demonstrates the family's correct understanding of DI?
    1. "The disease was probably brought on by a bad diet and little exercise."
    2. "Diabetes seems to run in my family, and that may be why my child has it."
    3. "My child will need to check blood sugar several times a day."
    4. "My child will have to use the bathroom more often than other children."

50. The nurse is interviewing the parent of a 9-year-old girl. The parent expresses concern because the daughter already has pubic hair and is starting to develop breasts. Which statements would be most appropriate?
    1. "Your daughter should get her period in approximately 6 months."
    2. "Your daughter is developing early and should be evaluated for precocious puberty."
    3. "Your daughter is experiencing body changes that are appropriate for her age."
    4. "Your daughter will need further testing to determine the underlying cause."
    5. "Your daughter will need sexual counseling now."

51. The nurse is taking care of a 10-year-old diagnosed with Graves disease. Which could the nurse expect this child to have recently had?
    1. Weight gain, excessive thirst, and excessive hunger.
    2. Weight loss, difficulty sleeping, and heat sensitivity.
    3. Weight gain, lethargy, and goiter.
    4. Weight loss, poor skin turgor, and constipation.

52. A 12-year-old with type 2 diabetes mellitus presents with a fever and a 2-day history of vomiting. The nurse observes that the child's breath has a fruity odor and breathing is deep and rapid. Which should the nurse do first?
    1. Offer the child 8 oz of clear noncaloric fluid.
    2. Test the child's urine for ketones.
    3. Prepare the child for an IV infusion.
    4. Offer the child 25 g of carbohydrates.

53. Which would the school nurse expect in a student who has an insulin-to-carbohydrate ratio of 1 : 10?
    1. The student administers 10 U of regular insulin for every gram of carbohydrate consumed.
    2. The student is trying to limit carbohydrate intake to 10 g per insulin dose.
    3. The student administers 1 U of regular insulin for every 10 grams of carbohydrate consumed.
    4. The student plans to eat 10 g of carbohydrate for every dose of insulin.

54. Which is the reason a student takes metformin (Glucophage) three times a day?
    1. Type 1 diabetes mellitus.
    2. Diabetes insipidus.
    3. Inflammatory bowel disease.
    4. Type 2 diabetes mellitus.

55. Which is the most likely reason an adolescent with diabetes has problems with low self-esteem?
    1. Managing diabetes decreases independence.
    2. Managing diabetes complicates perceived ability to "fit in."
    3. Obesity complicates perceived ability to "fit in."
    4. Hormonal changes are exacerbated by fluctuations in insulin levels.

56. The school nurse is talking to a 14-year-old about managing type 1 diabetes mellitus. Which statement indicates the student's understanding of the disease?
    1. "It really does not matter what type of carbohydrate I eat as long as I take the right amount of insulin."
    2. "I should probably have a snack right after gym class."
    3. "I need to cut back on my carbohydrate intake and increase my lean protein intake."
    4. "Losing weight will probably help me decrease my need for insulin."

57. The nurse is assigned to care for a newborn with goiter. The nurse's primary concern is which of the following?
    1. Reassuring the parents that the condition is only temporary and will be treated with medication.
    2. Maintaining a patent airway and preparing for emergency ventilation.
    3. Preparing the infant for surgery and initiating preoperative teaching with the parents.
    4. Obtaining a detailed history, particularly of medications taken during the mother's pregnancy.

58. A 13-year-old is being seen for an annual physical examination. The child has lost 10 lb despite reports of excellent appetite. Appearance is normal, except for slightly protruding eyeballs, and the parents report the child has had difficulty sleeping lately. The nurse should do which of the following?
1. Prepare the family for a neurology consult.
2. Explain the need for an ophthalmology consult.
3. Discuss the plan for thyroid function tests.
4. Explain the plan for an 8-hour fasting blood glucose test.

59. A 12-year-old with hyperthyroidism is being treated with standard antithyroid drug therapy. A parent calls the office stating that the child has a sore throat and fever. Which is the nurse's best response?
1. "Bring your child to the office or emergency department immediately."
2. "Slight fever and sore throat are normal side effects of the medication."
3. "Give your child the appropriate dose of ibuprofen and call back if symptoms worsen."
4. "Give your child at least 8 oz of clear fluids and call back if symptoms worsen."

Answer the next three questions with reference to the following figure:

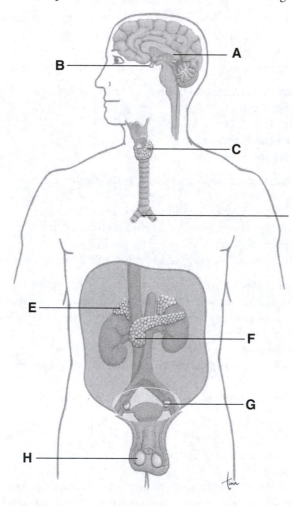

60. Hypofunction of which endocrine gland might cause type 2 diabetes mellitus?

_____

61. Hyperfunction of which endocrine gland might cause Cushing syndrome?

_____

62. Exophthalmic goiter is caused by hyperfunction of which endocrine gland?

_____

ANSWERS AND RATIONALES

The correct answer number and rationale for why it is the correct answer are given in **boldface blue type.** Rationales for why the other possible answer options are incorrect also are given, but they are not in boldface type.

1. 1. Height velocity is important to determine, not whether the measurement was incorrect at a previous visit.
   2. Expected adult height can be determined using a formula that takes into account the parents' height and can be calculated at any visit.
   3. **Height velocity is the most important aspect of a growth evaluation and can demonstrate deceleration in growth if it is present.**
   4. The dose of growth hormone replacement medication is based on weight.

   TEST-TAKING HINT: The health-care provider (HCP) is interested in height velocity over time. The need for multiple measurements ensures that there is measurable growth delay.

2. 1. Growth hormone levels elevate during sleep but cannot be used to determine a definitive diagnosis.
   2. Exercise increases growth hormone secretion but cannot be used for definitive diagnosis.
   3. Screening tests assist in determining in which direction further studies should be done.
   4. **The need for additional testing requires explanation. The abnormal IGF-1 and insulin-like growth factor binding protein require a definitive diagnosis when the levels are either abnormally high or low. Very young children do not secrete adequate levels of growth hormone to measure accurately and thus require challenge/stimulation testing.**

   TEST-TAKING HINT: The test taker should know that definitive diagnosis requires more specific testing.

3. 1. Although girls in the United States mature earlier than in previous decades, the lowest age at which puberty is considered normal is 7 years for white girls and 6 years for African American girls.
   2. **Dressing and acting appropriately for her chronological age should be encouraged for the well-being of the child.**
   3. Although she is fertile if she is pubescent, it is not developmentally necessary to consider the use of birth control at this time.
   4. The estrogen that is produced during puberty does assist in the closure of the epiphyseal plates. With proper medication management, however, the estrogen will be suppressed, and she will continue to grow.

   TEST-TAKING HINT: White girls sometimes enter puberty as early as 7 years of age. This is rare, however, and the extent of her pubertal development should prompt concern.

4. 2, 5.
   1. Although monitoring fluid intake is necessary, the child is on fluid restriction, and the amount of intake will be prescribed.
   2. **It is crucial to monitor and record urine output. The infant with DI has hyposecretion of ADH, and fluid restriction has little effect on urine formation. This infant is at risk for dehydration and for fluid and electrolyte imbalances.**
   3. It is a basic part of assessing the infant with fluid restriction to monitor skin turgor and the appearance of the mucous membranes, but they are not an absolute determination of overall well-being.
   4. It is a basic part of assessing the infant to check pulse and temperature (the infant can become very hyperthermic), but neither would be an absolute indicator of well-being.
   5. **As a result of DI the infant may have behavior changes such as lethargy and pain.**

   TEST-TAKING HINT: DI results from pituitary dysfunction. The posterior pituitary targets the renal tubules and acts on the distal and collecting tubules to make them permeable to water, thus increasing resorption and decreasing excretion of urine.

5. 1. Children with Graves disease have voracious appetites and lose weight.
   2. Encouraging school and continuation of typical activities is better in terms of long-term management. Gym class and after-school sports should be restricted until the child is euthyroid.
   3. Graves disease may go into remission after 2 or 3 years; there are some children, however, for whom it does not.

4. **Because the child is 12 years old, encouraging responsibility for health care is important. The child still needs family involvement and ongoing supervision but should not be completely dependent on family for care.**

TEST-TAKING HINT: The age of the patient is the key to answering the question.

6. 1. "Hashimoto thyroiditis" is a term that refers to hypothyroid disease. Laboratory tests would reveal a high TSH level.
   2. **Graves disease is hyperthyroidism and presents with low TSH levels, weight loss, and excessive nervousness.**
   3. Hypothyroidism is accompanied by a high TSH level.
   4. "Juvenile autoimmune thyroiditis" is a term referring to hypothyroid disease. Laboratory tests would reveal a high TSH level.

TEST-TAKING HINT: The clues to the answer are the low TSH level and the child's symptoms.

7. 1. The baby has hypocalcemia and is being treated for this condition by the team. This should be reviewed with the family.
   2. **Vitamin D toxicity (weakness, nausea, vomiting, and diarrhea) is a serious consequence of therapy and should be the top priority in teaching.**
   3. Reminding the family to give the medication as prescribed is helpful and should be a basic part of discharge care, but it is not the most important information.
   4. Giving the family the phone number for calling the clinic is part of basic care for discharge to home, but it is not the most important information.

TEST-TAKING HINT: Going over the side effects and risks of vitamin D treatment educates the family about what to watch for when giving the new medications.

8. 1. **The most common causes of secondary hyperparathyroidism are chronic renal disease and anomalies of the urinary tract. Blood studies indicate very high levels of calcium because the kidney is unable to process it.**
   2. Renal impairment causes phosphorus levels to become very high, and clients in CKD are often put on low-phosphorus diets to control the levels.
   3. Magnesium levels are elevated in CKD because magnesium is excreted in the urine. Magnesium is not regulated by the parathyroid gland.

4. Aluminum hydroxide keeps phosphorus mobilized so that it can be excreted.

TEST-TAKING HINT: CKD is caused by the kidneys' inability to process waste and excess minerals. Review which substances in excess cause which symptoms.

9. 1. Training *two* caretakers in the administration of the vasopressin reinforces the importance of the need to give the medication and ensures that medication can be given when the primary caretaker is unable to administer it. For someone on long-term injectable medication, two people need to know how to administer it for the preceding reason.
   2. Children should wear MedicAlert tags as soon as they are diagnosed.
   3. **Explaining that DI is different from DM is crucial to the parents' understanding of the management of the disease. DI is a rare condition that affects the posterior pituitary gland, whereas DM is a more common condition that affects the pancreas.**
   4. Children with DI do not grow out of their condition and will require close medical management and medications for the rest of their lives.

TEST-TAKING HINT: The term "diabetes" is commonly associated only with DM. As DI is an uncommon condition that is treated differently, families may easily confuse it with the more common condition DM.

10. 1. Bone age is a method of assessing skeletal maturity and does not give a diagnosis.
    2. The child with a delayed bone age may continue to grow. In many children with a delayed bone age, medication is required to help them continue to grow.
    3. **The bone age is a method of evaluating the epiphyseal growth centers of the bone using standardized, age-appropriate tables.**
    4. A bone age that is not delayed in a child of short stature is more concerning than if the growth were delayed. This means that further testing and evaluation are needed if the growth delay is to be reversed.

TEST-TAKING HINT: Explaining a bone age film clarifies for the family why the test is needed.

11. 1. Oily skin is not associated with a low serum thyroxine level. It is more consistent with hyperthyroidism.
    2. Pale, thickened patches of skin are not associated with hypothyroidism.

3. Moist skin and increased perspiration are characteristic of hyperthyroidism.
4. **Myxedema, associated with low serum thyroxine and raised thyrotropin levels, is characteristic of hypothyroid dysfunction and presents with swelling or puffiness of the limbs and face, sparse hair, and very dry skin. These signs may be accompanied by slowness of movements and mental dullness.**

TEST-TAKING HINT: Describing various assessments is integral to charting accurately. "Myxedema" is a term used to describe hypothyroid skin.

12. 1. **Initially, in the ED the child will be given an IV line, vital signs will be taken frequently, and seizure precautions will be taken.**
2. The child will be sent to the intensive care unit after being stabilized.
3. When children start to recover from an adrenocortical crisis, their progress is often very rapid, within 24 hours.
4. The child will present with headache, nausea and vomiting, high fever, high blood pressure, weakness, and abdominal pain. With prompt diagnosis and the institution of cortisol and fluids, a good recovery is likely.

TEST-TAKING HINT: The question is asking for the priority nursing intervention, which is starting an IV and taking VS.

13. **1, 5.**
1. **Keeping an extra month's supply of all medications, along with a prefilled syringe of hydrocortisone, will enable the family to treat an impending adrenal crisis before it becomes severe.**
2. Wearing a MedicAlert bracelet is advantageous and can be periodically mentioned to the family.
3. Children are more susceptible to infections when on a chronic anti-inflammatory medication such as cortisol.
4. Weight gain will occur over time, but with good diet and adequate exercise this can be controlled.
5. **Cortisol is an anti-inflammatory drug; with long-term use, it causes the child to be more susceptible to infections.**

TEST-TAKING HINT: Steroids are essential to life, so it is important to remind the family to have extra medication on hand at all times.

14. 1. Weight gain can and should be controllable with appropriate eating habits and adequate exercise.
2. The patient will quickly figure out that the medication tastes bitter and that the taste needs to be masked.
3. Excitability is not a common side effect.
4. **Cortisol should be taken with food to decrease gastric irritation.**

TEST-TAKING HINT: Administration of cortisol can cause serious gastric irritation. The nurse should teach the family to anticipate this problem and ensure that the medicine is taken with food.

15. 1. The baby should not be discharged from the hospital without a name, and never call the infant "it."
2. The fact that the gender is not known is difficult for families to accept, but the gender should be determined before discharge.
3. **Selecting a gender-neutral name enables the family and child to gradually accept and adjust to the baby's medical condition and sex.**
4. Calling the infant "baby" is akin to using the word "it."

TEST-TAKING HINT: The family needs to be given some positive way to cope with the fact that the infant's gender is in question.

16. 1. Cortisone increases the mobilization and utilization of fatty acids for energy, but it does not influence the hypertension.
2. **Cortisone suppresses the ACTH being secreted by the pituitary. Because very little, if any, cortisol is produced by the adrenal glands, the ACTH acts to increase cardiac activity and constrict the blood vessels, leading to hypertension.**
3. The adrenal glands synthesize and secrete cortisol.
4. Cortisone suppresses lymphocytes, eosinophils, and basophils, resulting in a decreased inflammatory and allergic response.

TEST-TAKING HINT: Regulation of hormonal secretions is based on negative feedback. The 21-hydroxylase deficiency is causing the adrenal gland to secrete too little cortisol. The pituitary is producing excess ACTH, trying to increase the adrenal secretion of cortisol, and causing the hypertension.

17. 1. **A pheochromocytoma is a rare tumor of the adrenal glands that secretes excess catecholamines, which are a group of amines secreted in the body that act as neurotransmitters. Examples include epinephrine, norepinephrine, and dopamine. Hypertension, headache, and decreased gastric motility are common with pheochromocytoma.**

2. A pheochromocytoma is a rare tumor of the adrenal glands that secretes excess catecholamines such as epinephrine, norepinephrine, and dopamine. Hypoglycemia and lethargy are not typical of pheochromocytoma. The excess catecholamines cause decreased gastric motility.

3. A pheochromocytoma is a rare tumor of the adrenal glands that secretes excess catecholamines such as epinephrine, norepinephrine, and dopamine. Bradycardia, diarrhea, and weight gain are not typical of pheochromocytoma.

4. A pheochromocytoma is a rare tumor of the adrenal glands that secretes excess catecholamines such as epinephrine, norepinephrine, and dopamine. These excess catecholamines cause hypertension, not hypotension. Although they can cause decreased gastrointestinal activity, anuria is not typical of pheochromocytoma.

TEST-TAKING HINT: The tumor arises from the adrenal medulla. The adrenal medulla secretes epinephrine and norepinephrine. Symptoms are those of excess hormones from the adrenal medulla.

18. 1. "Addison disease" is another term for "chronic adrenocortical insufficiency." Medications that replace normal glucocorticoids need to be increased, not decreased, in times of stress.

2. **Because the adrenal glands are not producing enough glucocorticoids, the dosage of both the cortisol and aldosterone must be increased and sometimes tripled in times of stress.**

3. "Addison disease" is another term for "chronic adrenocortical insufficiency." Both medications need to be continued.

4. "Addison disease" is another term for "chronic adrenocortical insufficiency." Oral medications should be increased in times of stress.

TEST-TAKING HINT: The adrenal gland is not able to produce enough hormone, especially during times of stress.

19. 1. First change the weight in pounds to kilograms by dividing the pounds by 2.2: 59.4 ÷ 2.2 = 27 kg. Determine the dosage of medication by multiplying 27 kg by the medication prescribed at 0.025 mg/kg. The total dosage needed is 0.675 mg.

2. **First change the weight in pounds to kilograms by dividing the pounds by 2.2: 59.4 ÷ 2.2 = 27 kg. Determine the dosage of medication by multiplying 27 kg by the medication prescribed at 0.025 mg/kg. The total dosage needed is 0.675 mg.**

3. First change the weight in pounds to kilograms by dividing the pounds by 2.2: 59.4 ÷ 2.2 = 27 kg. Determine the dosage of medication by multiplying 27 kg by the medication prescribed at 0.025 mg/kg. The total dosage needed is 0.675 mg.

4. First change the weight in pounds to kilograms by dividing the pounds by 2.2: 59.4 ÷ 2.2 = 27 kg. Determine the dosage of medication by multiplying 27 kg by the medication prescribed at 0.025 mg/kg. The total dosage needed is 0.675 mg.

TEST-TAKING HINT: Multiplying the milligrams per kilogram of weight by the patient's kilograms of weight yields the total milligrams dosage ordered.

20. 1. Determine the amount of solution by setting up an equation of 5 mg/5 mL as 0.675 mg/X mL = 0.0675 mL.

2. **Determine the amount of solution by setting up an equation of 5 mg/5 mL as 0.675 mg/X mL = 0.0675 mL.**

3. Determine the amount of solution by setting up an equation of 5 mg/5 mL as 0.675 mg/X mL = 0 .0675mL.

4. Determine the amount of solution by setting up an equation of 5 mg/5 mL as 0.675 mg/X mL = 0.0675mL.

TEST-TAKING HINT: The medication is mixed as 1 mg per each mL. Give 0.675 mL of the solution three times weekly.

21. 1. **EMLA cream works well for skin and cutaneous pain. Having the child assist in putting on the EMLA patch involves the child in the pain-relieving process.**

2. Because this is a monthly injection, it would not be appropriate to hold the child down forcefully, because this creates greater fear and anxiety.

3. Apply ice to the opposite side of the body.

4. Bribing children teaches them that the more they cry and fuss, the more they are rewarded.

TEST-TAKING HINT: Developing a trusting relationship with the child by allowing the child to help apply the EMLA cream gives the child some control in relieving the pain.

22. 1. 2.2 lb = 1 kg. Multiplying the kilograms by 2.2 yields 46.2 lb.
    2. 2.2 lb = 1 kg. Multiplying the kilograms by 2.2 yields 46.2 lb.
    3. 2.2 lb = 1 kg. Multiplying the kilograms by 2.2 yields 46.2 lb.
    4. 2.2 lb = 1 kg. Multiplying the kilograms by 2.2 yields 46.2 lb.

TEST-TAKING HINT: Parents frequently ask for "lay" terms of medical data. Knowing that there are 2.2 pounds in each kilogram enables determination of this number.

23. 1. Thyrotropin and somatotropin are secreted by the anterior pituitary but do not directly influence breast development.
    2. The gonadotropins stimulate the gonads to mature and produce sex hormones.
    3. Oxytocin is secreted by the *posterior* pituitary and targets the uterus and production of milk from the breasts.
    4. Thyrotropin and somatotropin are secreted by the anterior pituitary but do not directly influence breast development.

TEST-TAKING HINT: The anterior pituitary is responsible for stimulating and inhibiting the secretions from the various target organs.

24. **1. The posterior pituitary is responsible for the secretion of ADH and control of the renal tubules. The symptoms are those of DI.**
    2. The anterior pituitary functions as the master gland for growth, sexual function, and skin but does not directly influence the urinary system.
    3. The autonomic nervous system is not directly responsible for polyuria, polydipsia, and dehydration.
    4. The sympathetic nervous system is not directly responsible for polyuria, polydipsia, and dehydration.

TEST-TAKING HINT: The symptoms are classic for posterior pituitary dysfunction.

25. **2, 3, 4.**
    1. Thyroxine is secreted by the thyroid gland.
    2. Luteinizing hormone, prolactin, and ACTH are secreted by the anterior pituitary.
    3. Luteinizing hormone, prolactin, and ACTH are secreted by the anterior pituitary.
    4. Luteinizing hormone, prolactin, and ACTH are secreted by the anterior pituitary.
    5. Epinephrine is secreted by the adrenal medulla.
    6. Cortisol is secreted by the adrenal cortex.

TEST-TAKING HINT: The pituitary is the master gland and is responsible for stimulating and inhibiting target glands. The thyroid and the adrenal glands are target glands.

26. **1, 3.**
    1. Estrogen and progesterone are hormones secreted by the adrenal cortex that in excess would cause feminization of a young male child.
    2. Testosterone is secreted by the testes and does not result in feminization.
    3. Estrogen and progesterone are hormones secreted by the adrenal cortex that in excess would cause feminization.
    4. Cortisol is a glucocorticoid that is secreted by the adrenal cortex but does not result in feminization.
    5. Androgens are secreted by the adrenal cortex but would cause masculinization of the child.

TEST-TAKING HINT: The sex hormones influence the development of the reproductive organs and secondary sexual characteristics. Male feminization is a result of hypofunction of primarily the male sex hormones.

27. **3, 5.**
    1. A fasting blood glucose is helpful in determining the child's overall health but does not demonstrate excess cortisol production by the body.
    2. A thyroid panel is helpful in determining the child's overall health but does not demonstrate excess cortisol production by the body.
    3. A 24-hour urine for 17-hydroxycorticoids or a cortisone suppression test is used for diagnosing overproduction of cortisol by the body.
    4. Radiographic bone studies are helpful in determining the child's overall health but do not demonstrate excess cortisol production by the body.
    5. A 24-hour urine for 17-hydroxycorticoids or a cortisone suppression test is used for diagnosing overproduction of cortisol by the body.

6. A urine culture is helpful in determining the child's overall health but does **not** demonstrate excess cortisol production by the body.
7. A complete blood count is helpful in determining the child's overall health but does not demonstrate excess cortisol production by the body.

TEST-TAKING HINT: Cortisol levels can be measured with urine-specific testing.

28. 1. **Chvostek sign is a facial muscle spasm elicited by tapping on the facial nerve in the region of the parotid gland, indicates heightened neuromuscular activity, and leads the nurse to suspect hypoparathyroidism.**
2. Chvostek sign is a facial muscle spasm elicited by tapping on the facial nerve in the region of the parotid gland, indicates heightened neuromuscular activity, and leads the nurse to suspect hypoparathyroidism.
3. Chvostek sign is a facial muscle spasm elicited by tapping on the facial nerve in the region of the parotid gland, indicates heightened neuromuscular activity, and leads the nurse to suspect hypoparathyroidism.
4. Chvostek sign is a facial muscle spasm elicited by tapping on the facial nerve in the region of the parotid gland, indicates heightened neuromuscular activity, and leads the nurse to suspect hypoparathyroidism.

TEST-TAKING HINT: If a facial muscle spasm can be elicited, then the nurse would strongly suspect the child has hypothyroidism.

29. 1. The glands that line the gastrointestinal tract contain cells that produce hormones that control and coordinate secretion of digestive enzymes.
2. The thymus gland is well developed in infancy, attains its greatest size at puberty, and then is changed into fatty tissue.
3. The pituitary gland is the master gland for the body.
4. **The thymus acts to provide immunity to the very young body.**

TEST-TAKING HINT: The child wants information about the function of the thymus gland.

30. 1. Teens know their gender and may try on the roles of the opposite gender.
2. **Children 18 months to 30 months learn their gender from examining and touching their body parts and learning roles that are either male or female.**

3. Newborns do not identify with one gender or the other.
4. By 4 to 6 years of age, children have a clear understanding of their gender and the male or female roles that they are assigned.

TEST-TAKING HINT: Erikson's stages of psychosexual development define a 2-year-old as in the "autonomy vs. shame and doubt" stage. The 2-year-old explores the body and is given specific behaviors that indicate the gender.

31. 10th percentile.
The child would be in the 10th percentile in comparison with other boys the same age.

TEST-TAKING HINT: Mark the age of the child on the horizontal axis and find the weight in kilograms on the vertical axis; the weight-for-age percentile is where the two lines intersect.

32. 1. The data from the previous primary care provider are important for comparison purposes.
2. **The provider should be made aware of the decelerating weight for age. This pictorial information can then be reviewed with the parent.**
3. Failure to thrive is a diagnosis that can be organic, nonorganic, or idiopathic. Labeling a patient as having failure to thrive prior to the assessment is inappropriate.
4. Weighing toddlers can be a challenge because they are very active. The new weight should be obtained with only a diaper on the child. It should be recorded along with the previous provider's weights.

TEST-TAKING HINT: The nurse helps the health-care provider by identifying areas of concern.

33. 1. **TH;** the main physiological effect of TH is to regulate the basal metabolic rate and thereby control the process of growth and tissue differentiation.
2. **TH;** the main physiological effect of TH is to regulate the basal metabolic rate and thereby control the process of growth and tissue differentiation.
3. **TC;** the main effects that TC causes are related to lactation and menstrual flow.
4. **TC;** the main effects that TC causes are related to maintenance of blood calcium levels by decreasing calcium concentration in the blood.

5. **TH;** the main physiological effect of TH is to regulate the basal metabolic rate and thereby control the process of growth and tissue differentiation.

6. **TH;** the main physiological effect of TH is to regulate the basal metabolic rate and thereby control the process of growth and tissue differentiation.

TEST-TAKING HINT: TH is involved in many activities, and TC functions primarily to maintain calcium balance.

34. 1. The family should administer the reserve hydrocortisone injection intramuscularly immediately and then bring the child to the office.
  2. When children with adrenal insufficiency get influenza or are ill, the situation can be life threatening. The family should administer the reserve hydrocortisone injection intramuscularly and then bring the child to the office.
  3. **When children with adrenal insufficiency get influenza or are ill, the situation can be life threatening. The family should administer the reserve hydrocortisone injection intramuscularly and then bring the child to the office. There is no harm in giving extra hydrocortisone.**
  4. When children with adrenal insufficiency get influenza or are ill, the situation can be life threatening.

TEST-TAKING HINT: Because this child cannot produce hydrocortisone, the levels fall and cause abdominal pain, nausea, and vomiting. The child needs additional cortisol to recover.

35. **2, 3.**
  1. Dehydration is not a feature of SIADH.
  2. **ADH assists the body in retaining fluids and subsequently decreases serum osmolarity while the urine osmolarity rises. When serum sodium levels are decreased below 120 mEq/L, the child becomes symptomatic.**
  3. **ADH assists the body in retaining fluids and subsequently decreases serum osmolarity while the urine osmolarity rises. When serum sodium levels are decreased below 120 mEq/L, the child becomes symptomatic.**
  4. Hypoglycemia is not a feature of SIADH.
  5. Myxedema is not a feature of SIADH.

TEST-TAKING HINT: The posterior pituitary is responsible for secretion of ADH. SIADH is oversecretion of ADH.

36. **1, 2, 4, 5.**
  1. **Administering desmopressin acetate per nasal spray is a means of providing the necessary medication in a steady state, if it is given using the flexible nasal tube every 8 to 12 hours. This decreases nasal irritation.**
  2. **If the child becomes ill with rhinorrhea, the nasal spray will need to be administered via the buccal mucosa or rectum or the medication changed to tablets.**
  3. Administering desmopressin acetate per nasal spray is a means of providing the necessary medication in a steady state, if it is given using the flexible nasal tube every 8 to 12 hours.
  4. **Administering desmopressin acetate per nasal spray is a means of providing the necessary medication in a steady state, if it is given using the flexible nasal tube every 8 to 12 hours.**
  5. **Side effects of the desmopressin acetate are those of SIADH.**
  6. Administering desmopressin acetate per nasal spray is a means of providing the necessary medication in a steady state, if it is given using the flexible nasal tube every 8 to 12 hours.

TEST-TAKING HINT: Administering medication necessitates the parent be instructed in the technique, side effects, and what to do if the medication cannot be administered for some reason.

37. 1. Propylthiouracil is used to suppress thyroid function. One of the grave complications of the medication is leukopenia.
  2. **Propylthiouracil is used to suppress thyroid function. One of the grave complications of the medication is leukopenia.**
  3. Propylthiouracil is used to suppress thyroid function. One of the grave complications of the medication is leukopenia.
  4. Propylthiouracil is used to suppress thyroid function. One of the grave complications of the medication is leukopenia.

TEST-TAKING HINT: Side effects of a medication need to be assessed quickly. During the first few weeks of therapy, there is a risk of blood dyscrasias. The propylthiouracil prevents the conversion of iodine to its usable form.

38. 1. Glucagon is given only for severe hypoglycemia. The child's symptoms are those of mild hypoglycemia.
  2. **Milk is best to give for mild hypoglycemia, which would present with the symptoms described.**
  3. Insulin is appropriate for elevated blood glucose, but the symptoms listed are those of hypoglycemia, not hyperglycemia. It is important for the test taker to be able to distinguish between the two.
  4. Water is appropriate for mild hyperglycemia, but the symptoms listed are those of hypoglycemia.

TEST-TAKING HINT: The test taker should first determine hyper- or hypoglycemia, which should permit elimination of two choices, then choose the best answer. When describing symptoms of a diabetic patient, look for ways to determine either hypoglycemia or hyperglycemia.

39. 1. Growth hormone would be appropriate if the patient had panhypopituitarism.
  2. **The parathyroid is responsible for calcium reabsorption; therefore, supplemental calcium in the diet is the important point to be discussed in patient teaching.**
  3. Iodine is another important dietary supplement.
  4. Information about insulin injection is appropriate for diabetes mellitus, not parathyroid disorder.

TEST-TAKING HINT: The test taker needs to know the function of the parathyroid glands.

40. 1. Type 2 DM is best managed by diet, exercise, and oral medication.
  2. Proper diet and monitoring blood glucose are important in type 1 DM, but DM is characterized by insulin deficiency.
  3. Though insulin resistance can be one of the factors in type 1 DM, it is not the primary factor.
  4. **Individuals with type 1 DM do not produce insulin. If one does not produce insulin, type 1 DM is the diagnosis.**

TEST-TAKING HINT: The test taker should know the difference between type 1 and type 2 DM.

41. 1. **Risk for infection is a correct nursing diagnosis. Understanding DM is understanding the effect it has on peripheral circulation and impairment of defense mechanisms.**

2. Although many children with type 1 DM present with enuresis, impaired urinary elimination is not the best response.
3. Treatment includes injections, but this is not a risk for injury.
4. Type 1 DM, although lifelong, is not a terminal illness and can be well managed, so grieving is not an appropriate diagnosis.

TEST-TAKING HINT: The test taker needs to understand diabetes mellitus to choose correctly.

42. 1. Correct needle position is with the bevel facing upward.
  2. Injection is subcutaneous, so tissue is not spread as it would be for intramuscular injection.
  3. Aspiration for blood is not recommended for subcutaneous injections.
  4. **Skin tissue is elevated to prevent injection into the muscle when giving a subcutaneous injection. Insulin is only given subcutaneously.**

TEST-TAKING HINT: The test taker must understand that insulin is only given subcutaneously. Answers 2 and 3 can be eliminated by knowing how to give an intramuscular injection.

43. 1. Limiting fluids is appropriate for a child presenting with the symptoms of DI, not DM.
  2. Weight loss without the other presenting symptoms might be indicative of a need for a weight/nutrition consult.
  3. Strict intake and output monitoring is included in the care of a child with DI.
  4. **Frequent blood glucose testing is included in the care of a child with type 1 DM. The symptoms described in the question are characteristic of a child just prior to the diagnosis of type 1 DM.**

TEST-TAKING HINT: In a question that lists symptoms, it is important to determine the diagnosis. In this case, the test taker can anticipate type 1 DM and know that frequent glucose monitoring is part of the plan of care.

44. 1. Vasopressin is a medication used to treat the uncontrolled diuresis associated with DI.
  2. **Growth hormone is used to treat a child with hypopituitarism.**
  3. Hypopituitarism promotes short, not tall, stature.

4. Although hypoglycemia might be a factor when a child is undergoing diagnostic testing for hypopituitarism, blood sugar testing is not part of the treatment plan.

TEST-TAKING HINT: When presented with a question like this, the test taker must first consider the diagnosis and the clinical manifestations. Knowing that this diagnosis is considered primarily when a child presents with short stature and slowed growth curve, answer 2 is most appropriate.

45. 1. A child with hyperthyroidism displays increased activity.
    2. Thyroidectomy is not the first choice for treating hyperthyroidism, although it is considered if other treatments fail.
    3. **Because increased activity is characteristic of hyperthyroidism, providing opportunity for rest is a recommended nursing intervention.**
    4. Weight loss despite increased appetite and intake might be a symptom of hyperthyroidism. Just increasing calories is not the best option because the cause and treatment of the thyroid's hyperactivity needs to be addressed.

TEST-TAKING HINT: The test taker needs to know the signs and symptoms of hyperthyroidism to determine appropriate nursing interventions.

46. 1. Balanced diet, although important, is not determined by hemoglobin A1c.
    2. Anemia would be a correct choice if the question asked about hemoglobin, not hemoglobin A1c.
    3. **Hemoglobin A1c, or glycosylated hemoglobin, reflects average blood glucose levels over 2 to 3 months. Frequent high blood glucose levels would result in a higher hemoglobin A1c, suggesting that blood glucose needs to be in better control.**
    4. Presence of ketones in the blood, although associated with the absence of insulin and with high blood glucose levels, is not directly correlated with hemoglobin A1c.

TEST-TAKING HINT: The test taker needs to know the purpose of the hemoglobin A1c test.

47. 1. DI is caused by undersecretion of ADH (vasopressin). Replacement therapy with vasopressin is a long-term option, however, not a short-term one.

2. DI is not to be confused with DM, for which dietary planning is a large part of management.
3. **Vasopressin is the treatment of choice. It is important for patients and parents to understand that DI is a lifelong disease.**
4. Although a sign of DI is excessive urination, fluid replacement is needed, not restriction. Fluid restriction is only part of the diagnostic phase.

TEST-TAKING HINT: The test taker needs to understand the long-term implications of the diagnosis.

48. 1. Within 24 hours of fluid restriction, the urine becomes concentrated in a healthy child.
    2. Because the urine is not concentrated, the child is likely to have DI.
    3. Children should be carefully observed to make sure they are not sneaking fluids; however, the assumption that this child has been doing so should not be made.
    4. **Children with DI cannot concentrate urine.**

TEST-TAKING HINT: Understanding that DI causes uncontrolled diuresis, the test taker should choose answer 4. Answers 1 and 3 assume that there is something wrong with the diagnostic procedure and would be less likely to be correct. Answer 2 is the opposite of answer 4.

49. 1. The primary causes of DI are idiopathic, organic, and brain trauma, unlike the causes for type 2 DM, for which diet and exercise are major factors.
    2. DI does not have a hereditary factor.
    3. Blood sugar monitoring is important with DM, not DI.
    4. **Despite the use of vasopressin to treat the symptoms of DI, breakthrough urination is likely.**

TEST-TAKING HINT: The test taker needs to understand the difference between DI and DM.

50. 1. Menarche usually occurs within 2 years after the start of breast development.
    2. Age 9 is the average age of thelarche (breast bud development), which is followed shortly by the appearance of pubic hair.
    3. **The changes described in the question are normal for a healthy 9-year-old female.**
    4. No further testing is required because this is normal.

5. Sexual counseling does not need to be done now but in the future.

TEST-TAKING HINT: Understanding that the question describes a set of normal changes, the test taker could eliminate answers 2 and 5. Because the parent in the question is expressing concern, the most appropriate answer from the remaining three is the one offering reassurance, answer 3.

51. 1. Graves disease is a type of hyperthyroidism. Gradual weight loss, not weight gain, is a sign.
    2. Weight loss, increased activity, and heat intolerance can be expected when the thyroid gland is hyperfunctional.
    3. Weight gain as a symptom makes this answer incorrect.
    4. Constipation and dry skin with poor turgor are more likely in a patient with hypothyroidism.

TEST-TAKING HINT: The test taker needs to know the presenting signs and symptoms of Graves disease.

52. 1. The fruity odor is that of acetone. The patient is exhibiting signs of ketoacidosis. The history of vomiting and the Kussmaul breathing preclude oral rehydration.
    2. Although it is likely that ketones would be present, the child is in a life-threatening situation. Checking urine is not necessary.
    3. This patient needs fluid and electrolyte therapy to restore tissue perfusion prior to beginning IV insulin therapy.
    4. The patient is hyperglycemic, not hypoglycemic.

TEST-TAKING HINT: The patient's history of vomiting should clue the test taker to disregard choices for food or fluids by mouth, answers 1 and 4. Answer 2 might be possible, as the urine would test positive for ketones, but the deep and rapid breathing should help the test taker choose answer 3.

53. 1. An insulin-to-carbohydrate ratio refers to the amount of insulin given per gram of carbohydrate. A ratio of 1 : 10 means 1 U regular insulin for every 10 g carbohydrates. This dose would be appropriate if the child were planning a meal of 100 g of carbohydrates.
    2. Limiting carbohydrate intake is not a factor in managing type 1 DM.

3. **An insulin-to-carbohydrate ratio refers to the amount of insulin given per gram of carbohydrate. A ratio of 1 : 10 means 1 U regular insulin for every 10 g carbohydrates.**
4. An insulin-to-carbohydrate ratio refers to the amount of insulin given per gram of carbohydrate. A ratio of 1 : 10 means 1 U regular insulin for every 10 g carbohydrates.

TEST-TAKING HINT: The test taker needs to understand the insulin-to-carbohydrate ratio.

54. 1. Type 1 DM is managed with insulin, not oral agents.
    2. DDAVP, not metformin, is used to treat diabetes insipidus.
    3. Methylprednisolone (Medrol) can be used to treat inflammatory bowel disease.
    4. Metformin (Glucophage) is commonly used to manage type 2 DM.

TEST-TAKING HINT: Even being unfamiliar with the name "metformin," the test taker might guess that Glucophage would have something to do with destruction or digestion of glucose, thereby being able to correctly eliminate answers 2 and 3.

55. 1. Managing DM increases rather than decreases independence.
    2. Because the desire to fit in is so strong in adolescence, the need to manage one's diabetes can compromise the patient's perception of ability to do so. For example, an adolescent with type 1 DM has to plan meals and snacks, test blood sugar, limit choices of when and what to eat, and always be concerned with the immediate health consequences of actions as simple as eating. The fact that these limitations can negatively affect self-esteem is an essential concept for the nurse caring for adolescents with diabetes to understand.
    3. Obesity is not necessarily associated with type 1 DM.
    4. Hormone changes in adolescence often result in increasing insulin demands; however, increased insulin need not correlate with low self-esteem.

TEST-TAKING HINT: The test taker needs to understand normal development in the adolescent and that fitting in is extremely important.

56. 1. **A carbohydrate is a carbohydrate, and insulin dosing is based on blood sugar level and carbohydrates to be eaten.**
2. Snacks should be ingested before planned exercise rather than after.
3. Nutritional needs of children with DM do not differ from those without DM.
4. Weight loss is likely a factor in managing type 2 DM; type 1 DM is often preceded by dramatic weight loss. The nutritional needs of children with type 1 DM are essentially the same as those not affected.

TEST-TAKING HINT: The test taker needs to understand the basics of DM and how it is managed. Insulin and carbohydrates have to complement each other for good control.

57. 1. Goiter in a newborn can be life threatening and is usually treated by surgical removal or partial removal of the thyroid.
2. **Goiter in a newborn can cause tracheal compression, and positioning to help relieve pressure (i.e., neck hyperextension) is essential. Emergency precautions for ventilation and possible tracheostomy are also instituted.**
3. Although preparation for surgery might be necessary, the most important intervention is protecting the infant's airway.
4. Certain medications (antithyroid drugs) taken by the mother could predispose the infant to developing a goiter. Although the history is important, it is not the first priority for the nurse caring for this patient.

TEST-TAKING HINT: The test taker, if unsure of the correct response, should choose the one pertaining to the ABCs: airway, breathing, and cardiac status.

58. 1. The patient exhibits signs of Graves disease, a primary type of hyperthyroidism in children. A neurology consultation is not indicated.
2. Despite the exophthalmos, an eye consultation is not indicated.

3. **Diagnostic evaluation for hyperthyroidism is based on thyroid function tests. It is expected in this case that T4 and T3 levels would be elevated, because the thyroid gland is overfunctioning.**
4. Fasting blood glucose is used to help evaluate for other endocrine disorders, such as Cushing syndrome and DM.

TEST-TAKING HINT: One of the first nursing considerations is identifying children with hyperthyroidism.

59. 1. **A complication of antithyroid drug therapy is leukopenia. Fever and sore throat, therefore, need to be evaluated immediately. This is an essential component of discharge teaching for patients with Graves disease.**
2. Common side effects of antithyroid drugs include rash, nausea, vomiting, headache, drowsiness, but not sore throat.
3. This is a tempting choice for the test taker, because fever and sore throat appear to be fairly benign symptoms. Because the question includes information regarding Graves disease and medication therapy, however, the test taker should eliminate this answer.
4. It is most likely that medication, not fluid status, contributes to the child's symptoms.

TEST-TAKING HINT: The test taker needs to be familiar with adverse effects of all medications administered or that the family is taught about.

60. **F (pancreas).**

TEST-TAKING HINT: Type 2 DM can be caused by a slowed response of the pancreas.

61. **E (adrenal).**

TEST-TAKING HINT: Cushing syndrome results from too much circulating cortisol.

62. **C (thyroid).**

TEST-TAKING HINT: Hyperfunction of the thyroid may result in exophthalmic goiter.

Hematological/Oncology Disorders

KEYWORDS

The following words include English vocabulary, nursing/medical terminology, concepts, principles, or information relevant to content specifically addressed in the chapter or associated with topics presented in it. English dictionaries, your nursing textbooks, and medical dictionaries such as *Taber's Cyclopedic Medical Dictionary* are resources that can be used to expand your knowledge and understanding of these words and related information.

Aplastic anemia

Beta-thalassemia (Cooley anemia or thalassemia major)

Central nervous system prophylaxis

Chelation therapy

Factor VIII deficiency

Hemarthrosis

Hemophilia A

Hodgkin disease

Immunosuppressive

Intrathecal chemotherapy

Leukemia

Mucositis

Neuroblastoma

Neutropenia

Non-Hodgkin lymphoma

Osteosarcoma

Pancytopenia

Polycythemia

Polycythemia vera

Purpura

Reed-Sternberg cells

Sickle cell disease (sickle cell anemia)

Splenic sequestration

Thrombocytopenia

Vaso-occlusive crises

Von Willebrand disease

Wilms tumor

ABBREVIATIONS

Acute lymphoblastic leukemia (ALL)

Cytomegalovirus (CMV)

Idiopathic thrombocytopenia purpura (ITP)

Packed red blood cells (PRBCs)

Pneumocystis jiroveci pneumonia (PJP) (formerly pneumocystic pneumonia [PCP])

Severe combined immunodeficiency disease (SCID)

Vanillylmandelic acid (VMA)

QUESTIONS

1. The nurse is taking care of a child with sickle cell disease. The nurse is aware that which of the following problems is (are) associated with sickle cell disease? **Select all that apply.**
   1. Polycythemia.
   2. Hemarthrosis.
   3. Aplastic crisis.
   4. Thrombocytopenia.
   5. Vaso-occlusive crisis.

2. An 18-month-old male is brought to the clinic by his mother. His height is in the 50th percentile, and his weight is in the 80th percentile. The child is pale. The physical examination is normal, but his hematocrit level is 20%. Which of the following questions should assist the nurse in making a diagnosis? **Select all that apply.**
1. "How many bowel movements a day does your child have?"
2. "How much did your baby weigh at birth?"
3. "What does your child eat every day?"
4. "Has the child been given any new medications?"
5. "How much milk does your child drink per day?"

3. Which of the following factors need(s) to be included in a teaching plan for a child with sickle cell disease? **Select all that apply.**
1. The child needs to be taken to a physician when sick.
2. The parent should make sure the child sleeps in an air-conditioned room.
3. Emotional stress should be avoided.
4. It is important to keep the child well hydrated.
5. It is important to make sure the child gets adequate nutrition.

4. A nurse is caring for a 5-year-old with sickle cell vaso-occlusive crisis. Which of the following orders should the nurse question? **Select all that apply.**
1. Position the child for comfort.
2. Apply hot packs to painful areas.
3. Give meperidine (Demerol) 25 mg intravenously every 4 hours as needed for pain.
4. Restrict oral fluids.
5. Apply oxygen per nasal cannula to keep oxygen saturations above 94%.

5. A nurse is caring for a child with von Willebrand disease. The nurse is aware that which of the following is a clinical manifestation of von Willebrand disease? **Select all that apply.**
1. The child bruises easily.
2. Excessive menstruation.
3. The child has frequent nosebleeds.
4. Elevated creatinine levels.
5. Elevated blood pressure.

6. A child with hemophilia A fell and injured a knee while playing outside. The knee is swollen and painful. Which of the following measures should be taken to stop the bleeding? **Select all that apply.**
1. The extremity should be immobilized.
2. The extremity should be elevated.
3. Warm moist compresses should be applied to decrease pain.
4. Passive range-of-motion exercises should be administered to the extremity.
5. Factor VIII should be administered.

7. Which of the following activities should a nurse suggest for a client diagnosed with hemophilia? **Select all that apply.**
1. Swimming.
2. Golf.
3. Hiking.
4. Fishing.
5. Soccer.

8. Which of the following describes idiopathic thrombocytopenia purpura (ITP)? **Select all that apply.**
1. ITP is a congenital hematological disorder.
2. ITP causes excessive destruction of platelets.
3. Children with ITP have normal bone marrow.
4. Platelets are small in ITP.
5. Purpura is observed in ITP.

9. The nurse is caring for a child who is receiving a transfusion of PRBCs. The nurse is aware that if the child has a hemolytic reaction to the blood, the signs and symptoms would include which of the following? **Select all that apply.**
   1. Fever.
   2. Rash.
   3. Oliguria.
   4. Hypotension.
   5. Chills.

10. The nurse is caring for a child with leukemia. The nurse should be aware that children being treated for leukemia may experience which of the following complications? **Select all that apply.**
    1. Anemia.
    2. Infection.
    3. Bleeding tendencies.
    4. Bone deformities.
    5. Polycythemia.

11. Which of the following is a reason to perform a lumbar puncture on a child with a diagnosis of leukemia? **Select all that apply.**
    1. Rule out meningitis.
    2. Assess the central nervous system for infiltration.
    3. Give intrathecal chemotherapy.
    4. Determine increased intracranial pressure.
    5. Stage the leukemia.

12. Which of the following measures should the nurse implement to help with the nausea and vomiting caused by chemotherapy? **Select all that apply.**
    1. Give an antiemetic 30 minutes prior to the start of therapy.
    2. Continue the antiemetic as ordered until 24 hours after the chemotherapy is complete.
    3. Remove food that has a lot of odor.
    4. Keep the child on a nothing-by-mouth status.
    5. Wait until the nausea begins to start the antiemetic.

13. Which of the following can be a manifestation of leukemia in a child? **Select all that apply.**
    1. Leg pain.
    2. Fever.
    3. Excessive weight gain.
    4. Bruising.
    5. Enlarged lymph nodes.

14. Which of the following can lead to a possible diagnosis of human immunodeficiency virus (HIV) in a child? **Select all that apply.**
    1. Repeated respiratory infections.
    2. Intermittent diarrhea.
    3. Excessive weight gain.
    4. Irregular heartbeat.
    5. Poor weight gain.

15. A nurse is caring for a 15-year-old who has just been diagnosed with non-Hodgkin lymphoma. Which of the following should the nurse include in teaching the parents about this lymphoma? **Select all that apply.**
    1. The malignancy originates in the lymphoid system.
    2. The presence of Reed-Sternberg cells in the biopsy is considered diagnostic.
    3. Mediastinal involvement is typical.
    4. The disease is diffuse rather than nodular.
    5. Treatment includes chemotherapy and radiation.

16. The most important reason health-care providers prescribe a combination of antiretroviral drugs to children with HIV is to delay:
    1. Progression to AIDS.
    2. Enable treatment of multiple symptoms.
    3. Recurrence of symptoms.
    4. Drug resistance.

17. The nurse is caring for a child with sickle cell disease who is scheduled to have a splenectomy. What information should the nurse explain to the parents regarding the reason for a splenectomy?
    1. To decrease potential for infection.
    2. To prevent splenic sequestration.
    3. To prevent sickling of red blood cells.
    4. To prevent sickle cell crisis.

18. Which of the following is the most effective treatment for pain in a child with sickle cell crisis? **Select all that apply.**
    1. Meperidine (Demerol).
    2. Aspirin.
    3. Morphine.
    4. Behavioral techniques.
    5. Acetaminophen (Tylenol) with codeine.

19. The nurse is caring for a child with sickle cell disease who is scheduled to have an exchange transfusion. What information should the nurse teach the family?
    1. The procedure is done to prevent further sickling during a vaso-occlusive crisis.
    2. The procedure reduces side effects from blood transfusions.
    3. The procedure is a routine treatment for sickle cell crisis.
    4. Once the child's spleen is removed, it is not necessary to do exchange transfusions.

20. A nurse instructs the parent of a child with sickle cell disease about factors that might precipitate a pain crisis in the child. Which of the following factors identified by the parent as being able to cause a pain crisis indicates a need for further instruction?
    1. Infection.
    2. Overhydration.
    3. Stress at school.
    4. Cold environment.

21. A 10-year-old with severe factor VIII deficiency falls, injures an elbow, and is brought to the ED. The nurse should prepare which of the following?
    1. An IM injection of factor VIII.
    2. An IV infusion of factor VIII.
    3. An injection of desmopressin.
    4. An IV infusion of platelets.

22. Which of the following will be abnormal in a child with the diagnosis of hemophilia?
    1. Platelet count.
    2. Hemoglobin level.
    3. White blood cell count.
    4. Partial thromboplastin time (PTT).

23. The parent of a child with hemophilia is asking the nurse what caused the hemophilia. Which is the nurse's best response?
    1. It is an X-linked dominant disorder.
    2. It is an X-linked recessive disorder.
    3. It is an autosomal dominant disorder.
    4. It is an autosomal recessive disorder.

24. Which of the following measures should the nurse teach the parent of a child with hemophilia to do first if the child sustains an injury to a joint causing bleeding?
    1. Give the child a dose of acetaminophen (Tylenol).
    2. Immobilize the joint and elevate the extremity.
    3. Apply heat to the area.
    4. Administer factor per the home-care protocol.

25. Which of the following measures should be implemented for a child with von Willebrand disease who has a nosebleed?
    1. Apply pressure to the nose for at least 10 minutes.
    2. Have the child lie supine and quiet.
    3. Avoid packing of the nostrils.
    4. Encourage the child to swallow frequently.

26. A nurse educator is providing a teaching session for the nursing staff. Which of the following individuals is at greatest risk for developing beta-thalassemia (Cooley anemia)?
    1. A child of Mediterranean descent.
    2. A child of Mexican descent.
    3. A child whose mother has chronic anemia.
    4. A child who has a low intake of iron.

27. A nurse is doing discharge education with a parent who has a child with beta-thalassemia (Cooley anemia). The nurse informs the parent that the child is at risk for which of the following conditions?
    1. Hypertrophy of the thyroid.
    2. Polycythemia vera.
    3. Thrombocytopenia.
    4. Chronic hypoxia and iron overload.

28. The nurse is caring for a child diagnosed with thalassemia major who is receiving the first chelation therapy. What information should the nurse provide to the parent regarding the therapy? **Select all that apply.**
    1. Decreases the risk of bleeding.
    2. Eliminates excess iron.
    3. Prevents further sickling of the red blood cells.
    4. Provides an iron supplement.
    5. Hydration is necessary for the process to be effective.

29. Which of the following should the nurse expect to administer to a child with ITP and a platelet count of 5000/mm^3? **Select all that apply.**
    1. Platelets.
    2. Intravenous immunoglobulin.
    3. Packed red blood cells (PRBCs).
    4. White blood cells.
    5. Prednisolone.

30. Which test provides a definitive diagnosis of aplastic anemia?
    1. Complete blood count with differential.
    2. Bone marrow aspiration.
    3. Serum IgG levels.
    4. Basic metabolic panel.

31. The nurse is caring for a child with a diagnosis of ALL who is receiving chemotherapy. The nurse notes that the child's platelet count is 20,000/mm^3. Based on this laboratory finding, what information should the nurse provide to the child and parents?
    1. A soft toothbrush should be used for mouth care.
    2. Isolation precautions should be started immediately.
    3. The child's vital signs, including blood pressure, should be monitored every 4 hours.
    4. All visitors should be discouraged from coming to see the family.

32. A 5-year-old is admitted to the hospital with complaints of leg pain and fever. On physical examination, the child is pale and has bruising over various areas of the body. The health-care provider suspects that the child has ALL. The nurse informs the parent that the diagnosis will be confirmed by which of the following?
1. Lumbar puncture.
2. White blood cell count.
3. Bone marrow aspirate.
4. Bone scan.

33. The nurse is caring for a 10-year-old with leukemia who is receiving chemotherapy. The child is on neutropenic precautions. Friends of the child come to the desk and ask for a vase for the flowers they have brought with them. Which of the following is the best response?
1. "I will get you a special vase that we use on this unit."
2. "The flowers from your garden are beautiful but should not be placed in the room at this time."
3. "As soon as I can wash a vase, I will put the flowers in it and bring it to the room."
4. "Get rid of the flowers immediately. You could harm the child."

34. The nurse is discharging a child who has just received chemotherapy for neuroblastoma. Which of the following statements made by the child's parent indicates a need for additional teaching?
1. "I will inspect the skin often for any lesions."
2. "I will do mouth care daily and monitor for any mouth sores."
3. "I will wash my hands before caring for my child."
4. "I will take a rectal temperature daily and report a temperature greater than 101°F (38.3°C) immediately to the health-care provider."

35. Which intervention should be implemented after a bone marrow aspiration?
1. Ask the child to remain in a supine position.
2. Place the child in an upright position for 4 hours.
3. Keep the child nothing by mouth for 6 hours.
4. Administer analgesics as needed for pain.

36. Which of the following should be done to protect the central nervous system from the invasion of malignant cells in a child newly diagnosed with leukemia?
1. Cranial and spinal radiation.
2. Intravenous steroid therapy.
3. Intrathecal chemotherapy.
4. High-dose intravenous chemotherapy.

37. A child with leukemia is receiving chemotherapy and is complaining of nausea. The nurse has been giving the scheduled antiemetic. Which of the following should the nurse do when the child is nauseated?
1. Encourage low-protein foods.
2. Encourage low-caloric foods.
3. Offer the child's favorite foods.
4. Offer cool, clear liquids.

38. School-age children with cancer often have a body image disturbance related to hair loss, moon face, or debilitation. Which of the following interventions is (are) most appropriate? **Select all that apply.**
1. Encourage them to wear a wig similar to their own hairstyle.
2. Emphasize the benefits of the therapy they are receiving.
3. Have them play only with other children with cancer.
4. Use diversional techniques to avoid discussing changes in the body because of the chemotherapy.
5. Help them find a "special friend" who understands what they are experiencing.

39. The nurse receives a call from a parent of a child with leukemia in remission. The parent says the child has been exposed to chickenpox and has never had it. Which of the following responses is most appropriate for the nurse? **Select all that apply.**
   1. "You need to monitor the child's temperature frequently and call back if the temperature is greater than 101°F (38.3°C)."
   2. "The child has had two varicella immunizations as an infant but is no longer immune after chemotherapy."
   3. "You need to bring the child to the clinic for a varicella immunoglobulin vaccine."
   4. "Your child will need to be isolated for the next 2 weeks."
   5. "Your child may develop chicken pox lesions about 14 to 21 days after exposure."

40. The nurse is caring for a child being treated for ALL. Laboratory results indicate that the child has a white blood cell count of 5000/mm^3 with 5% polys and 3% bands. Which of the following analyses is most appropriate?
   1. The absolute neutrophil count is 400/mm^3, and the child is neutropenic.
   2. The absolute neutrophil count is 800/mm^3, and the child is neutropenic.
   3. The absolute neutrophil count is 4000/mm^3, and the child is not neutropenic.
   4. The absolute neutrophil count is 5800/mm^3, and the child is not neutropenic.

41. Which of the following is the best method to prevent the spread of infection to an immunosuppressed child?
   1. Administer antibiotics prophylactically to the child.
   2. Have people wash their hands prior to contact with the child.
   3. Assign the same nurses to care for the child each day.
   4. Limit visitors to family members only.

42. Which of the following is correct regarding prognostic factors for determining survival for a child newly diagnosed with ALL?
   1. The initial white blood cell count on diagnosis.
   2. The race of the child.
   3. The amount of time needed to initiate treatment.
   4. Children aged 12 to 15 years.

43. A child diagnosed with leukemia is receiving allopurinol (Zyloprim) as part of the treatment plan. The parents ask why their child is receiving this medication. What information about the medication should the nurse provide?
   1. Helps reduce the uric acid level caused by cell destruction.
   2. Helps make the chemotherapy more effective.
   3. Helps reduce the nausea and vomiting associated with chemotherapy.
   4. Helps decrease pain in the bone marrow.

44. Prednisone is given to children who are being treated for leukemia. Why is this medication given as part of the treatment plan?
   1. Enhances protein metabolism.
   2. Enhances sodium excretion.
   3. Increases absorption of the chemotherapy.
   4. Destroys abnormal lymphocytes.

45. Which of the following best describes the action of chemotherapeutic agents used in the treatment of cancer in children? **Select all that apply.**
   1. Suppress the function of normal lymphocytes in the immune system.
   2. Are alkylating agents and are cell-specific.
   3. Cause a replication of DNA and are cell-specific.
   4. Interrupt cell cycle, thereby causing cell death.
   5. Prednisone is a natural hormone.

46. A child has completed treatment for leukemia and comes to the clinic for a checkup with the parents. The parents express to the nurse that they are glad their child has been cured of cancer and is safe from getting cancer later in life. Which of the following should the nurse consider in responding?
    1. Childhood cancer usually instills immunity to all other cancers.
    2. Children surviving one cancer are at higher risk for a second cancer.
    3. The child may have a remission of the leukemia but is immune to all other cancers.
    4. As long as the child continues to take steroids, there will be no other cancers.

47. A teen is seen in clinic for a possible diagnosis of Hodgkin disease. The nurse is aware that which of the following symptoms should make the health-care provider suspect Hodgkin disease?
    1. Fever, fatigue, and pain in the joints.
    2. Anorexia with weight loss.
    3. Enlarged, painless, and movable lymph nodes in the cervical area.
    4. Enlarged liver with jaundice.

48. Which of the following confirms a diagnosis of Hodgkin disease in a 15-year-old?
    1. Reed-Sternberg cells in the lymph nodes.
    2. Blast cells in the blood.
    3. Lymphocytes in the bone marrow.
    4. VMA in the urine.

49. The parent of a teen with a diagnosis of Hodgkin disease asks what the child's prognosis will be with treatment. What information should the nurse give to the parent and child?
    1. Clinical staging of Hodgkin disease will determine the treatment; long-term survival for all stages of Hodgkin disease is excellent.
    2. There is a considerably better prognosis if the client is diagnosed early and is less than 5 years of age.
    3. The prognosis for Hodgkin disease depends on the type of chemotherapy.
    4. The only way to obtain a good prognosis is by chemotherapy and bone marrow transplant.

50. The nurse is caring for a child who is receiving extensive radiation as part of the treatment for Hodgkin disease. Which intervention should be implemented?
    1. Administer pain medication prior to the child's going to radiation therapy.
    2. Assess the child for neuropathy since this is a common side effect.
    3. Provide adequate rest, because the child may experience excessive malaise and lack of energy.
    4. Encourage the child to eat a low-protein diet while on radiation therapy.

51. The parent of a 4-year-old brings the child to the clinic and tells the nurse the child's abdomen is distended. After a complete examination, a diagnosis of Wilms tumor is suspected. Which of the following is most important when doing a physical examination on this child?
    1. Avoid palpation of the abdomen.
    2. Assess the urine for the presence of blood.
    3. Monitor vital signs, especially the blood pressure.
    4. Obtain an accurate height and weight.

52. The parent of a child diagnosed with Wilms tumor asks the nurse what the treatment plan will be. The nurse explains the usual protocol for this condition. Which information should the nurse give to the parent?
    1. The child will have chemotherapy and, after that has been completed, radiation.
    2. The child will need to have surgery to remove the tumor.
    3. The child will go to surgery for removal of the tumor and the kidney and will then start chemotherapy.
    4. The child will need radiation and later surgery to remove the tumor.

53. The nurse expects which of the following clinical manifestations in a child diagnosed with SCID?
1. Prolonged bleeding.
2. Failure to thrive.
3. Fatigue and malaise.
4. Susceptibility to infection.

54. What are the clinical manifestations of non-Hodgkin lymphoma?
1. Basically the same as those in Hodgkin disease.
2. Depends on the anatomical site and extent of involvement.
3. Nausea, vomiting, abdominal pain.
4. Behavior changes, jaundice, dry mouth.

55. When caring for a child with lymphoma, the nurse needs to be aware of which of the following?
1. The same staging system is used for lymphoma and Hodgkin disease.
2. Aggressive chemotherapy with central nervous system prophylaxis will give the child a good prognosis.
3. All children with lymphoma need a bone marrow transplant for a good prognosis.
4. Despite high-dose chemotherapy, the prognosis is very poor for most children.

56. Where is the primary site of origin of the tumor in children who have neuroblastoma?
1. Bone.
2. Kidney.
3. Abdomen.
4. Liver.

57. Which of the following is the most common opportunistic infection in children infected with human immunodeficiency virus (HIV)?
1. CMV.
2. Encephalitis.
3. Meningitis.
4. Pneumocystic pneumonia.

58. Which of the following laboratory tests will be ordered to determine the presence of the human immunodeficiency virus antigen in an infant whose mother is HIV+?
1. CD4 cell count.
2. Western blot.
3. IgG levels.
4. p24 antigen assay.

59. The nurse is instructing the parent of a child with HIV about immunizations. Which of the following should the nurse tell the parent? **Select all that apply.**
1. Hepatitis B vaccine will not be given to this child.
2. Members of the family should be cautioned not to receive the varicella vaccine.
3. The child will need to have a Western blot test done prior to all immunizations.
4. Pneumococcal and influenza vaccines are recommended.
5. Meningitis immunization.

60. The parent of a 2-year-old who is HIV+ questions the nurse about placing the child in day care. Which of the following is the best response?
1. The child should not go to day care until older, because there is a high risk for transmission of the disease.
2. The child can go to day care without restrictions and should be allowed to participate in all activities.
3. The child can go to day care but should avoid physical activity.
4. The child may go to day care, but the parent must inform all the parents at the day care that the child is HIV+.

The correct answer number and rationale for why it is the correct answer are given in **boldface blue type.** Rationales for why the other possible answer options are incorrect also are given, but they are not in boldface type.

1. **3, 5.**
   1. Polycythemia is seen in children with chronic hypoxia, such as cyanotic heart disease.
   2. Hemarthrosis, bleeding into a joint, is commonly seen in children with hemophilia.
   3. **Aplastic crisis, temporary cessation of red blood cell production, is associated with sickle cell anemia.**
   4. Thrombocytopenia is associated with idiopathic thrombocytopenia purpura, high altitude, medication side effects, and pregnancy.
   5. **Vaso-occlusive crisis is the most common problem in children with sickle cell disease.**

   TEST-TAKING HINT: Defining the terms will make the correct responses evident.

2. **3, 5.**
   1. Because the child has a low hematocrit level, the child most likely has anemia. Iron-deficiency anemia is the most common nutritional anemia. The number of bowel movements the child has is important information but not necessary to make the diagnosis of iron-deficiency anemia.
   2. Knowing birth weight can help determine whether the child is following his or her own curve on the growth chart.
   3. **A diet history is necessary to determine the nutritional status of the child and whether the child is getting sufficient sources of iron.**
   4. Knowing if the child is taking any new medication is not necessary to make the diagnosis of iron-deficiency anemia.
   5. **By asking how much milk the child consumes, the nurse can determine whether the child is filling up on milk and then not wanting to take food.**

   TEST-TAKING HINT: The most common anemia in children and in toddlers is iron-deficiency anemia, frequently the result of drinking too much milk and not eating enough iron-rich foods.

3. **1, 3, 4, 5.**
   1. **Seek medical attention for illness to prevent the child from going into a crisis.**
   2. A cold environment causes vasoconstriction, which needs to be prevented to get good tissue perfusion.
   3. **Stress can cause a depressed immune system, making the child more susceptible to infection and crisis. Parents and children are advised to avoid stress.**
   4. **The child needs good hydration and nutrition to maintain good health.**
   5. **The child needs good hydration and nutrition to maintain good health.**

   TEST-TAKING HINT: Focus on how to prevent a sickle cell crisis.

4. **3, 4, 5.**
   1. Medical treatment of sickle cell vaso-occlusive crises is directed toward preventing hypoxia. Tissue hypoxia is very painful, so placing the child in a position of comfort is important.
   2. Hot packs help relieve pain because they cause vasodilation, which allows increased blood flow and decreased hypoxia.
   3. **Tissue hypoxia is very painful. Narcotics such as morphine are usually given for pain when the child is in a crisis. Meperidine (Demerol) should be avoided because of the risk of Demerol-induced seizures.**
   4. **The child should receive hydration because when the child is in crisis, the abnormal S-shaped red blood cells clump, causing tissue hypoxia and pain.**
   5. **Oxygen is of little value unless the tissue is hypoxic. The objective of treatment is to minimize hypoxia.**

   TEST-TAKING HINT: Focus on the pathophysiology of a vaso-occlusive crisis. Keep in mind measures that decrease tissue hypoxia.

5. **1, 2, 3.**
   1. **Von Willebrand disease is a hereditary bleeding disorder characterized by deficiency of or defect in a protein. The disorder causes adherence of platelets to damaged endothelium and a mild deficiency of factor VIII. One of the manifestations of this disease is bleeding of the mucous membranes.**

2. **Excessive menstruation may be a manifestation of this disease.**
3. **Frequent nosebleeds are a common manifestation of this disease.**
4. There is no increase in creatinine in this disease.
5. There is no increase in blood pressure.

TEST-TAKING HINT: Von Willebrand disease is a minor factor VIII deficiency.

6. **1, 2, 5.**
   1. **Measures are needed to induce vasoconstriction and stop the bleeding, including immobilization of the extremity.**
   2. **Measures are needed to induce vasoconstriction and stop the bleeding. Treatment should include elevating the extremity.**
   3. Measures are needed to induce vasoconstriction and stop the bleeding. Treatment should include an application of cold compression. Warmth will slow the vasoconstriction and clotting process.
   4. Measures are needed to induce vasoconstriction and stop the bleeding. Passive ROM is not started until the bleeding has stopped.
   5. **Hemophilia A is a deficiency in factor VIII, which causes delay in clotting when there is a bleed. Giving a dose of Factor VIII concentrate will assist in the clotting process.**

TEST-TAKING HINT: Focus on the disease process and measures to stop bleeding.

7. **1, 2, 3, 4.**
   1. **Children with hemophilia should be encouraged to take part in noncontact activities that allow for social, psychological, and physical growth, such as swimming.**
   2. **Children with hemophilia should be encouraged to take part in noncontact activities that allow for social, psychological, and physical growth, such as golf.**
   3. **Children with hemophilia should be encouraged to take part in noncontact activities that allow for social, psychological, and physical growth, such as hiking.**
   4. **Children with hemophilia should be encouraged to take part in noncontact activities that allow for social, psychological, and physical growth, such as fishing.**

5. Contact sports like soccer should be discouraged.

TEST-TAKING HINT: Soccer is the only contact sport listed, so the other answers can be selected.

8. **2, 3, 5.**
   1. ITP is an acquired hematological condition that is characterized by excessive destruction of platelets, purpura, and normal bone marrow along with an increase in large, yellow platelets.
   2. **ITP is characterized by excessive destruction of platelets.**
   3. **The bone marrow is normal in children with ITP.**
   4. Platelets are large, not small.
   5. **ITP is characterized by purpura, which are areas of hemorrhage under the skin.**

TEST-TAKING HINT: Review the pathophysiology of ITP to determine the manifestations of the disease.

9. **1, 3, 4.**
   1. **Hemolytic reactions include fever, pain at insertion site, hypotension, renal failure, tachycardia, oliguria, and shock.**
   2. Febrile reactions are fever, rash, and chills. Allergic reactions include hives, itching, and respiratory distress.
   3. **Hemolytic reactions include fever, pain at insertion site, hypotension, renal failure, tachycardia, oliguria, and shock.**
   4. **Hemolytic reactions include fever, pain at insertion site, hypotension, renal failure, tachycardia, oliguria, and shock.**
   5. Febrile reactions are fever, chills, and rash. Allergic reactions include rash, hives, and respiratory distress.

TEST-TAKING HINT: Review the signs and symptoms of hemolytic reaction, febrile reaction, and allergic reaction. Understanding the causes of the reactions will help identify the symptoms.

10. **1, 2, 3.**
    1. **Anemia is caused by decreased production of red blood cells.**
    2. **Infection risk in leukemia is secondary to the neutropenia.**
    3. **Bleeding tendencies are from decreased platelet production.**
    4. There are no bone deformities with leukemia, but there is bone pain from the proliferation of cells in the bone marrow.
    5. Polycythemia is an increase in red blood cells.

TEST-TAKING HINT: Leukemia is cancer of the blood forming organs. Leukemia can be either acute or chronic. Review the pathophysiology of leukemia to determine the clinical problems.

11. **2, 3.**
1. There is no need to perform a spinal tap to rule out meningitis unless the patient has symptoms of meningitis.
2. **A lumbar puncture is done to determine whether the cancer cells have entered the CNS, but this would not be routine unless the child was symptomatic.**
3. **Chemotherapy can also be given through a lumbar puncture (spinal tap).**
4. ICP would be considered if the child had symptoms of headache, nausea, forceful vomiting, blurred or double vision, drowsiness, or seizure; an LP might then be performed.
5. Leukemia is not staged.

TEST-TAKING HINT: The primary site for leukemia involvement is the bone marrow. Rarely do children have CNS involvement.

12. **1, 2, 3.**
1. **The first dose should be given 30 minutes prior to the start of the therapy.**
2. **Antiemetic should be administered around the clock until 24 hours after the chemotherapy is completed.**
3. **It is also helpful to remove foods with odor so that the smell of the food does not make the child nauseated.**
4. The child should be allowed to take food and fluids as tolerated.
5. Antiemetics are most beneficial if given before the onset of nausea and vomiting.

TEST-TAKING HINT: These are measures to prevent nausea and vomiting.

13. **1, 2, 4, 5.**
1. **The proliferation of cells in the bone marrow can cause leg pain.**
2. **Fever is a result of the neutropenia.**
3. There is usually a decrease in weight because the child will feel sick and not as hungry.
4. **A decrease in platelets causes the bruising.**
5. **The lymph nodes are enlarged by the infiltration of leukemic cells.**

TEST-TAKING HINT: Review the consequences of depressed bone marrow and relate them to the clinical manifestations.

14. **1, 2, 5.**
1. **Symptoms of HIV include frequent respiratory infections. The symptoms present based on the underlying cellular immunodeficiency-related disease.**
2. **Symptoms of HIV include intermittent diarrhea. The symptoms present based on the underlying cellular immunodeficiency-related disease.**
3. Children with HIV are unable to create an immune response to infection. They develop recurrent bacterial infections and have poor weight gain. The symptoms present based on the underlying cellular immunodeficiency-related disease.
4. Irregular heartbeat is not associated with HIV.
5. **Symptoms of HIV include poor weight gain.**

TEST-TAKING HINT: Symptoms of HIV in children include lymphadenopathy, hepatosplenomegaly, chronic diarrhea, failure to thrive, and parotitis. Review common clinical signs and health conditions associated with the virus.

15. **1, 3, 4, 5.**
1. **Non-Hodgkin disease originates in the lymphoid system.**
2. Reed-Sternberg cells are diagnostic for Hodgkin disease and are not seen in non-Hodgkin lymphoma. Reed-Sternberg cells arise from "B" cells and are large, multinucleated cells.
3. **Mediastinal involvement is typical.**
4. **The disease is diffuse rather than nodular.**
5. **Treatment includes chemotherapy and radiation.**

TEST-TAKING HINT: The lymphomas are divided into Hodgkin disease (which primarily involves the lymph nodes with metastasis to extra lymphatic sites) and non-Hodgkin lymphoma (a heterogenous condition that has a variety of morphological, cytochemical, and immunological cell features).

16. 1. Indirectly the use of multiple antiretroviral medications does minimize progression to a diagnosis of AIDS, but each of the drugs alone cannot control the progression.
2. The symptoms of HIV will be resolved once the antiretroviral therapy begins to decrease the viral load.

3. There is no way to predict if and when recurrence will occur. Taking antiretroviral medications and maintaining a healthy life style is the best way to decrease the risk of the symptoms.

4. **A combination of antiretroviral medications is prescribed for a child who is HIV positive to delay development of drug resistance. HIV drugs work on different stages of the HIV life cycle to prevent reproduction of new virus particles.**

TEST-TAKING HINT: The importance of maintaining medications that assist in treatment and do not develop resistance is essential to controlling the virus.

17. 1. The cells involved with sickle cell disease are abnormal red blood cells, which do not decrease infections.
    2. **Splenic sequestration is a life-threatening situation in children with sickle cell disease. Once a child is considered to be at high risk of splenic sequestration or has had this in the past, the spleen will be removed.**
    3. Removal of the spleen will not prevent sickling, because it will not change the disease condition.
    4. The child will still have sickle cell disease and can still have sickle cell crises.

TEST-TAKING HINT: Review splenic sequestration and when a child can go into sickle cell crisis.

18. **3, 4, 5.**
    1. Meperidine (Demerol) should not be used because it may potentiate seizures.
    2. Aspirin should not be used in children because of the risk for Reye syndrome.
    3. **Morphine is the drug of choice for a child with sickle cell crises. Usually the child is started on oral doses of acetaminophen (Tylenol) with codeine. When that is not sufficient to alleviate pain, stronger narcotics are prescribed, such as morphine. Ketorolac (Toradol) may be indicated for short-term use for moderate-severe pain.**
    4. **Behavioral techniques such as positive self-talk, relaxation, distraction, and guided imagery are helpful when pain is occurring.**
    5. **Usually the child is started on oral doses of acetaminophen (Tylenol) with codeine when pain is described as mild to moderate.**

TEST-TAKING HINT: One needs to consider using narcotics when a child has sickle cell crises, because tissue hypoxia can cause severe pain.

19. 1. **Exchange transfusion reduces the number of circulating sickle cells and slows down the cycle of hypoxia, thrombosis, and tissue ischemia.**
    2. Exchange transfusion does not decrease risk of a transfusion reaction. Every time a transfusion is done, the child continues to be at risk for a reaction.
    3. This is not a routine procedure and is performed only when the number of sickle cells is elevated and the child is at high risk for thrombosis.
    4. After a splenectomy, transfusions still need to be done depending on the client's hemoglobin level.

TEST-TAKING HINT: Consider the reasons transfusions are given with sickle cell clients, one of which is exchanging the sickled red cells with non-sickled cells.

20. 1. An infection can cause a child to go into crisis.
    2. **Overhydration does not cause a crisis.**
    3. Emotional stress can cause a child to go into crisis.
    4. A cold environment causes vasoconstriction, which could lead to crisis.

TEST-TAKING HINT: Because a sickle cell crisis may be precipitated by infection, dehydration, trauma, hypoxia, or stress, use the process of elimination to determine the need for further instruction.

21. 1. Factor VIII is not given intramuscularly.
    2. **The child is treated with an IV infusion of factor VIII to replace the missing factor and help stop the bleeding.**
    3. Desmopressin is given to stimulate factor VIII production, and it is given intravenously.
    4. Platelets are not affected in hemophilia.

TEST-TAKING HINT: Focus on the diagnosis of hemophilia: A deficiency in factor VIII causes continued bleeding with an injury.

22. 1. Platelet function is normal in hemophilia.
    2. There is no change in hemoglobin with a diagnosis of hemophilia. The hemoglobin will drop with bleeding.
    3. The white blood cell count does not change with hemophilia.

4. **The abnormal laboratory results in hemophilia are related to decreased clotting function. Partial thromboplastin time is prolonged.**

TEST-TAKING HINT: Use the process of elimination to determine the test that indicates a decrease in clotting.

23. 1. Hemophilia is transmitted as an X-linked recessive disorder. About 60% of children have a family history of hemophilia. The usual transmission is by a female with the trait and an unaffected male.
   2. **Hemophilia is transmitted as an X-linked recessive disorder. About 60% of children have a family history of hemophilia. The usual transmission is by a female with the trait and an unaffected male.**
   3. Hemophilia is transmitted as an X-linked recessive disorder. About 60% of children have a family history of hemophilia. The usual transmission is by a female with the trait and an unaffected male.
   4. Hemophilia is transmitted as an X-linked recessive disorder. About 60% of children have a family history of hemophilia. The usual transmission is by a female with the trait and an unaffected male.

TEST-TAKING HINT: The test taker needs to know how hemophilia is transmitted.

24. 1. Acetaminophen (Tylenol) helps with the pain but does not stop the bleeding.
   2. Elevating and immobilizing the extremity are good interventions as they decrease blood flow. Factor should be administered first, however.
   3. Cold, not heat, should be applied to promote vasoconstriction.
   4. **Administration of factor should be the first intervention if home-care transfusions have been initiated.**

TEST-TAKING HINT: Treatment of hemophilia is to provide factor replacement as soon as possible after a bleed has started. Application of cold, elevation of extremities, and application of pressure for 10 to 15 minutes are all good interventions after the factor is given.

25. 1. **Applying pressure to the nose may stop the bleeding. In von Willebrand disease, there is an increased tendency to bleed from mucous membranes, leading to nosebleeds commonly from the anterior part of the nasal septum.**
   2. The child should sit up and lean forward to avoid aspiration of blood.

3. Packing the nose with cotton may stop bleeding, but be careful when the cotton is removed because it may dislodge the clot.
4. Swallowing will cause the child to swallow the blood, which then can cause vomiting.

TEST-TAKING HINT: Focus on the most common areas of bleeding in von Willebrand disease and on how to treat the bleeding.

26. 1. **Beta-thalassemia is an inherited recessive disorder that is found primarily in individuals of Mediterranean descent. The disease has also been reported in Asian and African populations.**
   2. It is not found often in the Mexican population.
   3. This is a hereditary disease that causes chronic anemia. The mother should have had thalassemia for this answer to be correct.
   4. This disorder has nothing to do with iron deficiency.

TEST-TAKING HINT: Use the process of elimination, knowing that the disorder is a hereditary disorder in those of Mediterranean descent.

27. 1. The thyroid is not involved in beta-thalassemia.
   2. Polycythemia vera is excessive red blood cell production, which can result in thrombosis.
   3. There is no increase in platelets in beta-thalassemia.
   4. **In beta-thalassemia, there is increased destruction of red blood cells, causing anemia. This results in chronic anemia and hypoxia. The children are treated with multiple blood transfusions, which can cause iron overload and damage to major organs.**

TEST-TAKING HINT: Focus on the pathophysiology of the disease. Then, by process of elimination, the effect of the disease on the body can be identified.

28. 2, 5.
   1. There are no bleeding tendencies in thalassemia major (beta-thalassemia or Cooley anemia), and chelation does not affect clotting.
   2. **Chelation therapy is used to rid the body of excess iron stores that result from frequent blood transfusions.**
   3. There is no sickling of red blood cells in thalassemia, and chelation therapy has no direct effect on red blood cells.

4. Chelation does not provide an iron supplement.
5. **Hydration is necessary for the process to be effective.**

TEST-TAKING HINT: Focus on the treatment of beta-thalassemia and how chelation therapy works.

29. **2, 5.**
    1. In ITP, destruction of platelets is caused from what is believed to be an immune response, so giving additional platelets would only result in new platelets being destroyed.
    2. **Intravenous immunoglobulin is given because the cause of platelet destruction is believed to be an autoimmune response to disease-related antigens. Treatment is usually supportive. Activity is restricted at the onset because of the low platelet count and risk for injury that could cause bleeding.**
    3. Red blood cells are not an effective treatment for ITP.
    4. Because this is a platelet deficiency, white blood cells are not an effective treatment for ITP. White blood cell infusion is rarely done with any disease process.
    5. **Treatment in the acute phase is often symptomatic, and prednisolone, IVIG, and anti-D antibody are often given. This tends to shorten the course because the disease tends to resolve over time. Focus on the cause of ITP and which cells are affected.**

30. 1. A complete blood count would show pancytopenia, which would lead the health-care provider to look for the cause of the blood abnormality.
    2. **Definitive diagnosis is determined from bone marrow aspiration, which demonstrates the conversion of red bone marrow to yellow, fatty marrow.**
    3. Serum IgG levels do not diagnose aplastic anemia, which does not seem to have an immune cause.
    4. A basic metabolic panel tests for metabolic disorders.

TEST-TAKING HINT: Focus on the fact that aplastic anemia is a failure in the bone marrow that causes pancytopenia, so analysis of the bone marrow would confirm the diagnosis.

31. 1. **Because the platelet count is decreased, there is a significant risk of bleeding, especially in soft tissue. The use of the soft toothbrush should help prevent bleeding of the gums.**

2. A low platelet count does not indicate a need to start isolation.
3. There is always a need to monitor the child frequently, but the low platelet count puts the child at risk for bleeding.
4. In caring for children, always screen visitors, but there is no need to restrict visitation unless something is found on the screening.

TEST-TAKING HINT: Identify that the platelet count is low and can cause bleeding. The plan of care should include measures to protect the child from bleeding.

32. 1. A lumbar puncture is done to look for blast cells in the spinal fluid, which indicate central nervous system disease. It is also done to administer intrathecal chemotherapy, because the chemotherapy that will be given does not pass through the blood–brain barrier.
    2. An altered white blood cell count occurs as a result of the disease, but it does not make the diagnosis, as many diseases can alter the white blood cell count.
    3. **The diagnostic test that confirms leukemia is microscopic examination of the bone marrow aspirate.**
    4. Bone scans do not confirm the diagnosis of a disease that occurs in the bone marrow.

TEST-TAKING HINT: The key to answering this question is the phrase "diagnosis will be confirmed."

33. 1. Flowers should not be kept in the room of the client who is neutropenic. There are no special vases that are used with these clients that can protect them from infection.
    2. **A neutropenic client should not have flowers in the room because the flowers may harbor *Aspergillus* or *Pseudomonas aeruginosa*. Neutropenic children are susceptible to infection. Precautions need to be taken so that the child does not come in contact with any potential sources of infection. Fresh fruits and vegetables can also harbor molds and should be avoided. Telling the friend that the flowers are beautiful but that the child cannot have them is a tactful way not to offend the friend.**
    3. Washing the vase will not change the reason for not having the flowers around the child.
    4. This could scare the visitors and make them feel guilty that they might harm the child in some way.

TEST-TAKING HINT: Review neutropenic precautions; then by process of elimination determine that answers 1 and 3 are incorrect. Answer 4 is not a professional way of interacting with visitors.

34. 1. Inspecting the skin is a good measure to monitor for infection and should be done.
    2. Mouth care is essential and should be done daily to help prevent infection. Chemotherapy puts the child at risk for mucositis.
    3. Washing the hands is one of the most important measures to prevent infection.
    4. **Monitoring the child's temperature and reporting it to the physician are important, but the temperature should not be taken rectally. The risk of injury to the mucous membranes is high. Rectal abscesses can occur in the damaged rectal tissue. The best method for taking the temperature is axillary, especially if the child has mouth sores.**

    TEST-TAKING HINT: Review home-care instructions for children who have just received chemotherapy. These are measures to protect the child from infection and to monitor for infection.

35. 1. There is no need to have the client remain supine after a bone marrow aspiration is done.
    2. The child can assume any position after a bone marrow aspiration.
    3. The child usually receives conscious sedation during the procedure and will have nothing by mouth prior to the procedure. Oral fluids can be resumed after the procedure is completed.
    4. **Children may experience minor discomfort after the procedure, and analgesics should be given as needed.**

    TEST-TAKING HINT: Review the procedure for doing a bone marrow aspiration and be aware of nursing care after the procedure. There should be no reason for the child to be in a specific position or to have fluids withheld after the procedure. Managing pain is always a priority need.

36. 1. Radiation should be done as part of therapy if there is metastasis.
    2. Steroids are given as part of the treatment protocol but do not need to be given intravenously. Steroids do not pass through the blood–brain barrier.

    3. **Giving chemotherapy via lumbar puncture allows the drugs to get to the brain and helps prevent metastasis of the disease.**
    4. Chemotherapy that is given intravenously will not pass through the blood–brain barrier.

    TEST-TAKING HINT: Oral and IV chemotherapies do not pass through the blood–brain barrier. Intrathecal chemotherapy needs to be done to protect the central nervous system from metastasis of the disease.

37. 1. It is better to provide high-protein nutritional supplements if the child can tolerate them.
    2. It is better to provide high-caloric nutritional supplements.
    3. Offering the child's favorite foods when the child is nauseated can create a later association with being sick; then the child may not want that food when not ill.
    4. **Cool, clear liquids are better tolerated. Milk-based products cause secretions to be thick and can cause vomiting.**

    TEST-TAKING HINT: With nausea and vomiting, it is important to consider nutritional status. Answers 1 and 2 do not improve nutrition. Supportive nutritional supplements should be offered. Review measures to prevent nausea and provide nutrition.

38. 1, 5.
    1. **Wearing a wig is a good way for the child to keep personal identity despite the loss of hair.**
    2. Just discussing the benefits of the therapy will not help the child with self-image.
    3. Having the child play only with other children with cancer could make the child feel even worse because of the inability to interact with friends. The child needs to find acceptance as appearance begins to change.
    4. Diverting the child's attention would be avoiding the truth and would not be dealing with the issues.
    5. **Children with cancer and body-image changes oftentimes need assistance in expressing themselves, which a "special friend" can help with.**

TEST-TAKING HINT: Review the side effects on the body from the chemotherapy and look at ways to help the child deal with body-image changes. Provide the child and family with accurate information of the side effects of the drugs, but also give the child ways to feel good.

39. **2, 3.**
    1. The temperature should always be monitored, but the child has been exposed to chickenpox. The child needs to be protected from getting the disease as it can be life threatening.
    2. **Chickenpox exposure is a real concern for a child who is immunocompromised, and action needs to be taken.**
    3. **The child should receive varicella zoster immune globulin within 96 hours of the exposure.**
    4. Starting isolation at this time does not protect the child.
    5. If the parent acts immediately and the child receives IVIG, the child will not develop the lesions of chicken pox.

    TEST-TAKING HINT: Review protective precautions that should be taken for immunocompromised children. Chickenpox can be deadly for these children.

40. 1. **The calculated absolute neutrophil count is 400/mm³ (0.08 × 5000), and the child is neutropenic because the count is less than 500/mm³.**
    2. The absolute neutrophil count is incorrectly calculated. The child would not be neutropenic with a count of 800/mm³.
    3. The absolute neutrophil count is incorrectly calculated. The child would not be neutropenic with a count of 4000/mm³.
    4. The absolute neutrophil count is incorrectly calculated. The child would not be neutropenic if the count were 5800/mm³.

    TEST-TAKING HINT: To calculate the absolute neutrophil count, multiply the white blood cell count by the percentage of neutrophils ("polys," "segs," and "bands"). For example: WBC = 1500/mm³, neutrophils = 7%, nonsegmented neutrophils (bands) = 7%. 7% + 7% = 14%. 0.14 × 1500 = 210/mm³ ANC. Precautions for infection should be used at all times with children who are immunosuppressed, but greater precautions must be taken when the ANC is less than 500/mm³.

41. 1. Antibiotics should be used only if the child has a bacterial infection.
    2. **Hand washing is the best method to prevent the spread of germs and protect the child from infection.**
    3. All nurses should use the same techniques in caring for the child. Assigning the same nurses may not be possible.
    4. Visitors should be screened for infection and communicable diseases, but visitors should not be limited to family members only.

    TEST-TAKING HINT: The first defense against infection is prevention. Strict hand-washing technique is a primary intervention to prevent the spread of infections. Review measures to protect the child from infection.

42. 1. **Children with a normal or low white blood cell count who do not have non-T, non-B acute lymphoblastic leukemia and who are CALLA-positive have a much better prognosis than those with high cell counts or other cell types.**
    2. Race is not a factor in prognosis of leukemia.
    3. The child should begin treatment as soon as diagnosed, but time in initiating treatment does not have an effect on prognosis.
    4. Children aged 2 to 9 years have the best prognosis. High-risk children include those under 1 year and over 10 years.

    TEST-TAKING HINT: Review the important prognostic factors that affect long-term survival for children with acute lymphoblastic leukemia.

43. 1. **Allopurinol (Zyloprim) reduces serum uric acid. When there is lysis of cells from chemotherapy, there will be an increase in serum uric acid.**
    2. There is no specific medication that makes chemotherapy more effective.
    3. Allopurinol (Zyloprim) is not an antiemetic.
    4. Allopurinol (Zyloprim) is not an analgesic.

    TEST-TAKING HINT: Review the effects of the tumor lysis syndrome that occurs when chemotherapy is started with children with leukemia.

44. 1. Prednisone does not enhance protein metabolism.
    2. Prednisone may cause retention of sodium.
    3. There is no drug that increases absorption of chemotherapy.
    4. **Prednisone is used in many of the treatment protocols for leukemia because there is abnormal lymphocyte production. Prednisone is thought to destroy abnormal lymphocytes.**

TEST-TAKING HINT: Prednisone is given in conjunction with chemotherapy. It helps modify the body's immune response.

45. **1, 4, 5.**
    1. **All chemotherapy is immunosuppressive, because most childhood cancers affect the immune system.**
    2. Not all chemotherapy drugs are alkylating agents.
    3. There is no replication of DNA with chemotherapy. Chemotherapy drugs such as the antimetabolites usually inhibit synthesis of DNA or RNA.
    4. **Mitotic inhibitors, such as vincristine (Oncovin), stop cell division but can also damage cells in all phases of the cell cycle.**
    5. **The corticosteroids are natural hormones that can be used to prevent nausea and allergic reactions. They are given with other chemotherapeutic agents.**

TEST-TAKING HINT: Review the function of each type of chemotherapeutic agent. Chemotherapy targets cells at different phases of the cell life cycle.

46. 1. There is no immunity to recurrent cancers with remission of the leukemia.
    2. **The most devastating late effect of leukemia treatment is development of secondary malignancy.**
    3. After the child is in remission, the child may relapse, but there is no immunity to other malignancy.
    4. The child will not receive steroid treatment after completing therapy.

TEST-TAKING HINT: Review late effects of treatment of childhood cancer. This should include chemotherapy as well as radiation treatments.

47. 1. Fever and pain may be some of the symptoms, but they can be caused by other forms of cancer. Joint pain is not a symptom of Hodgkin disease.
    2. Anorexia with weight loss can be a symptom of many other conditions.
    3. **Enlarged, painless, and movable lymph nodes in the cervical area are the most common presenting manifestations of Hodgkin disease.**
    4. Enlarged liver with jaundice is not a presenting symptom with Hodgkin disease.

TEST-TAKING HINT: Review the clinical manifestations of Hodgkin disease. Some of the manifestations are the same for many different cancers, so focus on the primary and most common manifestations.

48. 1. **A lymph node biopsy is done to confirm a histological diagnosis and staging of Hodgkin disease. The presence of Reed-Sternberg cells is characteristic of the disease.**
    2. Blast cells are usually seen with leukemia.
    3. A bone marrow aspiration is usually done to diagnose the type of leukemia.
    4. This test is done to diagnose neuroblastoma.

TEST-TAKING HINT: In reviewing Hodgkin disease, be aware of the specific cell identified to confirm diagnosis.

49. 1. **Long-term survival for all stages of Hodgkin disease is excellent. Early-stage disease can have a survival rate greater than 90%, with advanced stages having rates between 65% and 75%.**
    2. Hodgkin disease mostly affects adolescents.
    3. The treatment consists of chemotherapy and often radiation therapy and does not predict prognosis.
    4. Bone marrow transplant is not always necessary with the treatment of Hodgkin disease and will most likely worsen the prognosis.

TEST-TAKING HINT: Know the treatments for and the prognosis of Hodgkin disease.

50. 1. It should not be necessary to give pain medication, because radiation therapy should not be painful.
    2. Neuropathy is not a normal side effect of radiation therapy.
    3. **The most common side effect is extensive malaise, which may be from damage to the thyroid gland, causing hypothyroidism.**
    4. No diet restriction is required for the radiation therapy. Continue with nutritional supplements as needed to maintain adequate nutrition.

TEST-TAKING HINT: Review the side effects of radiation therapy. Lack of energy may be difficult emotionally in adolescents, because they want to keep up with their peers.

51. 1. **Palpating the abdomen of the child in whom a diagnosis of Wilms tumor is suspected should be avoided because manipulation of the abdomen may cause seeding of the tumor.**
    2. Hematuria is a clinical manifestation.
    3. Because the kidney is involved, hypertension should be assessed.
    4. Height and weight are always important to obtain, because they can be used to calculate doses of medications and chemotherapy.

TEST-TAKING HINT: All of the assessment data are important, but the key phrase is "most important." Seeding of the tumor could spread cancerous cells.

52. 1. Chemotherapy is started after tumor removal, and radiation is done depending on stage and histological pattern.
    2. Combination therapy of surgery and chemotherapy is the therapeutic management.
    3. **Combination therapy of surgery and chemotherapy is the primary therapeutic management. Radiation is done depending on clinical stage and histological pattern.**
    4. Radiation should be done after surgery and chemotherapy, depending on stage and histological pattern.

TEST-TAKING HINT: Staging and biopsy determine the treatment, but the child will always have the tumor and kidney removed, followed by chemotherapy.

53. 1. Prolonged bleeding indicates abnormalities of the clotting system.
    2. Failure to thrive is a consequence of a present illness.
    3. Fatigue and malaise result from decreases in red blood cells.
    4. **SCID is characterized by an absence of cell-mediated immunity, with the most common clinical manifestation being infection in children from age 3 months. These children do not usually recover from these infections.**

TEST-TAKING HINT: Review the clinical manifestations of SCID, keeping in mind that the word "immunodeficiency" should indicate infection, which is the key to getting the correct answer.

54. 1. The clinical manifestations are different from those of Hodgkin disease, because the enlarged lymph nodes usually occur in the cervical area.
    2. **The clinical manifestations include symptoms of involvement. Rarely is a single sign or symptom diagnostic. Metastasis to the bone marrow or central nervous system may produce manifestations of leukemia.**
    3. The manifestations are not just limited to the abdomen, and NHL is not usually seen in young children.
    4. Behavior changes, jaundice or dry mouth are not presenting signs of NHL.

TEST-TAKING HINT: Review the difference between Hodgkin disease and non-Hodgkin lymphoma.

55. 1. The clinical staging system used in Hodgkin disease is of little value in lymphoma. Other systems have been developed.
    2. **The use of aggressive combination chemotherapy has a major impact on the survival rates for children with a diagnosis of lymphoma. Because there is usually bone marrow involvement, there is a need for central nervous system prophylaxis.**
    3. Not all children receive a bone marrow transplant.
    4. Usually there is a good prognosis for lymphoma with aggressive chemotherapy.

TEST-TAKING HINT: Be careful not to answer a question with a response that has the word "all" in it, because rarely will something always occur.

56. 1. Tumor involvement in the bone is usually osteosarcoma.
    2. Tumors that are located in the kidney are most often a Wilms tumor.
    3. **Neuroblastoma tumors originate from embryonic neural crest cells that normally give rise to the adrenal medulla and the sympathetic nervous system. The majority of the tumors arise from the adrenal gland or from the retroperitoneal sympathetic chain. Therefore, the primary site is within the abdomen.**
    4. In most tumors in children, there is liver involvement when there is metastasis to the liver.

TEST-TAKING HINT: Review the origin of neuroblastoma to determine the tumor sites.

57. 1. CMV infection is one commonly associated with HIV infections in children, but it is not the most common.
    2. Encephalitis is not a specific opportunistic infection noted in HIV–infected children.
    3. Meningitis is not a specific opportunistic infection noted in HIV–infected children.
    4. *Pneumocystis jiroveci* **pneumonia is the most common opportunistic infection that can occur in HIV–infected children, and such children are treated prophylactically for this.**

TEST-TAKING HINT: Note the words "most common" in the question.

58.
1. The CD4 cell count indicates how well the immune system is working.
2. A Western blot test confirms the presence of HIV antibodies.
3. An IgG level samples the immune system.
4. **Detection of HIV in infants is confirmed by a p24 antigen assay, viral culture of HIV, or polymerase chain reaction.**

TEST-TAKING HINT: Review the laboratory tests for HIV-infected clients. The important word in the question is "infant."

59. 4, 5.
1. Hepatitis B vaccine is administered according to the immunization schedule.
2. The varicella vaccine is avoided in the child who is HIV-infected, not in the other members of the family.
3. A Western blot test is not done and is not necessary.
4. **Immunizations against childhood illnesses are recommended for children exposed to or infected with HIV. Pneumococcal and influenza vaccines are recommended at their scheduled times.**
5. **Meningococcal immunizations can be administered on the regular schedule.**

TEST-TAKING HINT: Review the immunization schedule, keeping in mind that HIV-infected children should not receive live viruses.

60.
1. The child can attend day care. The risk of transmission remains the same at any age.
2. **The child can attend day care without any limitations but should not attend with a fever.**
3. There is no need to restrict the child's activity.
4. There is no law that requires notification of the child's condition.

TEST-TAKING HINT: Review the modes of transmission of HIV infection in children. The day-care facility should practice universal precautions when caring for all its children.

Neuromuscular Disorders

KEYWORDS

The following words include English vocabulary, nursing/medical terminology, concepts, principles, or information relevant to content specifically addressed in the chapter or associated with topics presented in it. English dictionaries, your nursing textbooks, and medical dictionaries such as *Taber's Cyclopedic Medical Dictionary* are resources that can be used to expand your knowledge and understanding of these words and related information.

Atrophy

Congenital

Contracture

Dystrophy

ABBREVIATIONS

Cerebral palsy (CP)

Cerebrovascular accident (CVA)

Cerebrospinal fluid (CSF)

Computerized tomography (CT) scan

Cranial nerve (CN)

Emergency department (ED)

Guillain-Barré syndrome (GBS)

Individualized Education Plan (IEP)

Magnetic resonance imaging (MRI)

QUESTIONS

1. An adolescent presents with sudden-onset unilateral facial weakness with drooping of one side of the mouth. The teen is unable to close the eye on the affected side, but has no other symptoms and otherwise feels well. The nurse could summarize the condition by which of the following?
   1. The prognosis is poor.
   2. This may be a CVA.
   3. It is a fifth CN palsy.
   4. This is paralysis of the facial nerve.

2. The nurse is performing an admission assessment on a 9-year-old who has just been diagnosed with systemic lupus erythematosus. Which assessment findings should the nurse expect? **Select all that apply.**
   1. Headaches and nausea.
   2. Fever, malaise, and weight loss.
   3. A papular rash covering the trunk and face.
   4. Abdominal pain and dysuria.
   5. Joint pain, proteinuria, and lymphadenopathy.

3. The parents of a preschooler diagnosed with muscular dystrophy are asking questions about the course of their child's disease. Which should the nurse tell them? **Select all that apply.**
   1. "Muscular dystrophies usually result in progressive weakness."
   2. "The weakness that your child is having will probably not increase."
   3. "Your child will be able to function normally and not need any special accommodations."
   4. "The extent of weakness depends on doing daily physical therapy."
   5. "Your child may have pain in his legs with muscle weakness."

4. The nurse should tell the parents of a child with Duchenne (pseudohypertrophic) muscular dystrophy that some of the progressive complications include: **Select all that apply.**
   1. Dry skin and hair, hirsutism, protruding tongue, and mental retardation.
   2. Anorexia, gingival hyperplasia, dry skin and hair.
   3. Contractures, obesity, and pulmonary infections.
   4. Trembling, frequent loss of consciousness, and slurred speech.
   5. Increasing difficulty swallowing and shallow breathing.

5. Which can elicit the Gower sign? Have the child:
   1. Close the eyes and touch the nose with alternating index fingers.
   2. Hop on one foot and then the other.
   3. Bend from the waist to touch the toes.
   4. Walk like a duck and rise from a squatting position.

6. A 5-year-old has been diagnosed with pseudohypertrophic muscular dystrophy. Which nursing intervention(s) would be appropriate? **Select all that apply.**
   1. Discuss with the parents the potential need for respiratory support.
   2. Explain that this disease is easily treated with medication.
   3. Suggest exercises that will limit the use of muscles and prevent fatigue.
   4. Assist the parents in finding a nursing facility for future care.
   5. Encourage the parents to contact the school to develop an IEP.

7. Which foods would be best for a child with Duchenne muscular dystrophy? **Select all that apply.**
   1. High-carbohydrate, high-protein foods.
   2. No special food combinations.
   3. Extra protein to help strengthen muscles.
   4. Low-calorie foods to prevent weight gain.
   5. Thickened liquids and smaller portions that are cut up.

8. Which will help a school-age child with muscular dystrophy stay active longer? **Select all that apply.**
   1. Normal activities, such as swimming.
   2. Using a treadmill every day.
   3. Several periods of rest every day.
   4. Using a wheelchair upon getting tired.
   5. Sleeping as late as needed.

9. The mother of a child with Duchenne muscular dystrophy asks the nurse who in the family should have genetic screening. Who should the nurse say must be tested? **Select all that apply.**
   1. Mother.
   2. Sister.
   3. Brother.
   4. Aunts and all female cousins.
   5. Uncles and all male cousins.

10. The nurse knows that teaching was successful when a parent states which of the following are early signs of muscular dystrophy?
    1. Increased muscle strength.
    2. Difficulty climbing stairs.
    3. High fevers and tiredness.
    4. Respiratory infections and obesity.

11. The nurse is caring for a school-age child with Duchenne muscular dystrophy in the elementary school. Which would be an appropriate nursing diagnosis?
    1. Anticipatory grieving.
    2. Anxiety reduction.
    3. Increased pain.
    4. Activity intolerance.

12. The nurse knows that teaching has been successful when the parent of a child with muscle weakness states that the diagnostic test for muscular dystrophy is which of the following?
    1. Electromyelogram.
    2. Nerve conduction velocity.
    3. Muscle biopsy.
    4. Creatine kinase level.

13. Why does spinal cord injury without radiographic abnormality sometimes occur in children?
    1. Children can suffer momentary severe subluxation and trauma to the spinal cord.
    2. The immature spinal column in children does not allow for quality films.
    3. The hemorrhaging that occurs with injury obscures radiographic abnormalities.
    4. Radiographic abnormalities are not evident because of incomplete ossification of the vertebrae.

14. Which should a nurse in the ED be prepared for in a child with a possible spinal cord injury? **Select all that apply.**
    1. Severe pain.
    2. Elevated temperature.
    3. Respiratory depression.
    4. Increased intracranial pressure.
    5. Multiple sites of injury.

15. The nurse evaluates the teaching as successful when a parent states that which of the following can cause autonomic dysreflexia?
    1. Exposure to cold temperatures.
    2. Distended bowel or bladder.
    3. Bradycardia.
    4. Headache.

16. When assessing the neurological status of an 8-month-old, the nurse should check for which of the following? **Select all that apply.**
    1. Clarity of speech.
    2. Interaction with staff.
    3. Vision test.
    4. Romberg test.
    5. Ability to roll over and sit independently.

17. Which symptoms will a child suffering from complete spinal cord injury experience? **Select all that apply.**
    1. Loss of motor and sensory function below the level of the injury.
    2. Loss of interest in normal activities.
    3. Extreme pain below the level of the injury.
    4. Loss of some function, with sparing of function below the level of the injury.
    5. Loss of bowel and bladder control.

18. The nurse is planning care for a child with a T12 spinal cord injury. Which lifelong complication should the child and family know about? **Select all that apply.**
    1. Skin integrity.
    2. Incontinence.
    3. Loss of large and small motor activity.
    4. Loss of voice.
    5. Spasticity.

19. After spinal cord surgery, an adolescent suddenly complains of a severe headache. Which should be the nurse's first action?
    1. Check the blood pressure.
    2. Check for a full bladder.
    3. Ask if pain is present somewhere else.
    4. Ask if other symptoms are present.

20. An adolescent with a T4 spinal cord injury suddenly becomes dangerously hypertensive and bradycardic. Which intervention is appropriate?
    1. Call the neurosurgeon immediately, as this sounds like sudden intracranial hypertension.
    2. Check to be certain that the client's bladder is not distended.
    3. Administer diazoxide (Hyperstat) to treat the blood pressure.
    4. Administer atropine for bradycardia.

21. Which priority item should be placed at the bedside of a newborn with myelomeningocele? **Select all that apply.**
    1. A bottle of normal saline.
    2. A rectal thermometer.
    3. Extra blankets.
    4. A blood pressure cuff.
    5. Latex-free gloves.

22. The nurse is caring for an infant with myelomeningocele who is going to surgery later today for closure of the sac. Which would be a priority nursing diagnosis before surgery?
    1. Alteration in parent-infant bonding.
    2. Altered growth and development.
    3. Risk of infection.
    4. Risk for weight loss.

23. Which should the nurse include when teaching sexuality education to an adolescent with a spinal cord injury? **Select all that apply.**
    1. "You can enjoy a healthy sex life and most likely conceive children."
    2. "You will never be able to conceive if you have no genital sensation."
    3. "Development of secondary sex characteristics is delayed."
    4. "A few females have regular menstrual periods after injury."
    5. "You can get the same sexually transmitted infections that those without spinal cord injuries get."

24. A child with a repaired myelomeningocele is in the clinic for a regular examination. The child has frequent constipation and has been crying at night because of pain in the legs. After an MRI, the diagnosis of a tethered cord is made. Which should the nurse tell the parent?
    1. Tethered cord is a postsurgical complication.
    2. Tethered cord occurs during times of slow growth.
    3. Release of the tethered cord will be necessary only once.
    4. Offering laxatives and acetaminophen (Tylenol) daily will help control these problems.

25. Which intervention should be included in the plan of care for a newborn with a newly repaired myelomeningocele?
    1. Offer formula/breast milk every 3 hours.
    2. Turn the infant back to front every 2 hours.
    3. Place a wet dressing on the sac.
    4. Provide pain medication every 4 hours.

26. Which should the nurse do first when caring for an infant who just had a repair of a myelomeningocele?
    1. Weigh diapers for 24-hour urine output.
    2. Measure head circumference.
    3. Offer clear fluids.
    4. Assess for infection.

27. Which should be the priority nursing diagnosis for a 12-hour-old newborn with a myelomeningocele at L2?
    1. Altered bowel elimination related to neurological deficits.
    2. Potential for infection related to the physical defect.
    3. Altered nutrition related to neurological deficit.
    4. Disturbance in self-concept related to physical disability.

28. Over the past week, an infant with a repaired myelomeningocele has had a high-pitched cry and been irritable. Length, weight, and head circumference have been at the 50th percentile. Today, length is at the 50th percentile, weight is at the 70th percentile, and head circumference is at the 90th percentile. The nurse should do which of the following?
    1. Tell the parent this is normal for an infant with a repaired myelomeningocele.
    2. Tell the parent this might mean the baby has increased intracranial pressure.
    3. Suspect the baby's intracranial pressure is low because of a leak.
    4. Refer the baby to the neurologist for follow-up care.

29. Which should the nurse tell the parent of an infant with spina bifida?
    1. "Bone growth will be more than that of babies who are not sick because your baby will be less active."
    2. "Physical and occupational therapy will be helpful to stimulate the senses and improve cognitive skills."
    3. "Nutritional needs for your infant will be calculated based on activity level."
    4. "Fine motor skills will be delayed because of the disability."

30. Which gross motor skills should the nurse assess in a 3-month-old with spina bifida?
    1. Head control.
    2. Pincer grasp.
    3. Sitting alone.
    4. Rolling over.

31. A 15-year-old with spina bifida is seen in the clinic for a well-child checkup. The teen uses leg braces and crutches to ambulate. Which nursing diagnosis takes priority?
    1. Potential for infection.
    2. Alteration in mobility.
    3. Alteration in elimination.
    4. Potential body image disturbance.

32. A school-age child is admitted to the unit preoperatively for bladder reconstruction. The child is latex-sensitive. Which intervention should the nurse implement?
    1. Post a sign on the door and note in the chart that the child is latex-allergic.
    2. Use powder-free latex gloves when giving care.
    3. Keep personal items such as stuffed animals in a plastic bag to avoid latex contamination.
    4. Use a disposable plastic-covered blood pressure cuff that will stay in the child's room.

33. Which should the nurse prepare the parents of an infant for following surgical repair and closure of a myelomeningocele shortly after birth? The infant will:
    1. Not need any long-term management and should be considered cured.
    2. Not be at risk for urinary tract infections or movement problems.
    3. Have continual drainage of cerebrospinal fluid, needing frequent dressing changes.
    4. Need lifelong management of urinary, orthopedic, and neurological problems.

34. A newborn with a repaired myelomeningocele is assessed for hydrocephalus. Which would the nurse expect in an infant with hydrocephalus?
    1. Low-pitched cry and depressed fontanel.
    2. Low-pitched cry and bulging fontanel.
    3. Bulging fontanel and downwardly rotated eyes.
    4. Depressed fontanel and upwardly rotated eyes.

35. The nurse is developing a plan of care for a child recently diagnosed with cerebral palsy (CP). Which should be the nurse's priority goal?
    1. Ensure the ingestion of sufficient calories for growth.
    2. Decrease intracranial pressure.
    3. Teach appropriate parenting strategies for a special-needs child.
    4. Ensure that the child reaches full potential.

36. The nurse evaluates teaching of parents of a child newly diagnosed with CP as successful when the parents state that CP is which of the following?
    1. Inability to speak and uncontrolled drooling.
    2. Involuntary movements of lower extremities only.
    3. Involuntary movements of upper extremities only.
    4. An increase in muscle tone and deep tendon reflexes.

37. The parent of a toddler newly diagnosed with CP asks the nurse what caused it. The nurse should answer with which of the following?
    1. Most cases are caused by unknown prenatal factors.
    2. It is commonly caused by perinatal factors.
    3. The exact cause is not known.
    4. The exact cause is known in every instance.

38. Which developmental milestone should the nurse be concerned about if a 10-month-old cannot do it?
    1. Crawl.
    2. Cruise.
    3. Walk.
    4. Have a pincer grasp.

39. The parent of an infant asks the nurse what to watch for to determine whether the infant has CP. Which is the nurse's best response?
    1. "If the infant cannot sit up without support before 8 months."
    2. "If the infant demonstrates tongue thrust before 4 months."
    3. "If the infant has poor head control after 2 months."
    4. "If the infant has clenched fists after 3 months."

40. The parent of a young child with CP brings the child to the clinic for a checkup. Which parent's statement indicates an understanding of the child's long-term needs?
    1. "My child will need all my attention for the next 10 years."
    2. "Once in school, my child will catch up and be like the other children."
    3. "My child will grow up and need to learn to do things independently."
    4. "I'm the one who knows the most about my child and can do the most for my child."

41. A child with spastic CP had an intrathecal dose of baclofen (Lioresal) in the early afternoon. What is the expected result 3½ hours post-dose that suggests the child would benefit from a baclofen pump?
    1. The ability to self-feed.
    2. The ability to walk with little assistance.
    3. Decreased spasticity.
    4. Increased spasticity.

42. The nurse is doing a follow-up assessment of a 9-month-old. The infant rolls both ways, sits with some support, pushes food out of the mouth, and pushes away when held. The parent asks about the infant's development. The nurse responds by saying which of the following?
    1. "Your child is developing normally."
    2. "Your child needs to see the primary care provider."
    3. "You need to help your child learn to sit unassisted."
    4. "Push the food back when your child pushes food out."

43. Which would the nurse expect a child with spastic CP to demonstrate? **Select all that apply.**
    1. Increased deep tendon reflexes.
    2. Decreased muscle tone.
    3. Scoliosis.
    4. Contractures.
    5. Scissoring.
    6. Good control of posture.
    7. Good fine motor skills.

44. A 3-year-old child with CP is admitted for dehydration following an episode of diarrhea. The nurse's assessment follows: awake; pale, thin child lying in bed; multiple contractures; drooling; coughing spells noted when parent feeds. T 97.8°F (36.5°C), P 75, R 25, weight 7.2 kg, no diarrheal stool for 48 hours. Which nursing diagnosis is most important?
    1. Potential for skin breakdown: lying in one position.
    2. Alteration in nutrition: less than body requirements.
    3. Potential for impaired social support: parent sole caretaker.
    4. Alteration in elimination: diarrhea.

45. The parent of an infant with CP asks the nurse if the infant will be mentally retarded. Which is the nurse's best response?
    1. "Children with CP have some amount of mental retardation."
    2. "Approximately 20% of children with CP have normal intelligence."
    3. "Many children with CP have normal intelligence."
    4. "Mental retardation is expected if motor and sensory deficits are severe."

46. Parents bring their 2-month-old into the clinic with concerns that the baby seems "floppy." The parents say the baby seems to be working hard to breathe, eats very slowly, and seems to fatigue quickly. The nurse assesses intercostal retractions, although the baby is otherwise in no distress. The parents add there was a cousin whose baby had similar symptoms. The nurse would be most concerned with which possible complication?
    1. Respiratory compromise.
    2. Dehydration.
    3. Need for emotional support for the family.
    4. Feeding intolerance.

47. The mother of a newborn relates that this is her first child; the baby seems to sleep a lot and does not cry much. Which question would the nurse ask the mother?
    1. "How many ounces of formula does your baby take at each feeding?"
    2. "How many bowel movements does your baby have in a day?"
    3. "How much sleep do you get every night?"
    4. "How long does the baby stay awake at each feeding?"

48. The mother of an infant diagnosed with Werdnig-Hoffmann disease asks the nurse what she could have done during her pregnancy to prevent this. The nurse explains that the cause of Werdnig-Hoffmann is which of the following?
    1. Unknown.
    2. Restricted movement in utero.
    3. Inherited as an autosomal-recessive trait.
    4. Inherited as an autosomal-dominant trait.

49. The parents of a toddler diagnosed with Werdnig-Hoffmann disease ask the nurse what they can feed their child that would be quality food. Which would be good choices for the nurse to recommend?
    1. A hot dog and chips.
    2. Chicken and broccoli.
    3. A banana and almonds.
    4. A milkshake and a hamburger.

50. The parent of a child diagnosed with Werdnig-Hoffmann disease notes times of not being able to hear the child breathing. Which should the nurse do first?
    1. Check pulse oximetry on the child.
    2. Count the child's respirations.
    3. Listen to the child's lung sounds.
    4. Ask the parent if the child coughs at night.

51. A child presents with a history of having had an upper respiratory tract infection 2 weeks ago; complains of symmetrical lower extremity weakness, back pain, muscle tenderness; and has absent deep tendon reflexes in the lower extremities. Which is important regarding this condition?
    1. The disease process is probably bacterial.
    2. The recent upper respiratory infection is not important information.
    3. This may be an acute inflammatory demyelinating neuropathy.
    4. CN involvement is rare.

52. A child with GBS has had lots of oral fluids but has not urinated for 8 hours. Which is the nurse's first action?
    1. Check the child's serum blood urea nitrogen level.
    2. Check the child's complete blood count.
    3. Catheterize the child in and out.
    4. Run water in the bathroom to stimulate urination.

53. The nurse is planning care for a child who was recently admitted with GBS. Which is a priority nursing diagnosis?
1. Risk for constipation related to immobility.
2. Chronic sorrow related to presence of chronic disability.
3. Impaired skin integrity related to infectious disease process.
4. Activity intolerance related to ineffective cardiac muscle function.

54. Which should the nurse expect as an intervention in a child in the recovery phase of GBS? **Select all that apply.**
1. Assist with self-feeding skills.
2. Assist with grooming and dressing.
3. Arrange for in-home schooling.
4. Begin an active physical therapy program.
5. Begin active PT.

55. A child has a provisional diagnosis of myasthenia gravis. Which should the nurse expect in this child? **Select all that apply.**
1. Double vision, ptosis.
2. Tremors and seizures.
3. Coughing and choking.
4. Ascending paralysis.
5. Sensory disturbance.

56. The nurse judges teaching as successful when the parent of a child with myasthenia gravis states which of the following? **Select all that apply.**
1. "My child should play on the school's basketball team."
2. "My child should meditate every day."
3. "My child should be allowed to do what other kids do."
4. "My child should be watched carefully for signs of illness."
5. "My child should sleep in my room so that I can watch him better."

57. Which is the best advice to offer the parent of a 6-month-old with Werdnig-Hoffman disease on how to treat the infant's constipation?
1. Offer extra water every day.
2. Add corn syrup to two bottles a day.
3. Give the infant a glycerine suppository today.
4. Let the infant go 3 days without a stool before intervening.

58. Which should the nurse do for a 7-year-old living in a rural area who is missing school shots and who has sustained a puncture wound?
1. Administer TdaP vaccine.
2. Start the child on an antibiotic.
3. Clean the wound with hydrogen peroxide.
4. Send the child to the emergency department.

59. Which should the nurse expect in a 2-week-old with a brachial plexus injury? **Select all that apply.**
1. History of a normal vaginal delivery.
2. Small infant.
3. Absent Moro reflex on one side.
4. No sensory loss.
5. Associated clavicle fracture.

60. After surviving a motor vehicle accident but enduring a spinal cord injury, an adolescent is unable to walk but can use his arms, has no bowel or bladder control, and has no sensation below the nipple line. Referring to the following figure, identify the vertebral/spinal cord area most likely injured.

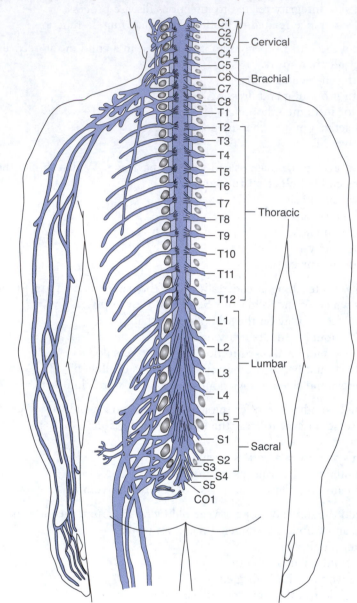

1. Cervical, C1–C5.
2. Cervical, C5–C7.
3. Thoracic, T1–T4.
4. Thoracic, T5–T12.
5. Lumbar, L2–L5.
6. Sacral, S1–S5.

61. Causes of autonomic dysreflexia include which of the following? **Select all that apply.**
1. Decrease in blood pressure.
2. Abdominal distention.
3. Bladder distention.
4. Diarrhea.
5. Tight clothing.
6. Hyperthermia.

ANSWERS AND RATIONALES

The correct answer number and rationale for why it is the correct answer are given in **boldface blue type**. Rationales for why the other possible answer options are incorrect also are given, but they are not in boldface type.

1. 1. Paralysis of the facial nerve (CN VII) generally resolves within 2 to 4 weeks and has a good prognosis. Treatment is supportive.
   2. It would be very unusual for a healthy adolescent to have a stroke. One would also expect other symptoms.
   3. CN V (the trigeminal nerve) innervates the muscles of mastication.
   4. **This client has Bell's palsy, which is an idiopathic mononeuritis of CN VII (the facial nerve) that innervates the face and muscles of expression.**

   TEST-TAKING HINT: The test taker must know CNs and their actions.

2. 2, 5.
   1. Neuropsychiatric symptoms include difficulty concentrating in school and emotional instability.
   2. **Fever, malaise, and weight loss are common presenting signs.**
   3. A rash is common, but with lupus it is usually a "butterfly" rash across the bridge of the nose. Maculopapular rashes are common but are usually on sun-exposed areas.
   4. Lupus nephritis requires urine output monitoring and is usually asymptomatic.
   5. **Joint pain, proteinuria, and lymphadenopathy are common presenting symptoms in children.**

   TEST-TAKING HINT: The test taker must know the presenting signs and symptoms of systemic lupus erythematosus.

3. 1, 5.
   1. **Muscular dystrophies are progressive degenerative disorders. The most common is Duchenne muscular dystrophy, which is an X-linked recessive disorder.**
   2. The weakness is progressive.
   3. The child will require assistance, and the need for it will increase with time and age.
   4. Daily therapy may be helpful in decreasing contractures, although it will not deter the disease progression.
   5. **The child may have pain due to loss of strength and muscle wasting.**

   TEST-TAKING HINT: The test taker should know that muscular dystrophy is a progressive degenerative disorder.

4. 3, 5.
   1. These symptoms are common with Down syndrome.
   2. Duchenne muscular dystrophy does not produce these symptoms.
   3. **The major complications of muscular dystrophy include contractures, disuse atrophy, infections, obesity, respiratory complications, and cardiopulmonary problems.**
   4. These symptoms are evidence of a possible head injury.
   5. **The muscles of a child with MD tend to show increasing weakness and atrophy over time. The children are at risk for swallowing, aspiration, and pneumonia.**

   TEST-TAKING HINT: The test taker should be able to identify signs and symptoms attributable to the loss of muscle function.

5. 1. This is the Romberg sign, which measures balance.
   2. This test measures balance and coordination.
   3. This test measures flexibility.
   4. **Children with muscular dystrophy display the Gower sign, which is great difficulty rising and standing from a squatting position because of the lack of muscle strength.**

   TEST-TAKING HINT: By eliminating cerebellar activities, the test taker would know that the Gower sign assists in measuring leg strength.

6. 1, 3, 5.
   1. **Muscles become weaker, including those needed for respiration, and a decision will need to be made about whether respiratory support will be provided.**
   2. This is a progressive disease, which medications do not treat.
   3. **Physical therapy will be part of the treatment plan, but respiratory support is a priority.**
   4. The parents need to decide eventually if they will keep the child home or cared for in a nursing facility, but that is not an immediate concern.

5. Parents should be encouraged to allow the child to go to school and participate in activities as tolerated.

TEST-TAKING HINT: Pseudohypertrophic muscular dystrophy is a progressive neuromuscular disease with no cure. Children can have a good quality of life if parents are guided in how to help their child.

7. 4, 5.
1. As the child with muscular dystrophy becomes less active, diet becomes more important. Attention should be paid to quality and quantity of food, so the child does not gain too much weight.
2. Good-quality foods are important as the child continues to grow.
3. Extra protein will not help the child recover from this disease.
4. **As the child becomes less ambulatory, moving the child will become more of a problem. It is not good for the child to become overweight for several health reasons in addition to decreased ambulation.**
5. **As the child loses muscle control, the need for thickened liquids and small, well-cut-up solids becomes essential.**

TEST-TAKING HINT: Nutrition is important for every child; as the child becomes less ambulatory, weight concerns arise.

8. 1, 3, 4.
1. **Swimming is an excellent exercise that uses many muscles and helps build strength. Children who are active are usually able to postpone use of a wheelchair. It is important to keep using muscles for as long as possible, and aerobic activity is good for a child.**
2. Use of a treadmill is not fun for children or adults, so keeping the child using the treadmill might be an issue.
3. **Any child with a chronic disease should be kept as active as possible for as long as possible; short rest periods built into the day are helpful in maintaining stamina.**
4. **Children with neuromuscular diseases oftentimes will use a wheelchair to conserve energy and increase mobility. The wheelchair acts as the child's means of getting to where they want to go as independently as possible.**
5. The child should be on a regular daily schedule including the same bedtime and getting up time. Rest times should be provided during the day.

TEST-TAKING HINT: Appropriate interventions for different kinds of chronically ill children can be similar, so think about what would be best for this child.

9. 1, 2, 4.
1. **Genetic counseling is important in all inherited diseases. Duchenne muscular dystrophy is inherited as an X-linked recessive trait, meaning the defect is on the X chromosome. Women carry the disease, and males are affected. All female relatives should be tested.**
2. **The X chromosome carries the disease, and males are affected. The sister should have genetic testing to determine whether she carries the gene and identify her risks for having male offspring with the disease.**
3. Because the disease is carried on the X chromosome, only females need to be genetically tested. Women carry the disease, and males are affected. All female relatives should be tested unless they are symptomatic.
4. **The X chromosome carries the disease and males are affected. All female relatives should be tested.**
5. The X chromosome carries the disease and males are affected. All female relatives should be tested.

TEST-TAKING HINT: Knowing that Duchenne muscular dystrophy is inherited as an X-linked trait excludes fathers, brothers, uncles, and male cousins as carriers.

10. 1. Muscles become enlarged from fatty infiltration, so they are not stronger.
2. **Difficulty climbing stairs, running, and riding a bicycle are frequently the first symptoms of Duchenne muscular dystrophy.**
3. High fevers and tiredness are not early signs of muscular dystrophy but could be later signs as complications become more common.
4. Respiratory infections and obesity are major complications as the disease progresses.

TEST-TAKING HINT: Early symptoms have to do with decreased ability to perform normal developmental tasks involving muscle strength.

11. 1. This diagnosis would relate to the family and not to the child.
2. This diagnosis would relate to the family and not to the child.
3. The child does not have pain with the muscular dystrophy process.

4. **The child would not be able to keep up with peers because of weakness, progressive loss of muscle fibers, and loss of muscle strength.**

TEST-TAKING HINT: Knowing that the child has decreased strength helps to answer the question.

12. 1. The electromyelogram is part of the diagnostic workup, but muscle biopsy results classify muscle disorders.
    2. Nerve conduction velocity is part of the diagnostic workup, but muscle biopsy results classify muscle disorders.
    3. **Muscle biopsy confirms the type of myopathy that the patient has.**
    4. Creatine kinase is in muscle tissue and is found in large amounts in muscular diseases.

TEST-TAKING HINT: Muscle biopsy is the definitive test for myopathies.

13. 1. **Spinal cord injury without radiographic abnormality results from the spinal cord sliding between the vertebrae and then sliding back into place without injury to the bony spine. It is thought to be the result of an immature spinal column that allows for reduction after momentary subluxation.**
    2. On x-ray the spinal cord and body structure appear normal. The edema of the cord and resulting ischemia can cause neurological dysfunction below the level of the injury.
    3. Hemorrhaging that occurs with the injury does not obscure radiographic findings.
    4. The vertebrae are adequately ossified for radiographic study to reveal abnormalities.

TEST-TAKING HINT: The test taker must understand the physiology of spinal cord injuries in children.

14. 3, 5.
    1. Severe pain is unlikely, but the child may have pain at the injury site.
    2. An elevated temperature is not common in a spinal cord injury. In fact, most trauma patients are hypothermic in spite of high ambient temperatures.
    3. **A spinal cord injury can occur at any level. The higher the level of the injury, the more likely the child is to have respiratory insufficiency or failure. The nurse should be prepared to support the child's respiratory system.**
    4. Spinal cord injury with an open or closed head injury does not cause an increase in intracranial pressure.

5. The nurse should expect that the child may have multiple injury sites as many spinal cord injuries are the result of trauma from falls from heights, violence, or sporting injuries. A complete head-to-toe assessment of the child should be performed.

TEST-TAKING HINT: The test taker must know the signs of a spinal cord injury.

15. 1. Exposure to cold temperatures does not trigger an episode of autonomic dysreflexia.
    2. **Autonomic dysreflexia results from an uncontrolled, paroxysmal, continuous lower motor neuron reflex arc due to stimulation of the sympathetic nervous system. It is a response that typically results from stimulation of sensory receptors such as a full bladder or bowel.**
    3. Symptoms of autonomic dysreflexia are bradycardia, headache, and potentially life-threatening hypertension.
    4. Symptoms of autonomic dysreflexia are bradycardia, headache, and potentially life-threatening hypertension.

TEST-TAKING HINT: The test taker must know what triggers autonomic dysreflexia and what the symptoms are.

16. 2, 5.
    1. The infant is preverbal, so assessing clarity of speech is not age-appropriate or developmentally appropriate.
    2. **Assessment for alteration in developmentally expected behaviors, such as stranger anxiety, is helpful. Interaction with staff is not to be expected due to stranger anxiety.**
    3. Vision testing is not the priority assessment.
    4. An 8-month-old infant is not tested with the Romberg test.
    5. **Sitting and rolling over are two skills that an 8-month-old infant should be able to accomplish.**

TEST-TAKING HINT: The test taker must know what is appropriate infant development.

17. 1, 5.
    1. **Children with complete spinal cord injury lose motor and sensory function below the level of the injury as a result of interruption of nerve pathways.**
    2. Although spinal cord–injured children may suffer depression, it is not correct to state that all of them lose interest in normal activities.

3. Pain is absent below the level of the injury because of loss of sensory function.

4. When injury is in the lumbar region (L1–L5), the child loses control and sensation of the hips, thighs, and feet. This affects all motor activities such as walking and sitting,

5. **The nerves to the perineal are affected when injuries occur to the lumbar region. The child develops a neurogenic bladder and bowel.**

TEST-TAKING HINT: A spinal cord injury causes loss of motor and sensory function below the level of the injury.

18. **1, 2, 3, 5.**
   1. **Spinal cord–injury clients experience many issues because of the loss of innervation below the level of the injury. Skin integrity and incontinence are issues because of immobility and loss of pain receptors below the level of the injury.**
   2. **Skin integrity and incontinence are issues because of immobility and loss of pain receptors below the level of the injury.**
   3. **Loss of motor activity is also a result of loss of innervation below the level of the injury.**
   4. Loss of voice is not a complication of T12 injury.
   5. **With incomplete severing of the spinal cord, flaccid spasticity occurs initially as a result of the injury and shock, but oftentimes converts to muscle spasticity during the rehabilitation stage.**

TEST-TAKING HINT: The test taker must know the long-term effects of spinal cord injuries.

19. 1. The autonomic nervous system responds with arteriolar vasospasm, which results in an uncontrolled increase in blood pressure. The parasympathetic nervous system (vagus nerve) sends a stimulus to the heart resulting in bradycardia and vasodilation.
   2. **The sympathetic nervous system responds to a full bladder or bowel resulting from an uncontrolled, paroxysmal, continuous lower motor neuron reflex arc. This response is usually from stimulation of sensory receptors (e.g., distended bladder or bowel). Because the efferent pulse cannot pass through the spinal cord, the vagus nerve is not "turned off," and profound symptomatic bradycardia may occur.**

3. Pain is not usually felt below the level of the injury, and pain elsewhere does not cause a severe headache.

4. In autonomic dysreflexia, the patient does not experience other symptoms.

TEST-TAKING HINT: Autonomic dysreflexia is usually caused by a full bladder or bowel.

20. 1. Sudden hypertension and bradycardia are symptoms of autonomic dysreflexia. The nurse needs to make assessments of the fullness of the bowel and bladder, take the blood pressure, and relieve the bowel or bladder before calling the doctor.
   2. **The first assessment is of the bladder and bowel to check for fullness. The presence of either could trigger autonomic dysreflexia.**
   3. The first intervention is to assess the bladder for fullness before administering any medication.
   4. The first intervention is to assess the bladder for fullness before administering any medication.

TEST-TAKING HINT: The test taker must know which symptoms are suggestive of autonomic dysreflexia.

21. **1, 5.**
   1. **Before the surgical closure of the sac, the infant is at risk for infection. A sterile dressing is placed over the sac to keep it moist and help prevent it from tearing. Because the dressings dry out at least every hour, it is important to assess them frequently and apply saline as needed. Good hand washing is also important.**
   2. The infant's temperature will be taken, but prevention of infection is the priority.
   3. Infants with myelomeningocele intact are often naked and placed in an incubator for warmth. Temperature does need to be maintained and the infant protected from sick people.
   4. Blood pressure is difficult to monitor in the newborn period, especially if the baby is lying on the abdomen. Prevention of infection is the priority.
   5. **Latex-free clean gloves would be used for all care of this infant. A box should be kept at the infant's bedside. Children with spina bifida are at risk for latex allergy and should not be exposed to latex.**

TEST-TAKING HINT: The test taker should focus on the care and potential complications of an infant with spina bifida to answer the question correctly.

22. 1. Because of the infant's prolonged hospitalization, there can be alterations in parental bonding. Because the myelomeningocele is unrepaired, the major risk is infection.
    2. Altered growth and development may occur, but in the preoperative period, risk of infection is the priority. The long-term diagnosis of altered growth and development will be addressed at each well-child visit.
    3. **The unrepaired myelomeningocele is oftentimes a thin membrane that covers the neural contents of the spine. A normal saline dressing is placed over the sac to prevent tearing. The tearing would allow the CSF to escape and microorganisms to enter. The infant is at high risk for spinal cord infections. The priority nursing diagnosis is risk of infection.**
    4. It is normal in the first 2 weeks of life to lose up to 10% of birth weight. In fact, this infant may lose more weight because of surgery, but the priority is risk of infection.

    TEST-TAKING HINT: The preoperative priority is risk of infection, especially when effort is necessary to keep a sterile saline dressing on the sac.

23. **1, 4, 5.**
    1. **The reproductive system continues to function properly after a spinal cord injury. Much sexual activity and response occurs in the brain as well.**
    2. Conception does not depend on sensation in the genitals.
    3. Secondary sex characteristics develop normally.
    4. **Females may have irregular periods after the injury, but most return to their normal cycles.**
    5. **Those with spinal cord injuries can acquire sexually transmitted infections and need to use safe sex practices.**

    TEST-TAKING HINT: Spinal cord injuries have little effect on reproduction.

24. 1. **Tethered cord is caused by scar tissue formation from the surgical repair of the myelomeningocele and may affect bowel, bladder, or lower extremity functioning. As the child grows, this will affect continence and mobility.**
    2. Tethered cord occurs during growth spurts.
    3. Often the release of the tether will again become necessary.

    4. Laxatives and acetaminophen are temporary remedies, and they treat only the symptoms.

    TEST-TAKING HINT: Tethering is caused by scar tissue from any surgical intervention and may recur as the child grows.

25. 1. **Following surgery, a newborn may want formula/breast milk every 2 to 4 hours. Be sure to monitor intake and output.**
    2. Following surgery, the infant should not be positioned on the back. Monitor respirations when the infant is on the abdomen.
    3. Before surgery, priority care for an infant with a myelomeningocele is to protect the sac.
    4. Infants with myelomeningocele do not have pain because of lack of nerve innervations below the level of the defect.

    TEST-TAKING HINT: Realizing the defect is on the back eliminates answer 2. After surgery, the sac is repaired, so there is no need for a wet dressing, which eliminates answer 3.

26. 1. Weighing diapers for 24-hour urine output totals is important, but it is not the first thing to do following surgery.
    2. **Hydrocephalus occurs in about 90% of infants with myelomeningocele, so measuring the head circumference daily and watching for an increase are important. Accumulation of cerebrospinal fluid can occur after closure of the sac.**
    3. Clear fluids are offered after the infant is fully awake and there is no vomiting.
    4. Assessing for infection is important, but infection is not usually seen in the initial postoperative period.

    TEST-TAKING HINT: The dynamics of the cerebrospinal fluid change after closure of the sac.

27. 1. Infants with myelomeningocele have altered bowel elimination as a result of their defect, but this is not the priority.
    2. **Because this infant has not had a repair, the sac is exposed. It could rupture, allowing organisms to enter the CSF, so this is the priority.**
    3. These infants usually eat normally.
    4. The infant is too young to have a self-concept disturbance.

    TEST-TAKING HINT: Before surgery, the myelomeningocele is exposed, so risk of infection is much higher.

28. 1. The fact that the head circumference has changed so much might indicate increased intracranial pressure.
  2. **The increase in head size is one of the first signs of increased intracranial pressure; other signs include high-pitched cry and irritability.**
  3. The increase in head size is one of the first signs of increased intracranial pressure; other signs include high-pitched cry and irritability.
  4. This infant should be referred to the neurosurgeon, not the neurologist, and a CT scan should be obtained to determine the cause of the increase.

TEST-TAKING HINT: The test taker should know that the head size of an infant grows only 0.5 in. (1.3 cm) a month for the first 6 months. Having the infants' head size cross percentiles after only 1 to 2 days is an alarming finding.

29. 1. Bone growth is related to weight-bearing as well as to secretion of the growth hormone. Decreased activity usually results in less bone growth.
  2. **Children with decreased activity due to illness or trauma are helped by physical and occupational therapy. The varied activities stimulate the senses.**
  3. This is partially true. Nutritional needs in children are also calculated based on growth needs.
  4. Many children with myelomeningocele have low-level defects, usually in the lumbar area, which do not affect upper body fine motor skills.

TEST-TAKING HINT: The test taker should know normal growth and development patterns.

30. 1. **A 3-month-old should have good head control.**
  2. Pincer grasp occurs at about 9 months.
  3. Sitting alone occurs at about 6 months.
  4. Rolling over occurs at about 4 months.

TEST-TAKING HINT: The test taker must know normal developmental milestones.

31. 1. This is certainly a possibility, especially as the teen uses braces and can have some skin irritation.
  2. **This is a nursing diagnosis that affects many aspects of the teen's life. Mobility is important in all aspects of their lives. Braces and crutches enable him to more fully participate in activities and maintain some degree of independence.**

3. Because the teen is ambulatory, the teen probably has a lower-level defect, but even lower-level defects have some type of elimination issues.
  4. As an adolescent on crutches and wearing braces, the teen would have the issue of body image disturbance, which must be addressed after alteration in mobility.

TEST-TAKING HINT: The test taker must know normal development.

32. 1. **Posting a sign on the door and charting that the child has a latex allergy is important so that others will be aware of the allergy.**
  2. Do not use latex gloves with a child who has a latex allergy.
  3. Keeping personal items in a plastic bag does not keep latex away from the child.
  4. A plastic cover for the blood pressure cuff is proper to use but is not related to the latex allergy.

TEST-TAKING HINT: The test taker must know which supplies have latex and about contact allergies.

33. 1. Children with myelomeningocele have ongoing, lifelong, complex health-care needs.
  2. Children with myelomeningocele may have frequent urinary tract infections and mobility concerns.
  3. The surgical closure prevents the leakage of cerebrospinal fluid; dressing changes are necessary only during the postoperative period.
  4. **Although immediate surgical repair decreases infection, morbidity, and mortality rates, these children will require lifelong management of neurological, orthopedic, and elimination problems.**

TEST-TAKING HINT: The test taker can eliminate answer 1 owing to the complexity of myelomeningocele.

34. 1. An alteration in the circulation of the cerebrospinal fluid causes hydrocephalus. The anterior fontanel bulges because of an increase in CSF, and an increase in intracranial pressure causes a high-pitched cry in infants and downward deviation of the eyes, also called sunset eyes.
  2. An alteration in the circulation of the cerebrospinal fluid causes hydrocephalus. The anterior fontanel bulges because of an increase in cerebrospinal fluid, and an increase in intracranial pressure causes a high-pitched cry in infants and downward deviation of the eyes, also called sunset eyes.

3. An alteration in the circulation of the cerebrospinal fluid causes hydrocephalus. The anterior fontanel bulges because of an increase in cerebrospinal fluid, and an increase in intracranial pressure causes a high-pitched cry in infants and downward deviation of the eyes, also called sunset eyes. With sunset eyes, the sclera can be seen above the iris.

4. An alteration in the circulation of the cerebrospinal fluid causes hydrocephalus. The anterior fontanel bulges because of an increase in cerebrospinal fluid, and an increase in intracranial pressure causes a high-pitched cry in infants and downward deviation of the eyes, also called sunset eyes.

TEST-TAKING HINT: The test taker must know the difference in clinical signs of hydrocephalus in infants and older children. Infants' heads expand, whereas older children's skulls are fixed. The anterior fontanel closes between 12 and 18 months.

35. 1. Adequate calories are an appropriate goal, but the priority for a special-needs child is that the child develop to full potential.
2. Children with CP do not have increased intracranial pressure.
3. **Teaching appropriate parenting strategies for a special-needs child is important and is done so that the child can maximize her personal skills and minimize her limitation.**
4. A child with CP needs a health-care team that can aid the family in helping them grow and develop to their full potential. The priority for all children is to develop to their full potential.

TEST-TAKING HINT: All of these are important goals, but determining the priority goal for a special-needs child is the key.

36. 1. Children may also have pseudobulbar involvement, which creates swallowing difficulties and recurrent aspiration.
2. Involuntary movements of the lower extremities would be classified as spastic diplegia. These children do have some upper motor neuron involvement but not to the same degree as the lower motor involvement.
3. Depending on the type of CP, the abnormal involuntary movements of the upper extremities indicate a more diffuse injury to the entire brain.

4. The primary disorder is of muscle tone, but there may be other neurological disorders such as seizures, vision disturbances, and impaired intelligence. Spastic CP is the most common type and is characterized by a generalized increase in muscle tone, increased deep tendon reflexes, and rigidity of the limbs on both flexion and extension.

TEST-TAKING HINT: The test taker must know the definition of CP.

37. 1. CP is defined as a non-progressive (static) injury to an infant either before birth, during birth, or after birth. Depending on the presenting symptoms and the results of diagnostic testing, the etiology of the brain injury can be fairly accurately determined.
2. **It is generally thought that the majority of infants with CP had an insult in utero. Some of the causes of perinatal insult include hypoxia, trauma, infections, or genetic abnormalities.**
3. With current diagnostic testing for genetic abnormalities and MRIs, the etiology of the brain insult can be more often determined.
4. Frequently, the exact cause can be determined by history and physical and diagnostic studies.

TEST-TAKING HINT: The test taker must know the latest information to answer this question correctly.

38. 1. **Most infants are able to crawl unassisted by 8 months.**
2. Infants learn to cruise (walk around holding on to furniture) at about 9 to 10 months.
3. Walking occurs on average at about 12 months.
4. Pincer grasp (thumb and forefinger) occurs at about 9 to 10 months.

TEST-TAKING HINT: The test taker must know developmental milestones.

39. 1. Children with CP frequently have developmental delays, including not being able to sit alone by 8 months. Sitting alone usually occurs by 6 months, so 8 months would be the outer limit of normal development and cause for concern.
2. Tongue thrust is common in infants younger than 6 months, but if it goes on after 6 months it is of concern.
3. Good head control is normally attained by 3 months.
4. **Clenched fists after 3 months of age may be a sign of upper motor injury and CP.**

TEST-TAKING HINT: The test taker must know normal developmental milestones to identify those that are abnormal.

40. 1. There is no magic age when the child with special needs becomes independent and no longer needs parental assistance. The child may need some type of assistance for the rest of his life.
2. With appropriate therapy and good parental support, the child has the potential to maximize his abilities and minimize his limitations. The parent's best approach is to help the child achieve as much independence as possible given his particular disability.
3. **The parent of a child with a disability should have the goal of assisting the child in achieving as much self-care as he is capable of, given his particular limitations.**
4. At times, parents have tremendous grief and need to care totally for the child. It is important for the parent to be guided in helping the child achieve his potential.

TEST-TAKING HINT: The test taker must understand the goals for children with chronic illnesses or disorders. One goal is to ensure that the child be diagnosed as early as possible so that interventions can be started. Another is to help the child realize as much potential as possible.

41. 1. The expected benefit from intrathecal baclofen (Lioresal) is less spasticity, which allows the child to have more muscle control. This leads to more fine motor control and ambulation. The onset of action is 30 minutes, and it peaks in 6 hours.
2. The expected benefit from intrathecal baclofen (Lioresal) is less spasticity, which allows the child to have more muscle control. This leads to more fine motor control and ambulation. The onset of action is 30 minutes, and it peaks in 6 hours.
3. **If baclofen (Lioresal) were to work for this child, one could tell because spasticity would be decreased.**
4. Baclofen (Lioresal) should decrease, not increase, spasticity.

TEST-TAKING HINT: The test taker must know the purpose of baclofen (Lioresal).

42. 1. A 9-month-old should be able to sit alone, crawl, pull up, not push food out of the mouth (tongue thrust), and push away when held when wanting to get down. This child is not developing normally and must see the primary care provider.
2. **A 9-month-old should be able to sit alone, crawl, pull up, not push food out of the mouth (tongue thrust), and push away when held when wanting to get down. The developmental screening the child received should be followed by a complete history, physical exam, and more specific developmental testing.**
3. Children with developmental delay benefit from occupational, physical, and speech therapies. The therapist can teach the parent how to work with the child to help him learn to sit independently.
4. The occupational therapist can evaluate the child's ability to suck, swallow, and chew. The therapist can also teach the parent ways to assist the child to eat "normally."

TEST-TAKING HINT: The test taker must know normal developmental milestones. Rolling occurs at about 4 months, sitting alone occurs at 6 months, and pushing food out of the mouth decreases by 4 months when the tongue thrust reflex wanes.

43. 1, 3, 4, 5.
1. **Children with spastic CP have increased deep tendon reflexes.**
2. Children with spastic CP have increased muscle tone.
3. **Children with spastic CP have scoliosis.**
4. **When children with spastic CP have quadriplegia, they can also develop contractures of the Achilles tendons, knees, and adductor muscles.**
5. **Children with spastic CP have scissoring when walking.**
6. Depending on the amount of body involvement, children with spastic CP may have poor control of posture. It takes a lot of muscle control to stand up straight and maintain posture in space.
7. Children with spastic quadriplegic CP may have poor fine motor skills. There are varying degrees of severity of CP depending on the amount of brain injury.

TEST-TAKING HINT: The test taker must know the typical signs of CP.

44. 1. This child is definitely at risk for skin breakdown, but alteration in nutrition is the priority. The child weighs 15 pounds, which is normal for a 4-month-old. The child is severely underweight. The parent needs help to manage the coughing spells while the child is being fed.

2. **This child is severely underweight
   and malnourished for a 3-year-old.
   The coughing episodes while feeding
   put the child at risk for aspiration and
   pneumonia. A thorough history, physical
   examination, and a feeding study should
   be performed to determine whether it is
   even safe to feed the child orally. This
   is the priority nursing diagnosis for this
   severely underweight child. Weight is
   average for a 4-month-old. The coughing
   episodes while feeding may indicate
   aspiration. The parent needs help to
   learn how to feed so that less coughing
   occurs.**

3. The parent needs support in caring for
   this child, but alteration in nutrition is the
   priority. The child weighs 15 pounds, which
   is normal for a 4-month-old. The child is
   severely underweight, and the parent needs
   help to manage the coughing spells while the
   child is being fed.

4. The child has not had a diarrheal stool for
   48 hours, so the assumption is safe that the
   illness is over. The child weighs 15 pounds,
   which is normal for a 4-month-old. The
   child is severely underweight, and the parent
   needs help to manage the coughing spells
   while the child is being fed.

**TEST-TAKING HINT: The test taker should
convert the weight in kilograms to pounds
to have a better understanding of it.
Knowing what a 3-year-old should weigh
helps with answering this question.**

45. 1. Children with CP have a range of intellectual
       abilities, from being profoundly retarded to
       having a high intelligence quotient. Many
       have normal intelligence. If a child has severe
       speech problems, some may assume that the
       child's intelligence is severely affected when
       that may not be true.

    2. Children with CP have a range of intellectual
       abilities, from being profoundly retarded to
       having a high intelligence quotient. Many
       have normal intelligence. If a child has severe
       speech problems, some may assume that the
       child's intelligence is severely affected when
       that may not be true.

    3. **Many children with CP have normal
       intelligence.**

    4. Children with CP have a range of intellectual
       abilities, from being profoundly retarded to
       having a high intelligence quotient. Many
       have normal intelligence. If a child has severe
       speech problems, some may assume that the
       child's intelligence is severely affected when
       that may not be true.

**TEST-TAKING HINT: Children with CP have a
wide range of intellectual abilities.**

46. 1. **This baby may have Werdnig-Hoffman
       disease, which is characterized by
       progressive generalized muscle weakness
       that eventually leads to respiratory
       failure. Respiratory compromise is the
       most important complication.**

    2. There is no history of being unable to ingest
       oral fluids; the baby is just a slow feeder.

    3. This is important, but respiratory
       compromise is a priority in this situation.

    4. There is no indication of feeding intolerance;
       the baby is just a slow feeder.

**TEST-TAKING HINT: Consider the ABCs in
this situation: airway, breathing, and cardiac
status. These are priorities when caring for
clients.** ·

47. 1. **Babies can lose up to 10% of birth weight
       but should regain it by 2 weeks of age.
       Knowing how much the baby eats can
       help the nurse determine whether the
       infant is receiving adequate nutrition.**

    2. The number of bowel movements will also
       indicate whether the infant receives enough
       formula.

    3. If the infant does not awaken during the
       night, then the mother may sleep all night.
       Most 2-week-olds feed every 2 to 4 hours
       day and night.

    4. How long the infant stays awake is not the
       most important information. Most infants
       sleep about 20 hours per day.

**TEST-TAKING HINT: The "red flags" in this
question are that the baby sleeps a lot and
does not cry much, both unusual behaviors.
Follow-up questions need to be asked to
determine whether the infant is gaining
weight as expected.**

48. 1. Werdnig-Hoffmann disease is inherited as
       an autosomal-recessive trait. There is an
       affected gene from both mother and father
       passed to the baby.

    2. Werdnig-Hoffmann disease is inherited as
       an autosomal-recessive trait. There is an
       affected gene from both mother and father
       passed to the baby.

    3. **Werdnig-Hoffmann disease is inherited
       as an autosomal-recessive trait. There is
       an affected gene from both mother and
       father passed to the baby.**

    4. Werdnig-Hoffmann disease is inherited as
       an autosomal-recessive trait. There is an
       affected gene from both mother and father
       passed to the baby.

TEST-TAKING HINT: The test taker needs to know how infants get this progressive disease.

49. 1. Hot dogs and chips are too high in sodium and fat.
2. **Chicken is a good source of protein, and broccoli is a good choice for naturally occurring vitamins. The parent may have to chop the food up for the infant to safely eat.**
3. A banana is a food toddlers usually like. A child under 5 years should not eat nuts because they are a choking hazard for a child who does not chew food well.
4. A milkshake has a high amount of fat, as does a hamburger.

TEST-TAKING HINT: The test taker must know good-quality foods that should be offered to children.

50. 1. Pulse oximetry measures the oxygen percentage in the blood. It can be assessed after the child's vital signs are determined.
2. **The first intervention is to check the respiratory rate of the child to see if it is abnormal, then listen to the lung sounds, and then check pulse oximetry.**
3. The first intervention is to check the respiratory rate of the child to see if it is abnormal, then listen to the lung sounds, and then check pulse oximetry.
4. The first intervention is to check the respiratory rate of the child to see if it is abnormal, then listen to the lung sounds, and then check pulse oximetry. Asking if the child coughs at night would be helpful information as well.

TEST-TAKING HINT: The test taker would first count respirations to determine whether the rate is normal for a child that age. Auscultation comes next, then pulse oximetry if needed.

51. 1. When children present with recurring respiratory symptoms, the disease etiology is frequently viral.
2. When children present with neurological symptoms after a viral respiratory illness, the nurse should consider the symptoms to be a complication of the viral illness until proved otherwise.
3. **This child probably has GBS, which is an acute inflammatory demyelinating neuropathy.**
4. When neurological symptoms follow an acute viral illness, the CNs are frequently involved.

TEST-TAKING HINT: Having a prior upper respiratory infection usually means this condition is not caused by bacteria, which eliminates answers 1 and 2. That leaves the choice between answers 3 and 4.

52. 1. Children with GBS frequently have urinary retention, so catheterization is necessary. Complications of GBS are usually respiratory and swallowing difficulties. Checking the serum blood urea nitrogen can be done but would take too long. Eight hours is quite a lengthy time for the child not to have voided.
2. The complete blood count does not provide helpful information about urinary retention.
3. **The child must be in-and-out catheterized to avoid the possibility of developing a urinary tract infection from urine left in the bladder for too long.**
4. Running water in the bathroom is a strategy used frequently to encourage patients to void. It takes time for it to work, however, and sometimes it does not have the intended results.

TEST-TAKING HINT: Urinary retention occurs with GBS, and catheterization is necessary in a child who has had lots of fluids but not voided in 8 hours.

53. 1. The goal is to prevent complications related to immobility. Efforts include maintaining skin integrity, maintaining respiratory function, and preventing contractures. Constipation is a concern, but not the primary concern.
2. Most children recover completely, so there is no chronic sorrow.
3. **The goal is to prevent complications related to immobility. Efforts include maintaining skin integrity, maintaining respiratory function, and preventing contractures.**
4. GBS is a disease affecting the peripheral nervous system, not the cardiac muscle.

TEST-TAKING HINT: The test taker must have a basic understanding of GBS and know that it affects the peripheral nervous system.

54. 3, 5.
1. Referral to OT would have been done depending on the degree of fine motor involvement.
2. Because grooming and dressing are life skills the child may need to relearn, referral to PT would be appropriate and done earlier in the course of treatment.

3. Working with the child's teacher and the school staff to keep the child at the same pace as his classmates is crucial for the healthy recovery of the child.
4. GBS does not affect cognitive functioning.
5. Beginning active physical therapy is important for helping muscle recovery and preventing contractures.

TEST-TAKING HINT: The test taker must know the normal progress of the disease, which may take weeks or months for recovery to occur. A hint is provided by the word "recovery" in the question.

55. **1, 3.**
1. Symptoms in a child with myasthenia gravis include fatigue, double vision, ptosis, and difficulty swallowing and chewing. This is an autoimmune disease triggered by a viral or bacterial infection. Antibodies attack acetylcholine receptors and block their functioning.
2. Tremors and seizures are not generally seen in myasthenia gravis.
3. Symptoms in a child with myasthenia gravis include fatigue and difficulty swallowing and chewing.
4. The paralysis tends to wax and wane but is not the result of an ascending paralysis. The paralysis is first noticed in the eye muscles and eyelids and then progresses. It is the result of the neuromuscular junction not being able to send the acetylcholine to the muscle.
5. Myasthenia gravis does not cause any sensory disturbances.

TEST-TAKING HINT: The test taker must know the signs and symptoms of myasthenia gravis in children. This is an autoimmune disease triggered by a viral infection in which antibodies attack acetylcholine receptors and block their functioning.

56. **3, 4.**
1. Children with myasthenia gravis should not play strenuous sports. The increased stress from being in a competitive sport tends to negatively impact children, and they should learn strategies to decrease stress.
2. It is important that children with myasthenia gravis have activities they can participate in without causing stress. Activities such as board games, horseback riding, and hiking should be encouraged. Some children would benefit from meditation but may take time to appreciate the results.

3. Children with myasthenia gravis can do many things other children do. They should be advised not to play strenuous sports, and they should learn how to control stress.
4. Children are watched for signs of illness because of the exacerbation of signs of myasthenia gravis.
5. It's not recommended that children sleep in the same bedroom as their parents unless it can't be avoided.

TEST-TAKING HINT: The test taker must know the physiology of the illness and consider that this is a chronic disease. The child is first a child, so he will have all the growth and development issues children without a chronic disease have.

57. **1.** Constipation means hard stools and infrequent passage. Adding extra water to the diet helps make the stool softer in a child of this age.
2. It is not recommended to add corn syrup or honey to the bottle of a child younger than 12 months because of the danger of botulism.
3. It is not recommended to give an infant a glycerine suppository for hard, infrequent stools; constipation should be managed with dietary changes.
4. Regular bowel elimination minimizes abdominal pain and the typical 6-month-old has two or three soft stools a day. Adding additional water daily is the easiest first step in handling constipation.

TEST-TAKING HINT: The test taker must know how to treat constipation in an infant, which is different from treating it in a child.

58. **1.** A 7-year-old child who is not fully immunized and has a tetanus-prone wound should receive TdaP vaccine to prevent tetanus. Tetanus-prone wounds include puncture wounds and those contaminated with dirt, feces, or soil.
2. An antibiotic probably will be started, but administering TdaP vaccine is the priority.
3. Wounds are routinely cleansed with soap and water. Hydrogen peroxide does not clean better.
4. This child can be cared for in the clinic.

TEST-TAKING HINT: The test taker must know about wound care and which wounds are considered contaminated.

59. 3, 4, 5.

1. A brachial plexus injury in an infant (resulting from tearing or stretching of a nerve) usually occurs with large babies and breech delivery.
2. A brachial plexus injury in an infant (resulting from tearing or stretching of a nerve) usually occurs with large babies and breech delivery.
3. **The infant will have an absent Moro reflex on one side and no sensory loss.**
4. **The infant will have an absent Moro reflex on one side and no sensory loss.**
5. **The injury may be associated with a fractured clavicle.**

TEST-TAKING HINT: The test taker must know what a brachial plexus is and how an injury would affect it.

60.
1. C1–C5 is too high, because the patient has the use of the arms and sensation to the nipple line.
2. C5–C7 is too high, because the patient still has the use of the arms.
3. **Damage at T1–T4 manifests at or just below the nipple line. Every area below would be affected.**
4. Sensation ends at the nipple line, so T5–T12 is too low.
5. L2–L5 is too low, because the patient has sensation only to the nipple line.
6. S1–S5 is too low.

TEST-TAKING HINT: Deficits occur at and below the level of injury.

61. 2, 3, 5.
1. A decrease in blood pressure does not contribute to autonomic dysreflexia. Increased blood pressure usually occurs with autonomic dysreflexia.
2. **Autonomic dysreflexia may be caused by abdominal pressure from a fecal impaction.**
3. **An distended bladder is usually the precipitating factor causing an increase in abdominal pressure.**
4. Fecal impaction and constipation, not diarrhea, can be causes of autonomic dysreflexia.
5. **Tight clothing can increase pressure to the central core of the body.**
6. Hyperthermia does not cause autonomic dysreflexia.

TEST-TAKING HINT: Autonomic dysreflexia most often occurs because of an irritating stimulus within the body below the level of spinal cord injury.

Orthopedic Disorders

12

KEYWORDS

The following words include English vocabulary, nursing/medical terminology, concepts, principles, or information relevant to content specifically addressed in the chapter or associated with topics presented in it. English dictionaries, your nursing textbooks, and medical dictionaries such as *Taber's Cyclopedic Medical Dictionary* are resources that can be used to expand your knowledge and understanding of these words and related information.

Abduction

Adduction

Growth plate

Osteomyelitis

Pavlik harness

Pes cavus

Pes planus

Synovial fluid

ABBREVIATIONS

Developmental dysplasia of the hip (DDH)

Intravenous fluids (IVF)

Juvenile rheumatoid arthritis (JRA)

Nonsteroidal anti-inflammatory drugs (NSAIDs)

Osteogenesis imperfecta (OI)

Patient-controlled analgesia (PCA)

Slipped capital femoral epiphysis (SCFE)

Systemic lupus erythematosus (SLE)

QUESTIONS

1. Which would the nurse expect to assess on a 3-week-old infant with developmental dysplasia of the hip (DDH)? **Select all that apply.**
   1. Excessive hip abduction.
   2. Femoral lengthening of an affected leg.
   3. Asymmetry of gluteal and thigh folds.
   4. Pain when lying prone.
   5. Positive Ortolani test.

2. Which should the nurse stress to the parents of an infant in a Pavlik harness for treatment of developmental dysplasia of the hip (DDH)?
   1. Put socks on over the foot pieces of the harness to help stabilize the harness.
   2. Use lotions or powder on the skin to prevent rubbing of straps.
   3. Remove harness during diaper changes for ease of cleaning diaper area.
   4. Check under the straps at least two to three times daily for red areas.

3. Which can occur in untreated developmental dysplasia of the hip (DDH)? **Select all that apply.**
   1. Duck gait.
   2. Pain.
   3. Osteoarthritis in adulthood.
   4. Osteoporosis in adulthood.
   5. Increased flexibility of the hip joint in adulthood.

4. The nurse is teaching about congenital clubfoot in infants. The nurse evaluates the teaching as successful when the parent states that clubfoot is best treated when?
   1. Immediately after diagnosis.
   2. At age 4 to 6 months.
   3. Prior to walking (age 9 to 12 months).
   4. After walking is established (age 15 to 18 months).

5. Which is the definition of "talipes varus"?
   1. An inversion or bending inward of the foot.
   2. An eversion or bending outward of the foot.
   3. A high arch of the foot.
   4. A turning in of the forefoot.

6. The nurse tells the parent that other conditions can be associated with congenital clubfoot. **Select all that apply.**
   1. Myelomeningocele.
   2. Cerebral palsy.
   3. Diastrophic dwarfism.
   4. Breech position in utero.
   5. Prematurity.
   6. Fetal alcohol spectrum disorder.

7. When planning a rehabilitative approach for a child with osteogenesis imperfecta (OI), the nurse should prevent which of the following? **Select all that apply.**
   1. Positional contractures and deformities.
   2. Bone infection.
   3. Muscle weakness.
   4. Osteoporosis.
   5. Misalignment of lower extremity joints.

8. Which classification of osteogenesis imperfecta (OI) is lethal in utero and in infancy?
   1. Type I.
   2. Type II.
   3. Type III.
   4. Type IV.

9. When counseling the parents of a child with osteogenesis imperfecta (OI), the nurse should include which of the following? **Select all that apply.**
   1. Discourage future children because the condition is inherited.
   2. Provide education about the child's physical limitations.
   3. Give the parents a letter signed by the primary care provider explaining OI.
   4. Provide information on contacting the Osteogenesis Imperfecta Foundation.
   5. Encourage the parents to treat the child like their other children.
   6. Encourage use of calcium to decrease risk of fractures.

10. Which factor is associated with slipped capital femoral epiphysis (SCFE)? **Select all that apply.**
    1. Obesity.
    2. Female gender.
    3. Family history of SCFE.
    4. Age of 5 to 9 years.
    5. Pubertal hormonal changes.
    6. Endocrine disorders.

11. Which should be obtained to make a diagnosis of slipped capital femoral epiphysis (SCFE)?
    1. A history of hip trauma.
    2. A physical examination of hip, thigh, and knees.
    3. A complete blood count.
    4. A radiographic examination of the hip.

12. Which should be included in teaching a family about postsurgical care for slipped capital femoral epiphysis (SCFE)? **Select all that apply.**
    1. The client will receive help with weight-bearing ambulation 24 to 48 hours after surgery.
    2. Monitoring of pain medication to prevent drug dependence.
    3. Instruction on pin site care.
    4. Offering low-calorie meals to encourage weight loss.
    5. Correct use of crutches by the client.
    6. Exercises to strengthen hip and leg muscles.

13. Which would the nurse assess in a child diagnosed with osteomyelitis? **Select all that apply.**
    1. Unwillingness to move affected extremity.
    2. Severe pain.
    3. Fever.
    4. Previous closed fracture of an extremity.
    5. Redness and swelling at the site.

14. The parent of a child diagnosed with osteomyelitis asks how the child acquired the illness. Which is the nurse's best response?
    1. "Direct inoculation of the bone from stepping barefoot on a sharp stick."
    2. "An infection from a scratched mosquito bite carried the infection through the bloodstream to the bone."
    3. "The blood supply to the bone was disrupted because of the child's diabetes."
    4. "An infection of the upper respiratory tract."

15. A 10-year-old with osteomyelitis has been on intravenous antibiotics for 48 hours. The child is allergic to amoxicillin. Vital signs are T 101.8°F (38.8°C), BP 100/60, P 96, R 24. Which is the primary reason for surgical treatment?
    1. Young age.
    2. Drug allergies.
    3. Nonresponse to intravenous antibiotics.
    4. Health-care provider preference.

16. The nurse expects the blood culture report of an 8-year-old with septic arthritis to grow which causative organism?
    1. *Streptococcus pneumoniae.*
    2. *Escherichia coli.*
    3. *Staphylococcus aureus.*
    4. *Neisseria gonorrhoeae.*

17. Which instruction should the nurse give the parents of an adolescent with slipped capital femoral epiphysis (SCFE)? **Select all that apply.**
    1. Continue upper body exercises to limit loss of muscle strength.
    2. Do not turn the teen in bed when complaining of pain.
    3. Provide homework, computer games, and other activities to decrease boredom.
    4. Do most activities of daily living for the teen.
    5. Expect expressions of anger and hostility.
    6. Continue setting limits on behavior.

18. The parent of a 3-week-old states that the infant was recasted this morning for clubfoot and has been crying for the past hour. Which intervention should the nurse suggest the parent do first?
    1. Give pain medication.
    2. Reposition the infant in the crib.
    3. Check the neurocirculatory status of the foot.
    4. Use a cool blow-dryer to blow into the cast to control itching.

19. Which should the nurse include in the teaching plan for a child who had surgery to correct bilateral clubfeet and had the casts removed? **Select all that apply.**
    1. "Your child will need to wear a brace on the feet 23 hours a day for 12 months."
    2. "Your child should see an orthopedic surgeon regularly until the age of 18 years."
    3. "Your child will not be able to participate in sports that require a lot of running."
    4. "Your child may have a recurrence of clubfoot in a year or more."
    5. "Most children treated for clubfeet develop feet that appear and function normally."
    6. "Most children treated for clubfeet require surgery at puberty."

20. Which part(s) of the body should the nurse assess on a child in a spica cast? List the relevant label(s) from the following figure. _____

21. When a child is suspected of having osteomyelitis, the nurse can prepare the family to expect which of the following? **Select all that apply.**
    1. Pain medication is contraindicated so that symptoms are not masked.
    2. Blood cultures will be obtained.
    3. Pus will be aspirated from the subperiosteum.
    4. An intravenous line with antibiotics will be started.
    5. Surgery will be necessary.

22. Where should the top of the crutch bar be in relation to the axilla?

    _____

23. Select the number of inches lateral to the heel where a crutch should be placed.
    1. 1 to 3.
    2. 4 to 5.
    3. 6 to 8.
    4. 9 to 10.

24. Which is most important when teaching a parent about preventing osteomyelitis?
    1. Parents can stop worrying about bone infection once their child reaches school age.
    2. Parents need to clean open wounds thoroughly with soap and water.
    3. Children will always get a fever if they have osteomyelitis.
    4. Children should wear long pants when playing outside because their legs might get scratched.

25. The nurse caring for a child with osteomyelitis assesses poor appetite. Which intervention is most appropriate for this child? **Select all that apply.**
    1. Offer high-calorie liquids.
    2. Offer favorite foods.
    3. Do not worry about intake, because appetite loss is expected.
    4. Suggest removal of the intravenous line to encourage oral intake.
    5. Decrease pain medication that might cause nausea.
    6. Offer frequent small meals.

26. The nurse on the pediatric floor is receiving a child with the possible diagnosis of septic arthritis of the elbow. Which would the nurse expect on assessment? **Select all that apply.**
    1. Resistance to bending the elbow.
    2. Nausea and vomiting.
    3. Fever.
    4. Bruising of the elbow.
    5. Swelling of the elbow.
    6. A history of nursemaid's elbow as a toddler.

27. A 12-year-old diagnosed with scoliosis is to wear a brace for 23 hours a day. What is the most likely reason the child will not wear it for that long?
    1. Pain from the brace.
    2. Difficulty in putting the brace on.
    3. Self-consciousness about appearance.
    4. Not understanding what the brace is for.

28. A spinal curve of less than _____ degrees that is nonprogressive does not require treatment for scoliosis.

29. A 13-year-old just returned from surgery for scoliosis. Which nursing intervention is appropriate in the first 24 hours? **Select all that apply.**
    1. Assess for pain.
    2. Logroll to change positions.
    3. Get the teen to the bathroom 12 to 24 hours after surgery.
    4. Check neurological status.
    5. Monitor blood pressure.

30. A 9-year-old is in a spica cast and complains of pain 1 hour after receiving intravenous opioid analgesia. What should the nurse do first?
    1. Give more pain medication.
    2. Perform a neuromuscular assessment.
    3. Call the surgeon for orders.
    4. Change the child's position.

31. A 14-year-old with osteogenesis imperfecta (OI) is confined to a wheelchair. Which nursing interventions will promote normal development? **Select all that apply.**
    1. Encourage participation in groups with teens who have disabilities or chronic illness.
    2. Encourage decorating the wheelchair with stickers.
    3. Encourage transfer of primary care to an adult provider at age 18 years.
    4. Allow the teen to view the radiographs.
    5. Help the teen set realistic goals for the future.
    6. Discourage discussion of sexuality, because the child is not likely to date.

32. After the birth of an infant with clubfoot, the nursery nurse should do which of the following when instructing the parents? **Select all that apply.**
    1. Speak in simple language about the defect.
    2. Avoid the parents unless providing direct care so that they can grieve privately.
    3. Keep the infant's feet covered at all times.
    4. Present the infant as precious; emphasize the well-formed parts of the body.
    5. Tell the parent that defects could be much worse.
    6. Be prepared to answer questions multiple times.

33. The nurse should be suspicious of which condition in the following figure?

34. Name the harness in the following figure.

35. Which condition is the harness used for in the following figure?

36. When instructing a family about care of an orthosis, the nurse should emphasize which of the following?
1. Clean the brace with diluted bleach.
2. Dry the brace over a heater or in the sun.
3. Clean the brace weekly with mild soap and water.
4. Return the brace to the orthopedic surgeon for cleaning.

37. When teaching parents about osteosarcoma, the nurse knows instruction has been successful when a parent says that this type of cancer is common in which age-group?
    1. Infants.
    2. Toddlers.
    3. School-age children.
    4. Adolescents.

38. A child with osteosarcoma is going to receive chemotherapy before surgery. Which statement by the parents indicates they understand the side effect of neutropenia?
    1. "My child will be more at risk for diarrhea."
    2. "My child will be more at risk for infection."
    3. "My child's hair will fall out."
    4. "My child will need to drink more."

39. Which is most important to discuss with an adolescent who is going to have a leg amputation for osteosarcoma?
    1. Pain.
    2. Spirituality.
    3. Body image.
    4. Lack of coping.

40. Which would be the best nursing intervention for a child with phantom pain after an amputation?
    1. Tell the child that the pain does not exist.
    2. Request a PCA pump from the physician for pain management.
    3. Encourage the child to rub the stump.
    4. Provide amitriptyline (Elavil) to help with pain.

41. Use the following labels to name the places on the bone in the following figure.
    1. Epiphysis.
    2. Diaphysis.
    3. Epiphyseal plate.
    4. Medullary cavity.
    5. Calcaneus bone.
    6. Compact bone.

42. The nurse is teaching an adolescent about Ewing sarcoma and indicates which as a common site?
    1. Shaft.
    2. Growth plate.
    3. Ball of the femur.
    4. Bone marrow.

43. Which nursing diagnosis is most important for a child with Ewing sarcoma who will be undergoing chemotherapy?
    1. Risk for fluid volume deficit.
    2. Potential for chronic pain.
    3. Risk for skin impairment.
    4. Ineffective airway clearance.

44. A child is going to receive radiation for Ewing sarcoma. Which of the following is the best nursing intervention to prevent skin breakdown during therapy?
    1. Advise the child to wear loose-fitting clothes to minimize irritation.
    2. Advise the child to use emollients to prevent dry skin.
    3. Apply cold packs nightly to reduce the warmth caused by the treatments.
    4. Apply hydrocortisone to soothe itching from dry skin.

45. A child with Ewing sarcoma is undergoing a limb salvage procedure. Which statement indicates the parents understand the procedure?
    1. "Our child will have a bone graft to save the limb."
    2. "Our child will need follow-up lengthening procedures."
    3. "Our child will need shorter shirt sleeves."
    4. "Our child will not need chemotherapy."

46. A child with Ewing sarcoma is receiving chemotherapy and is experiencing severe nausea. The nurse has to administer lorazepam (Ativan) at 0.04 mg/kg, and the child weighs 65 lb. What dose should the nurse administer? _____

47. The nurse is explaining rhabdomyosarcoma cancer to an adolescent. From which of the following muscles does the cancer arise?
    1. Skeletal.
    2. Cardiac.
    3. Striated.
    4. Connective.

48. A child is diagnosed with stage IV rhabdomyosarcoma, and the parent asks what that means. The nurse provides which of the following explanations?
    1. The tumor is limited to the organ site.
    2. There is regional disease from the organ involved.
    3. There is distant metastatic disease.
    4. The disease is limited to the lymph nodes.

49. The nurse evaluates teaching as successful when the parent explains that an excisional biopsy is done for which reason?
    1. To find metastatic disease.
    2. To remove all metastatic disease.
    3. To confirm the type of metastatic disease.
    4. To treat metastatic disease.

50. It is recommended that a child with metastatic rhabdomyosarcoma undergo a bone marrow transplant. Education regarding life-threatening side effects should include:
    1. Diarrhea.
    2. Fever.
    3. Skin breakdown.
    4. Tumor shrinkage.

51. Which of the following applies to the care of a child with a retroperitoneal rhabdomyosarcoma? **Select all that apply.**
    1. Acute pain.
    2. Risk for impaired urinary elimination.
    3. Impaired gas exchange.
    4. Self-care deficit.
    5. Risk for constipation.

52. The nurse is teaching the parent of a child newly diagnosed with juvenile idiopathic arthritis (JIA). The nurse would evaluate the teaching as successful when the parent is able to say that the disorder is caused by the:
    1. Breakdown of osteoclasts in the joint space causing bone loss.
    2. Loss of cartilage in the joints.
    3. Buildup of calcium crystals in joint spaces.
    4. Immune-stimulated inflammatory response in the joint.

53. Which would the nurse teach an adolescent is a complication of corticosteroids used in the treatment of juvenile idiopathic arthritis (JIA)?
    1. Fat loss.
    2. Adrenal stimulation.
    3. Immune suppression.
    4. Hypoglycemia.

54. Which would the nurse teach a patient when NSAIDs are prescribed for treating juvenile idiopathic arthritis (JIA)?
    1. Take with food.
    2. Take on an empty stomach.
    3. Blood levels are required for drug dosages.
    4. Good oral hygiene is needed.

55. Why are chemotherapeutic agents such as methotrexate (Trexall) and cyclophosphamide (Cytoxan) sometimes used to treat juvenile idiopathic arthritis (JIA)?
    1. Are effective against cancer-like JIA.
    2. Suppress the immune system.
    3. Are similar to NSAIDs.
    4. Are absorbed into the synovial fluid.

56. One nursing diagnosis for juvenile idiopathic arthritis (JIA) is impaired physical mobility. **Select all that apply.**
    1. Give pain medication prior to ambulation.
    2. Assist with range-of-motion activities.
    3. Encourage the child to eat a high-fat diet.
    4. Provide oxygen as necessary.
    5. Use nonpharmacological methods, such as heat.

57. The nurse is teaching the parent of a child diagnosed with systemic lupus erythematosus (SLE). The nurse evaluates the teaching as effective when the parent states:
    1. "The cause is unknown."
    2. "There is no genetic involvement."
    3. "Drugs are not a trigger for the illness."
    4. "Antibodies improve disease outcome."

58. A child is admitted to the pediatric unit with the diagnosis of systemic lupus erythematosus (SLE). On assessment, the nurse expects the child to have which of the following signs and symptoms? **Select all that apply.**
    1. Oral ulcers.
    2. Malar rash.
    3. Weight gain.
    4. Heart failure.
    5. Anemia

59. Which is an important nursing intervention to teach about photosensitivity to the parents of a child with systemic lupus erythematosus (SLE)?
    1. Regular clothing is appropriate for sun exposure.
    2. Sunscreen application is necessary for protection.
    3. Teenage patients cannot participate in outdoor sports.
    4. Uncovered fluorescent lights offer no danger.

60. Which is an important nursing intervention to monitor in a child with systemic lupus erythematosus (SLE) and renal involvement?
    1. Monitor weight.
    2. Check for uric salts in urine.
    3. Watch for hypotension.
    4. Check for protein in urine.

61. Because estrogen is a possible trigger for a systemic lupus erythematosus (SLE) flare, advice for a teenage girl who may become sexually active includes which of the following? **Select all that apply.**
    1. Use Ortho Tri-Cyclen.
    2. Use Depo-Provera.
    3. Practice abstinence.
    4. Use condoms.
    5. Use Ortho Evra.

62. A 6-year-old involved in a bicycle crash has a spleen injury and a right tibia/fibula fracture that has been casted. Which is an early sign of compartment syndrome in this child? **Select all that apply.**
    1. Edema.
    2. Numbness.
    3. Severe pain.
    4. Weak pulse.
    5. Anular rash.

63. Nursing care of a child with a fractured extremity in whom there is suspected compartment syndrome includes which of the following? **Select all that apply.**
    1. Assess pain.
    2. Assess pulses.
    3. Elevate extremity above the level of the heart.
    4. Monitor capillary refill.
    5. Provide pain medication as needed.

64. Which is the nurse's best explanation to the parent of a toddler who asks what a greenstick fracture is?
    1. It is a fracture located in the growth plate of the bone.
    2. Because children's bones are not fully developed, any fracture in a young child is called a greenstick fracture.
    3. It is a fracture in which a complete break occurs in the bone, and small pieces of bone are broken off.
    4. It is a fracture that does not go all the way through the bone.

65. A nurse is caring for a 5-year-old who has a fracture of the tibia involving the growth plate. When providing information to the parents, the nurse should indicate that:
    1. This is a serious injury that could cause long-term growth issues.
    2. The fracture usually heals within 6 weeks without further complications.
    3. The child will never be able to play contact sports.
    4. Fractures involving the growth plate require pain medication.

The correct answer number and rationale for why it is the correct answer are given in **boldface blue type**. Rationales for why the other possible answer options are incorrect also are given, but they are not in boldface type.

1. **3, 5.**
   1. In DDH, a newborn can have excessive hip adduction.
   2. In DDH, an appearance of femoral shortening is frequently present on the affected side.
   3. **In DDH, asymmetrical thigh and gluteal folds are frequently present.**
   4. Infants do not experience pain from this condition.
   5. **The Ortolani maneuver moves a disclocated hip back into the socket with a distinct clunk.**

   TEST-TAKING HINT: If the test taker knows that DDH decreases smooth movement of the femoral head, then answers 1 and 2 can be eliminated because they indicate increased movement of the femur.

2. 1. Socks should be put on under the straps to prevent rubbing of the skin. The harness is stable if fitted correctly.
   2. Lotions and powders tend to cake and irritate under the straps. Their use is not recommended.
   3. The harness is not to be removed except in specific conditions and after instruction on removal and refitting. Diapering is easily done with the harness in place.
   4. **Checking under straps frequently is suggested to prevent skin breakdown.**

   TEST-TAKING HINT: The test taker can eliminate answer 1 because the question is about skin redness and irritation, not harness fit.

3. **1, 2, 3.**
   1. **Due to abnormal hip joint function, the client's gait is stiff and waddling.**
   2. **Due to abnormal femoral head placement, the client may experience pain and decreased flexibility in adulthood.**
   3. **Due to abnormal femoral head placement, the client may experience osteoarthritis in the hip joint in adulthood.**
   4. There is no increased risk for osteoporosis.
   5. There is no increased flexibility of the hip joint in adulthood.

   TEST-TAKING HINT: If the test taker knows that untreated DDH leads to decreased smooth movement of hip joint, then answer 5 can be eliminated.

4. 1. **The best outcomes for clubfoot are seen if casting begins as soon as the diagnosis is made, usually at birth.**
   2. Although casting helps if started in the newborn period, the delay of even 4 to 6 months postpones the positive outcome.
   3. Infants of 9 months are already pulling up to stand and taking steps. Clubfoot puts weight on surfaces of the feet that are not meant for weight-bearing.
   4. Clubfoot does not allow for normal gait, and the delay will decrease the likelihood of a successful outcome.

   TEST-TAKING HINT: The general principle of early treatment of orthopedic problems should lead to the correct answer.

5. 1. **"Talipes varus" is an inversion of the entire foot.**
   2. "Talipes valgus" is an eversion of the foot.
   3. "Pes cavus" is a high arch of the foot.
   4. Inversion of the forefoot is "metatarsus adductus."

   TEST-TAKING HINT: The test taker must know the definition of terms. "Varus" is defined as turning inward toward the body. "Valgus" means turning outward or going away from the midline.

6. **1, 2, 3.**
   1. **There is an association between myelomeningocele and congenital clubfoot.**
   2. **There is an association between some forms of cerebral palsy and congenital clubfoot.**
   3. **There is an association between diastrophic dwarfism and congenital clubfoot.**
   4. Breech position is not associated with congenital clubfoot. It is associated with DDH.
   5. There is no association between prematurity and congenital clubfoot.
   6. Fetal alcohol spectrum disorder is not associated with clubfoot.

   TEST-TAKING HINT: The test taker could look at other congenital deformities to gain a clue to an association to clubfoot.

7. **1, 3, 4, 5.**
   1. **A long-term goal in caring for a child with OI is to prevent contractures and deformities.**
   2. There is no increased risk for bone infection in OI.
   3. **A long-term goal in caring for a child with OI is to prevent muscle weakness.**
   4. **A long-term goal in caring for a child with OI is to prevent osteoporosis.**
   5. **A long-term goal in caring for a child with OI is to prevent misalignment of lower extremity joints.**

   TEST-TAKING HINT: The test taker should think about general nursing considerations for children with fractures and choose answers 1, 3, 4, and 5.

8. 1. Type I is the most common form. It is characterized by little deformity, variable fractures, blue sclera, hearing loss common in the 20s, and a normal life span.
   2. **Type II is lethal in utero and in infancy because of multiple fractures and deformities and underdeveloped lungs.**
   3. Type III is characterized by fractures, deformities, and short stature. Patients rarely live to age 30 years.
   4. Type IV is similar to type I but not associated with blue sclera.

   TEST-TAKING HINT: The test taker might be tempted to choose type IV, thinking that the higher number (IV) is the most severe form of OI.

9. **2, 3, 4.**
   1. Genetic counseling should be provided as part of long-term care so that the parents can make an informed decision about future children.
   2. **The nurse should provide education about the child's physical limitations so that physical therapy and appropriate activity can be encouraged.**
   3. **OI is frequently confused with child abuse. Carrying a letter stating that the child has OI and what that condition looks like can ease the stressors of an emergency department visit.**
   4. **The Osteogenesis Imperfecta Foundation is an organization that can provide information and support for a family with a child with the condition.**
   5. Children with OI must be treated with careful handling and cannot be allowed to participate in all activities that unaffected siblings are allowed.

6. There is no support for the use of additional calcium to decrease fractures.

   TEST-TAKING HINT: The test taker can eliminate answer 1 because it is based on the nurse's values, not necessarily those of the parents.

10. **1, 3, 5, 6.**
    1. **Obesity increases the risk of SCFE by stressing the epiphyseal plate.**
    2. SCFE is more common in males.
    3. **Risk factors include a family history of SCFE.**
    4. SCFE is most common from the ages of 10 to 16 years.
    5. **SCFE is most common during pubertal hormonal changes.**
    6. **SCFE is associated with endocrine disorders such as hyperthyroidism.**

    TEST-TAKING HINT: If the test taker knows that SCFE is most common during rapid growth, answer 4 can be eliminated, and answer 5 can be chosen.

11. 1. In most cases of SCFE, there is no history of trauma to the hip. There is sudden onset of pain, often after a fall.
    2. Physical examination may reveal some restriction of rotation of the hip, but it is not diagnostic.
    3. There is no change in blood laboratory values with SCFE. Radiographic examination is the only definitive tool for diagnosis of SCFE.
    4. **Radiographic examination is the only definitive diagnostic tool for SCFE.**

    TEST-TAKING HINT: The most definitive tool in assessing a hip is radiographic examination.

12. **3, 5, 6.**
    1. Ambulation is to be non-weight-bearing with crutches until range of motion is painless. This is usually 4 to 8 weeks.
    2. Pain medication is to be administered regularly during hospitalization to provide comfort to the patient and encourage cooperation with daily activities and ambulation. Drug dependence for the postoperative patient is not a significant concern.
    3. **The parents will be assessing pin sites for infection and stability upon discharge. Instructions on care should be demonstrated for and then by the parents.**

4. Although obesity is often a factor in SCFE, the patient requires adequate caloric intake for healing and recovery postoperatively. Obesity issues can be addressed after surgical recovery.
5. **Instruction on crutch usage will be given prior to discharge. Crutch walking will not be done during the early postoperative stage.**
6. **The physical therapist will give the client exercises to strengthen the hip and leg muscles.**

TEST-TAKING HINT: The test taker should be able to rule out answer 2 by understanding the safe use of pain medication in the immediate postoperative period.

13. **1, 2, 3, 5.**
    1. **Pain in an extremity leads to resistance to movement.**
    2. **Pain is frequently severe in osteomyelitis.**
    3. **Fever is present in the acute phase of the illness.**
    4. Osteomyelitis can sometimes be seen after a direct inoculation of an open fracture. There is no increased risk after a closed fracture.
    5. **Redness and swelling occur because of the infection.**

TEST-TAKING HINT: The test taker can rule out answer 4 if it is understood that a closed fracture does not increase the risk of bone infection.

14. 1. Although osteomyelitis can occur from direct inoculation, inoculation is not the most common cause.
    2. **Infection through the bloodstream is the most likely cause of osteomyelitis in a child.**
    3. Although osteomyelitis can occur because of blood supply disruption, that is more likely to occur in older adults. Diabetes does increase the risk of osteomyelitis, but diabetes is more common in older adults.
    4. A viral upper respiratory infection is not the most likely cause.

TEST-TAKING HINT: The age of the patient is important in choosing the most likely cause of the disease.

15. 1. All children with osteomyelitis are treated initially with intravenous antibiotics, regardless of age.
    2. Although drug allergies are a concern, antibiotic choices can be made to accommodate clients with specific drug allergies.

3. **If a client does not respond to an appropriate antibiotic within 48 hours, surgery may be indicated.**
4. Although there is some difference of opinion about the use of surgery in the treatment of osteomyelitis, the standard initial treatment is intravenous antibiotics.

TEST-TAKING HINT: Answer 4 should be eliminated because client treatment should be based on evidence.

16. 1. *S. pneumoniae* is more common in children younger than age 5 years, but it is not the most common organism.
    2. *E. coli* is more common in neonates, but it is also not the most common cause.
    3. ***S. aureus* is a common organism found on the skin and is frequently the cause of septic arthritis.**
    4. *N. gonorrhoeae* should be considered in sexually active patients, but it is not the most common organism.

TEST-TAKING HINT: The age of the child is important in choosing the correct answer.

17. **1, 3, 5, 6.**
    1. **Immobilization can lead to a decrease in muscle strength. Upper body exercises should be continued soon after surgery.**
    2. Although turning the client in bed after surgery may be painful, it is essential that parents and the client know that it is necessary to prevent skin ulcerations and promote healing.
    3. **It is important for this client to continue as many normal activities as possible. This should include schoolwork and leisure activities.**
    4. To promote independence that is essential for a teenager, this client should be encouraged to continue activities of daily living.
    5. **Some expressions of anger and hostility are normal, because this adolescent is losing some independence with this immobility.**
    6. **Continuation of setting limits on behavior is important to keep as much normality as possible.**

TEST-TAKING HINT: The test taker needs to understand the developmental need for independence in this age-group.

18. 1. The cause of the crying needs to be determined prior to administering pain medication.
    2. Although this is a good choice, it is not the first intervention.

3. Checking the neurocirculatory status of the foot is the highest priority.
4. Although this is a good choice for cast discomfort, it is not the first choice.

TEST-TAKING HINT: The test taker should prioritize nursing interventions and know that safety needs are paramount.

19. 1, 2, 4, 5.
1. After the final casting, bracing is required for 12 months. This decreases the likelihood of a recurrence.
2. Because clubfoot can recur, it is important to have regular follow-up with the orthopedic surgeon until age 18 years.
3. After treatment, most children are able to participate in any sport.
4. Even with proper bracing, there may be a recurrence.
5. Most children treated for clubfeet develop normally appearing and functioning feet.
6. Most children do not require surgery at puberty.

TEST-TAKING HINT: If the test taker is aware that clubfoot can recur, providing instruction that includes long-term follow-up care will help in selecting answers.

20. C, D.
The nurse needs to assess areas under the cast for drainage through the cast and assess neurocirculatory status of the feet.

TEST-TAKING HINT: The test taker should know to check for neurocirculatory status and wound drainage.

21. 2, 3, 4.
1. Medication will be given regularly to help with the pain.
2. Blood cultures will be obtained to determine the organism causing the infection.
3. Pus will be aspirated from the subperiosteum.
4. Antibiotics will be given via an intravenous line.
5. Surgery is indicated only when medication fails.

TEST-TAKING HINT: If the test taker is unsure of specific care for osteomyelitis, standard nursing care for infection can lead to correct choices.

22. The crutch bar should not put pressure on nerves in the axilla.

TEST-TAKING HINT: The axillae do not rest on the crutch bar.

23. 1. This position does not provide the best protection for balance and stability.
2. This position does not provide the best protection for balance and stability.
3. This position provides the best protection for balance and stability.
4. This position does not provide the best protection for balance and stability.

TEST-TAKING HINT: Consider the stance that is best for balance when standing.

24. 1. Osteomyelitis can occur in children older than school age.
2. Because bacteria from an open wound can lead to osteomyelitis, thorough cleaning with soap and water is the best prevention.
3. Children with osteomyelitis do not always have a fever.
4. It is not necessary to require children to wear long pants whenever playing outside.

TEST-TAKING HINT: The test taker can eliminate answers 1 and 3 because they do not address prevention.

25. 1, 2, 6.
1. High-calorie liquids are sometimes received better when the child has a poor appetite.
2. Offering favorite foods can sometimes tempt the child to eat, even with a poor appetite.
3. Although decreased appetite is expected, it is something that needs nursing intervention in order to promote healing.
4. An intravenous line is necessary for antibiotics, so it cannot be removed to encourage oral intake.
5. Although some pain medications cause nausea, their use is important. If clients are in pain, they are not likely to want to eat.
6. Frequent small meals might increase daily caloric intake.

TEST-TAKING HINT: Using routine nursing interventions for decreased appetite can lead to the correct answers.

26. 1, 2, 3, 5.
1. Infection of the elbow joint can cause pain that leads to protecting the joint and resisting movement.
2. Infection of the elbow may cause generalized nausea and vomiting.
3. Infection of the elbow frequently causes fever.

4. There is no bruising with septic arthritis.
5. **Septic arthritis can cause swelling of the joint.**
6. There is no increased risk with a history of nursemaid's elbow.

TEST-TAKING HINT: The test taker can rule out answer 6, because risk of infection is not related to past injury.

27. 1. Wearing the brace is not painful.
2. Putting on the brace is not difficult.
3. **Children this age are very conscious of their appearance and fitting in with their peers, so they might be very resistant to wearing a brace.**
4. Although a child this age might not fully understand how the brace helps the condition, that would not be the most likely cause of noncompliance.

TEST-TAKING HINT: The test taker must understand the development of children.

28. 20.
A 20-degree spinal curve that is nonprogressive will not disfigure or interfere with normal functioning, so it is not treated with bracing or surgery.

TEST-TAKING HINT: The test taker must know about treatment for scoliosis.

29. 1, 2, 4, 5.
1. **General postoperative nursing interventions include assessing for pain.**
2. **Specific to scoliosis surgery, logrolling is the means of changing positions.**
3. Patients may not be upright less than 24 hours postoperatively.
4. **It is essential to check neurological status in a patient who just had scoliosis surgery.**
5. **General postoperative nursing interventions include assessing vital signs.**

TEST-TAKING HINT: The test taker can use general postoperative care principles to lead to several correct answers.

30. 1. The nurse needs to assess the child prior to giving more pain medication.
2. **The nurse looks for the source of the pain by performing a neuromuscular assessment.**
3. If the neuromuscular assessment is normal, the nurse might need to call the surgeon for further orders.
4. The child's position should be changed to determine whether that helps with pain management after the neuromuscular assessment is performed.

TEST-TAKING HINT: The surgeon should be called only after an assessment of the client and a change of position is done. The test taker can rule out answer 3.

31. 1, 2, 4, 5.
1. **This client is trying to become more independent and trying to fit in with the peer group. Encouraging socializing with peers who face similar challenges alleviates feelings of isolation.**
2. **Decorating the wheelchair encourages the client to assume independence in self-care.**
3. It is not necessarily appropriate to transfer health care at age 18 years. If the teen is with a provider who has known the client and family most of the teen's life, it might be best to remain with that provider for several more years.
4. **Allowing the patient to view radiographs encourages the patient to assume self-care.**
5. **Helping the patient set realistic goals for the future encourages independence.**
6. It is appropriate for the nurse to discuss sexuality with this client. Being confined to a wheelchair does not preclude dating or becoming intimate.

TEST-TAKING HINT: The test taker can use knowledge of normal growth and development to help choose correct answers.

32. 1, 4, 6.
1. **The parents will likely be shocked immediately after the birth of the child. To facilitate their understanding, the nurse should speak in simple terms.**
2. Avoiding the parents is not therapeutic.
3. The baby should be shown to the parents as are all newborns, without hiding the clubfoot.
4. **The baby should be shown to the parents as are all newborns, emphasizing the well-formed parts of the body.**
5. Negating the parents' grieving is not therapeutic.
6. **Information may need to be repeated as the family begins to absorb the information.**

TEST-TAKING HINT: The test taker can draw on therapeutic communication skills to choose correct answers.

33. **DDH.**
The asymmetry of the thigh folds suggests DDH.

TEST-TAKING HINT: When assessing the infant's hips/legs the asymmetry of the thigh folds suggests DDH.

34. **Pavlik harness.**
The Pavlik harness is used to treat DDH diagnosed in the newborn period.

TEST-TAKING HINT: The harness places the hip joints in abduction.

35. **It is used for DDH.**
The Pavlik harness is used to treat DDH in neonates.

TEST-TAKING HINT: Being able to answer previous questions correctly can sometimes help with later questions.

36. 1. The use of bleach can damage the brace.
2. Drying the brace in direct sunlight or on a heater can warp it.
3. **An orthosis should be cleaned weekly with mild soap and water.**
4. The brace can be safely cleaned at home.

TEST-TAKING HINT: The test taker can rule out answer 4 because equipment care would not be confined to a physician's office.

37. 1. Osteosarcoma is a common cancer of adolescents.
2. Osteosarcoma is a common cancer of adolescents.
3. Osteosarcoma is a common cancer of adolescents.
4. **Osteosarcoma is a common cancer of adolescents.**

TEST-TAKING HINT: The test taker must remember that pediatric cancers usually develop during times of peak growth. Adolescence is the time of peak bone growth.

38. 1. Diarrhea is a side effect of chemotherapy, not neutropenia.
2. **Neutropenia makes a child more at risk for infection because the immune system is compromised by the chemotherapy.**
3. Alopecia is a side effect of chemotherapy, not neutropenia.
4. Dehydration is a potential side effect of chemotherapy, not neutropenia.

TEST-TAKING HINT: Knowledge of word parts can help in choosing the correct answer. "Neutropenia" consists of *neutro-* (meaning "neutrophils," a subset of the white blood cells) and *-penia* (meaning "low or decreased").

39. 1. Pain is a common concern, but adolescents are more concerned about their body image.

2. In general, adolescents are more concerned with their body image and not with spirituality.
3. **Body image is a developmental issue for adolescents and influences their acceptance of themselves and by peers.**
4. Body image is more of a concern for adolescents and should be addressed first by the nurse. Lack of coping is not a priority at this time.

TEST-TAKING HINT: The question asks for specific versus general anticipatory guidance issues.

40. 1. This is not a helpful intervention.
2. PCA is not necessary for phantom pain.
3. Rubbing the stump is not helpful and possibly harmful to healing.
4. **Amitriptyline (Elavil) is a medication for nerve pain that is helpful in relieving phantom pain.**

TEST-TAKING HINT: Knowing that phantom pain is due to nerve pain from the lost limb enables elimination of answer 2.

41.

Calcaneus bone
Epiphysis
Epiphyseal plate
Medullary cavity
Diaphysis
Compact bone

TEST-TAKING HINT: The test taker should look at each word and think about the parts of the bone. Separate the parts of the words and think about what their stems mean to help with locations.

42. 1. **Ewing sarcoma is a bone tumor that affects the shafts of long bones.**
2. Pediatric bone sarcomas do not affect the growth plate.

3. This is a specific location of a specific bone. Ewing sarcoma can affect multiple bones.
4. The bone marrow is a site for hematological cancers.

TEST-TAKING HINT: It is important to be familiar with the physiology of bones to understand how bone sarcomas affect them. Ewing sarcoma is a rare cancer that affects a different part of the bone relative to osteosarcoma.

43. 1. **Chemotherapy can cause nausea, vomiting, and possibly diarrhea, which contribute to fluid volume deficit.**
2. Chemotherapy itself does not cause chronic pain.
3. Radiation therapy has the potential for skin impairment.
4. This is not an acute problem with chemotherapy.

TEST-TAKING HINT: This is a general question asking for basic side effects of chemotherapy.

44. 1. **Loose clothing helps reduce irritation on the sensitive irradiated skin.**
2. Emollients are contraindicated during radiation because they can reflect the rays.
3. Irradiated skin is very sensitive to extreme temperatures; a cold pack could cause pain.
4. Hydrocortisone is not helpful for the radiation-induced itching; it is for atopic itching.

TEST-TAKING HINT: The test taker must know what is most helpful for relieving irritation caused by radiation. The question asks for what to do during therapy.

45. 1. Bone grafts are not part of limb salvage.
2. **Limb salvage requires lengthening procedures to encourage the bone to continue to grow so that the child will not have a short limb.**
3. This does not indicate understanding by the parents.
4. Having a limb salvage does not mean the child will never require chemotherapy as part of the treatment.

TEST-TAKING HINT: A limb salvage means the limb is saved, but that is not the end of treatment for the child.

46. 1.2 mg.
Change pounds to kilograms (2.2 lb = 1 kg: 65/2.2 = 29.5 kg). Then multiply kilograms by the dose of 0.04 mg/kg: 29.5 × 0.04 = 1.18 mg or round to 1.2 mg.

TEST-TAKING HINT: Divide 65 lb by 2.2 to determine kilograms.

47. 1. Striated muscle is in many organs and sites of the body, thus leading to the multiple sites of the disease.
2. Striated muscle is in many organs and sites of the body, thus leading to the multiple sites of the disease.
3. **Striated muscle is in many organs and sites of the body, thus leading to the multiple sites of the disease.**
4. There is no such muscle.

TEST-TAKING HINT: The test taker must understand the basic locations for each muscle listed.

48. 1. This is stage I disease.
2. This is stage II disease.
3. **Stage IV disease means there is distant metastatic disease.**
4. Lymph node involvement is not used as part of staging for rhabdomyosarcoma.

TEST-TAKING HINT: The test taker must be familiar with the basic staging of cancers.

49. 1. Metastatic disease is confirmed by a combination of tests.
2. A biopsy removes only a small piece of the tumor.
3. **A biopsy confirms the histology of the tumor.**
4. Chemotherapy, radiation, and surgery are required for treatment.

TEST-TAKING HINT: A biopsy is used to get the basic information of any solid cancer. Additional tests and procedures are part of treatment and more extensive diagnosis.

50. 1. Diarrhea can be a side effect of chemotherapy, but it is not usually life threatening.
2. **Fever indicates infection that can be life threatening after a bone marrow transplant.**
3. Skin breakdown is usually not life threatening.
4. Tumor shrinkage is expected with treatment, but it is not life threatening.

TEST-TAKING HINT: The test taker must understand what a bone marrow transplant involves and how bone marrow suppression can have life-threatening effects.

51. 1, 2, 5.
1. **Pain occurs because of pressure on the organs in the lower abdomen.**

2. **A retroperitoneal tumor affects the organs of the lower abdomen, including the bowel and bladder.**
3. A retroperitoneal tumor affects the organs of the lower abdomen, including the bowel and bladder. This tumor does not affect the lungs.
4. There is no indication the child cannot administer self-care.
5. **Because this tumor is in the lower abdomen, it puts pressure on the bowel, causing constipation.**

TEST-TAKING HINT: The test taker must understand the anatomy of the body. Having an idea of the organs involved will indicate possible problems that can arise when a tumor is in those locations.

52. 1. This is part of the normal breakdown and buildup of bone in the body.
2. This is part of the process for osteoarthritis.
3. This is the pathophysiology of calcium chondrosis.
4. **JIA is caused by an immune response by the body on the joint spaces.**

TEST-TAKING HINT: The test taker must understand JIA is an immune-modulated disorder in which the body attacks itself, causing destruction of the joint spaces.

53. 1. Long-term corticosteroid use causes fat deposits, especially in the back, face, and trunk.
2. With the use of corticosteroids, there is adrenal suppression because the exogenous steroid causes the body to lower production of its own steroids.
3. **Steroids cause immune suppression, which is the reason behind its use in JIA; it reduces the body's attack on itself.**
4. Steroids cause hyperglycemia.

TEST-TAKING HINT: The test taker must understand how immune system diseases work in order to know how treatments will be helpful. Consider how steroids work and their complications. Each answer listed, except the correct answer, is the opposite of the true side effects.

54. 1. **NSAIDs can cause gastric bleeding with long-term use; food helps to reduce the exposure of the drug on the stomach lining.**
2. NSAIDs can cause gastric bleeding with long-term use; food helps to reduce the exposure of the drug on the stomach lining.
3. NSAIDs do not require a blood level because they are available over the counter.

4. NSAIDs do not interfere with the oral cavity; however, other medications used for JIA cause oral ulcers.

TEST-TAKING HINT: The test taker must know what NSAIDs are and that they are available over the counter.

55. 1. JIA is not a type of cancer.
2. **These drugs affect the immune system to reduce its ability to attack itself, as in the case of JIA.**
3. These medications are not the same as NSAIDs.
4. They are not absorbed into the synovial fluid to treat JIA; they suppress the immune system.

TEST-TAKING HINT: There are some drugs that are used for other reasons outside of their usual use, such as chemotherapeutic agents. Many drugs have multiple uses.

56. 1, 2, 5.
1. **Providing pain medication prior to ambulation helps decrease pain during ambulation.**
2. **Children with JIA need to do range-of-motion exercises to prevent joint stiffness.**
3. A high-fat diet is not helpful for mobility.
4. Oxygen is usually not necessary with the diagnosis of JIA.
5. **Using nonpharmacological methods such as heat helps with flexibility and pain.**

TEST-TAKING HINT: By understanding the disease process of JIA, the test taker will know what interventions are needed to help alleviate pain and disability.

57. 1. **SLE is a complex disease; there are many triggers, but how the disease develops is not known.**
2. There is some correlation with family history.
3. There are multiple triggers for SLE, including prescription drugs.
4. Antibodies have nothing to do with SLE outcome.

TEST-TAKING HINT: Not all diseases have a known cause.

58. 1, 2, 5.
1. **Oral ulcers are a common early symptom. Typically, at least four symptoms must be present for the diagnosis of SLE.**
2. **The "butterfly," or malar, rash is the most common manifestation of SLE.**
3. Weight loss, not weight gain, is a symptom of SLE.

4. Heart failure is not a common manifestation, but it can occur after long-term disease that affects the heart muscle.
5. **Anemia is often a presenting symptom of SLE.**

TEST-TAKING HINT: By understanding the pathophysiology of SLE, the test taker will be able to find the correct answer.

59. 1. Sun-protective clothing is important, including hats.
2. **Sunscreen helps reduce accelerated burning due to sensitivity.**
3. Participating in sports is important for normality and should be encouraged.
4. Protection from uncovered fluorescent lights is as important as protection from ultraviolet A and B light.

TEST-TAKING HINT: In general, sunscreen is important for every question regarding sun exposure and photosensitivity.

60. 1. For renal impairment due to SLE, monitoring the child's weight is important, but checking the urine is a priority.
2. Uric salts are a normal concentrate of urine.
3. Hypertension, not hypotension, is a problem with renal involvement.
4. **Protein in urine is a sign of renal impairment, even in nephrotic syndrome, in which the kidneys are losing protein.**

TEST-TAKING HINT: The test taker must understand what can happen to the body when organs, such as the kidneys, fail.

61. **2, 3, 4.**
1. Ortho Tri-Cyclen contains estrogen; therefore, it is contraindicated.
2. **Depo-Provera contains progesterone and is the only contraceptive that is approved for use in sexually active women with SLE.**
3. **Abstinence is always recommended to prevent pregnancy.**
4. **Condoms are always recommended.**
5. Ortho Evra ("the patch") contains estrogen and is therefore not recommended.

TEST-TAKING HINT: The test taker must be familiar with the types of contraceptives and know which contain combination hormones versus progesterone only.

62. **1, 3.**
1. **Edema and pain are early signs of compartment syndrome.**
2. Numbness and tingling are late signs of compartment syndrome.

3. **Edema and pain are early signs of compartment syndrome.**
4. A weak pulse is a late sign of compartment syndrome.
5. There is no rash with early compartment syndrome.

TEST-TAKING HINT: The test taker can eliminate answers 2 and 5 because numbness, tingling and rash are not signs of early compartment syndrome.

63. **1, 2, 4, 5.**
1. **In a recent fracture, the nurse should assess pain and provide treatment.**
2. **Pain, pallor, and weak or absent pulses are all signs of compartment syndrome.**
3. Elevating the extremity is important to decrease edema prior to the onset of compartment syndrome. However, once compartment syndrome is suspected, the extremity should be kept at the level of the heart to facilitate arterial and venous flow.
4. **Weak or absent pulse is a sign of compartment syndrome, so monitoring capillary refill is important in assessment.**
5. **Pain, pallor, and weak or absent pulses are signs of compartment syndrome. Pain should be treated.**

TEST-TAKING HINT: The test taker can eliminate answer 3 because it is important to keep the affected extremity at heart level to help arterial and venous blood flow.

64. 1. It is a fracture that does not go all the way through the bone.
2. It is a fracture that does not go all the way through the bone.
3. It is a fracture that does not go all the way through the bone.
4. **It is a fracture that does not go all the way through the bone.**

TEST-TAKING HINT: The test taker must know the definition of a greenstick fracture.

65. 1. **Fractures of the growth plate are serious because they can disrupt the growth process.**
2. Long-term follow-up is usually needed to evaluate limb discrepancies and potential joint abnormalities.
3. The ability to participate in contact sports depends on many potential complications.
4. The amount of pain medication needed in all fractures is determined by the client.

TEST-TAKING HINT: The test taker must know that fractures that affect the growth plate are serious.

Neurological Disorders

KEYWORDS

The following words include English vocabulary, nursing/medical terminology, concepts, principles, or information relevant to content specifically addressed in the chapter or associated with topics presented in it. English dictionaries, your nursing textbooks, and medical dictionaries such as *Taber's Cyclopedic Medical Dictionary* are resources that can be used to expand your knowledge and understanding of these words and related information.

Absence seizure

Akinetic seizure

Anencephaly

Anterior fontanel

Apgar

Atonic seizure

Brachycephaly

Brudzinski sign

Cerebellum

Consciousness

Craniosynostosis

Cushing triad

Decerebrate posturing

Decorticate posturing

Delirium

Encephalitis

Epidural hematoma

Epilepsy

Hemiplegia

Hydrocephalus

Kernig sign

Ketogenic diet

Leukemia

Malignancy

Meningitis

Myelomeningocele

Neuroblastoma

Neurogenic bladder

Neurogenic shock

Neurological checks

Nuchal rigidity

Obtunded

Pancytopenia

Posturing

Reye syndrome

Seizure

Spina bifida occulta

Subdural hematoma

Ventricle

Ventriculoperitoneal shunt

ABBREVIATIONS

Cerebral palsy (CP)

Cerebrospinal fluid (CSF)

Diabetes insipidus (DI)

Electroencephalogram (EEG)

Intracranial pressure (ICP)

Motor vehicle accident (MVA)

Pediatric intensive care unit (PICU)

Shaken baby syndrome (SBS)

Ventriculoperitoneal (VP)

QUESTIONS

1. The nurse is caring for a child who has been in a motor vehicle accident (MVA). The child falls asleep unless her name is called or she is gently shaken. This state of consciousness is referred to as:
   1. Coma.
   2. Delirium.
   3. Obtunded.
   4. Confusion.

2. The nurse is caring for a 3-year-old with an altered state of consciousness. The nurse determines that the child is oriented by asking the child to:
   1. Name the president of the United States.
   2. Identify her parents and state her own name.
   3. State her full name and phone number.
   4. Identify the current month but not the date.

3. The parents of a child with altered consciousness ask if they can stay during the morning assessment. Select the nurse's best response.
   1. "Your child is more likely to answer questions and cooperate with any procedures if you are not present."
   2. "Most children feel more at ease when parents are present, so you are more than welcome to stay at the bedside."
   3. "It is our policy to ask parents to leave during the first assessment of the shift."
   4. "Many children fear that their parents will be disappointed if they do not do well with procedures, so we recommend that no parents be present at this time."

4. The mother of an unconscious child has been calling her name repeatedly and gently shaking her shoulders in an attempt to wake her up. The nurse notes that the child is flexing her arms and wrists while bringing her arms closer to the midline of her body. The child's mother asks, "What is going on?" Select the nurse's best response.
   1. "I think your daughter hears you, and she is attempting to reach out to you."
   2. "Your child is responding to you; please continue trying to stimulate her."
   3. "It appears that your child is having a seizure."
   4. "Your child is demonstrating a reflex that indicates she is overwhelmed with the stimulation she is receiving."

5. Which signs best indicate increased intracranial pressure (ICP) in an infant? **Select all that apply.**
   1. Sunken anterior fontanel.
   2. Complaints of blurred vision.
   3. High-pitched cry.
   4. Increased appetite.
   5. Sleeping more than usual.

6. Which of the following would be included in the plan of care for a hospitalized newborn following surgical repair of a myelomeningocele? **Select all that apply.**
   1. Skull x-rays.
   2. Daily head circumference measurements.
   3. MRI scan.
   4. Vital signs every 6 hours.
   5. Holding to breastfeed.

7. A child with a ventriculoperitoneal (VP) shunt complains of headache and blurry vision and now experiences irritability and sleeping more than usual. The parents ask the nurse what they should do. Select the nurse's best response.
1. "Give her some acetaminophen (Tylenol), and see if her symptoms improve. If they do not improve, bring her to the health-care provider's office."
2. "It is common for girls to have these symptoms, especially prior to beginning their menstrual cycle. Give her a few days, and see if she improves."
3. "You are probably worried that she is having a problem with her shunt. This is very unlikely because it has been working well for 9 years."
4. "You should immediately take her to the emergency department because these may be symptoms of a shunt malfunction."

8. Which position initially is most beneficial for an infant who has just returned from having a ventriculoperitoneal (VP) shunt placed?
1. Semi-Fowler in an infant seat.
2. Flat in the crib.
3. Trendelenburg.
4. In the crib with the head elevated to 90 degrees.

9. The nurse is aware that cloudy cerebrospinal fluid (CSF) most likely indicates:
1. Viral meningitis.
2. Bacterial meningitis.
3. No infection, because CSF is usually cloudy.
4. Sepsis.

10. A child is being admitted with the diagnosis of meningitis. Select the procedure the nurse should do first:
1. Administration of intravenous antibiotics.
2. Administration of maintenance intravenous fluids.
3. Placement of a Foley catheter.
4. Send the spinal fluid and blood samples to the laboratory for cultures.

11. The nurse is caring for a 6-month-old infant diagnosed with meningitis. When the child is placed in the supine position and flexes his neck, the nurse notes he flexes his knees and hips. This is referred to as:
1. Brudzinski sign.
2. Cushing triad.
3. Kernig sign.
4. Nuchal rigidity.

12. Select the best room assignment for a newly admitted child with bacterial meningitis.
1. Semiprivate room with a roommate who also has bacterial meningitis.
2. Semiprivate room with a roommate who has bacterial meningitis but has received intravenous antibiotics for more than 24 hours.
3. Private room that is dark and quiet with minimal stimulation.
4. Private room that is bright and colorful and has developmentally appropriate activities available.

13. Which order would the nurse question for a child just admitted with the diagnosis of bacterial meningitis?
1. Maintain isolation precautions until 24 hours after receiving intravenous antibiotics.
2. Intravenous fluids at 1½ times regular maintenance.
3. Neurological checks every hour.
4. Administer acetaminophen (Tylenol) for temperatures higher than 38°C (100.4°F).

14. The nurse is caring for a 1-year-old who has just been diagnosed with viral encephalitis. The parents ask if their child will be admitted to the hospital. Select the nurse's best response.
    1. "Your child will likely be sent home because encephalitis is usually caused by a virus and not bacteria."
    2. "Your child will likely be admitted to the pediatric floor for intravenous antibiotics and observation."
    3. "Your child will likely be admitted to the PICU for close monitoring and observation."
    4. "Your child will likely be sent home because she is only 1 year old. We see fewer complications and a shorter disease process in the younger child."

15. The nurse knows further education is needed about Reye syndrome when a mother states:
    1. "I will have my children immunized against varicella and influenza."
    2. "I will make sure not to give my child any products containing aspirin."
    3. "I will give aspirin to my child to treat a headache."
    4. "Children with Reye syndrome are admitted to the hospital."

16. A child with Reye syndrome is described in the nurse's notes as follows: 1200—comatose with sluggish pupils; when stimulated, demonstrates decerebrate posturing. 1400—unchanged except that now demonstrates decorticate posturing when stimulated. The nurse concludes that the child's condition is:
    1. Worsening and progressing to a more advanced stage of Reye syndrome.
    2. Worsening, and the child may likely experience cardiac and respiratory failure.
    3. Improving and progressing to a less advanced stage of Reye syndrome.
    4. Improving because the child's posturing reflexes are similar.

17. To treat a common manifestation of Reye syndrome, which medication would the nurse expect to have readily available?
    1. Furosemide (Lasix).
    2. Insulin.
    3. Glucose.
    4. Morphine.

18. A child diagnosed with meningitis is having a generalized tonic-clonic seizure. Which should the nurse do first?
    1. Administer blow-by oxygen and call for additional help.
    2. Reassure the parents that seizures are common in children with meningitis.
    3. Call a code and ask the parents to leave the room.
    4. Assess the child's temperature and blood pressure.

19. A child with a seizure disorder has been having episodes during which she drops her pencil and simply appears to be daydreaming. This is most likely a/an:
    1. Absence seizure.
    2. Akinetic seizure.
    3. Non-epileptic seizure.
    4. Simple spasm seizure.

20. A preschooler has been having periods during which he suddenly falls and appears to be weak for a short time after the event. The preschool teacher asks what she should do. Select the nurse's best response.
    1. "Have the parents follow up with his health-care provider because this is likely an atonic seizure."
    2. "Find out if there have been any new stressors in his life because it could be attention-seeking behavior."
    3. "Have the parents follow up with his health-care provider because this is likely an absence seizure."
    4. "The preschool years are a time of rapid growth, and many children appear clumsy. It would be best to watch him and see if it continues."

21. The diet that produces anticonvulsant effects from ketosis consists of:
1. High-fat and low-carbohydrate foods.
2. High-fat and high-carbohydrate foods.
3. Low-fat and low-carbohydrate foods.
4. Low-fat and high-carbohydrate foods.

22. Which medication should the nurse anticipate administering first to a child in status epilepticus?
1. Establish an intravenous line and administer intravenous lorazepam (Ativan).
2. Administer rectal diazepam (Valium).
3. Administer an oral glucose gel to the side of the child's mouth.
4. Administer oral diazepam (Valium).

23. The nurse is providing discharge teaching to the parents of a toddler who experienced a febrile seizure. The nurse knows clarification is needed when the mother says:
1. "My child will likely have another seizure."
2. "My child's 7-year-old brother is also at high risk for a febrile seizure."
3. "I'll give my child acetaminophen (Tylenol) when ill to prevent the fever from rising too high too rapidly."
4. "Most children with febrile seizures do not require seizure medicine."

24. A child recently diagnosed with epilepsy is being evaluated for anticonvulsant medication therapy. The child will likely be placed on which type of regimen?
1. Two to three oral anticonvulsant medications so that dosing can be low and side effects minimized.
2. One oral anticonvulsant medication to observe effectiveness and minimize side effects.
3. One rectal gel to be administered in the event of a seizure.
4. A combination of oral and intravenous anticonvulsant medications to ensure compliance.

25. Which activity should an adolescent just diagnosed with epilepsy avoid?
1. Swimming, even with a friend.
2. Being in a car at night.
3. Participating in any strenuous activities.
4. Returning to school right away.

26. Which is the best action for the nurse to take during a child's seizure?
1. Administer the child's rescue dose of oral diazepam (Valium).
2. Loosen the child's clothing, and call for help.
3. Place a tongue blade in the child's mouth to prevent aspiration.
4. Carry the child to the infirmary to call 911 and start an intravenous line.

27. Brain damage in a child who sustained a closed-head injury can be caused by which factor?
1. Increased perfusion to the brain and increased metabolic needs of the brain.
2. Decreased perfusion to the brain and decreased metabolic needs of the brain.
3. Increased perfusion to the brain and decreased metabolic needs of the brain.
4. Decreased perfusion of the brain and increased metabolic needs of the brain.

28. A child fell off his bike and sustained a closed-head injury. The child is currently awake and alert, but his mother states that he "passed out" for approximately 2 minutes. The mother appears highly anxious and is very tearful. The child was not wearing a helmet. Which is a priority for the triage nurse to say at this time?
1. "Was anyone else injured in the accident?"
2. "Tell me more about the accident."
3. "Did he vomit, have a seizure, or display any other behavior that was unusual when he woke up?"
4. "Why was he not wearing a helmet?"

29. The nurse is caring for an unconscious 6-year-old who has had a severe closed-head injury and notes the following changes: Heart rate has dropped from 120 to 55, blood pressure has increased from 110/44 to 195/62, and respirations are becoming more irregular. Which should the nurse do first after calling the physician?
    1. Call for additional help and prepare to administer mannitol (Osmitrol).
    2. Continue to monitor the patient's vital signs and prepare to administer a bolus of isotonic fluids.
    3. Call for additional help and prepare to administer an antihypertensive.
    4. Continue to monitor the patient and administer supplemental oxygen.

30. A child in the PICU with a head injury is comatose and unresponsive. The parent asks if he needs pain medication. Select the nurse's best response.
    1. "Pain medication is not necessary because he is unresponsive and cannot feel pain."
    2. "Pain medication may interfere with his ability to respond and may mask any signs of improvement."
    3. "Pain medication is necessary to make him comfortable."
    4. "Pain medication is necessary for comfort, but we use it cautiously because it increases the demand for oxygen."

31. The nurse is caring for a child with a skull fracture who is unconscious and has severely increased intracranial pressure (ICP). The nurse notes the child's temperature to be 104°F (40°C). Which should the nurse do first?
    1. Place a cooling blanket on the child.
    2. Administer acetaminophen (Tylenol) via nasogastric tube.
    3. Administer acetaminophen (Tylenol) rectally.
    4. Place ice packs in the child's axillary areas.

32. The nurse is caring for an adolescent who remains unconscious 24 hours after sustaining a closed-head injury in a motor vehicle accident (MVA). She responds to deep, painful stimulation with decorticate posturing and has an intracranial monitor that shows periodic increased ICP. All other vital signs remain stable. Select the most appropriate nursing action.
    1. Encourage the teen's peers to visit and talk to her about school and other pertinent events.
    2. Encourage the teen's parents to hold her hand and speak loudly to her in an attempt to help her regain consciousness.
    3. Attempt to keep a normal day/night pattern by keeping the teen in a bright, lively environment during the day and dark quiet environment at night.
    4. Attempt to keep the environment dark and quiet and encourage minimal stimulation.

33. A 2-month-old infant is brought to the emergency department after experiencing a seizure. The infant appears lethargic with very irregular respirations and periods of apnea. The parents report the baby is no longer interested in feeding and, before the seizure, rolled off the couch. What additional testing should the nurse immediately prepare for?
    1. Computed tomography (CT) scan of the head and dilation of the eyes.
    2. Computed tomography (CT) scan of the head and electroencephalogram (EEG).
    3. X-rays of the head.
    4. X-rays of all long bones.

34. The nurse knows that young infants are at risk for injury from shaken baby syndrome (SBS) because:
    1. The anterior fontanel is open.
    2. They have insufficient musculoskeletal support and a disproportionate head-to-body ratio.
    3. They have an immature vascular system with veins and arteries that are more superficial.
    4. There is immature myelination of the nervous system in a young infant.

35. An infant is born with a sac protruding through the spine, containing cerebrospinal fluid (CSF), a portion of the meninges, and nerve roots. This condition is referred to as:
    1. Meningocele.
    2. Myelomeningocele.
    3. Spina bifida occulta.
    4. Anencephaly.

36. Which is the nurse's best response to the parents of a neonate with a meningocele who ask what can they expect?
    1. "After initial surgery to close the defect, most children experience no neurological dysfunction."
    2. "Surgery to close the sac will be postponed until the infant has grown and has enough skin to form a graft."
    3. "After the initial surgery to close the defect, the child will likely have motor and sensory deficits."
    4. "After the initial surgery to close the defect, the child will likely have future problems with urinary and bowel continence."

37. The nurse is caring for an infant with a myelomeningocele. The parents ask the nurse why the nurse keeps measuring the baby's head circumference. Select the nurse's best response:
    1. "Babies' heads are measured to ensure growth is on track."
    2. "Babies with a myelomeningocele are at risk for hydrocephalus, which shows up as an increase in head size."
    3. "Because your baby has an opening on the spinal cord, your infant is at risk for meningitis, which can show up as an increase in head size."
    4. "Many infants with myelomeningocele have microcephaly, which can show up as a decrease in head size."

38. A parent of a newborn diagnosed with myelomeningocele asks what is/are common long-term complication(s)? The nurse's best response is which of the following? **Select all that apply.**
    1. Learning disabilities.
    2. Urinary tract infections.
    3. Hydrocephalus.
    4. Decubitus ulcers and skin breakdown.
    5. Nutrition issues.
    6. Attention deficit disorders

39. Which is included in the plan of care for a newborn who has a myelomeningocele?
    1. Place the infant in the prone position with a sterile dry dressing over the defect. Slowly begin oral gastric feeds to prevent the development of necrotizing enterocolitis.
    2. Place the infant in the prone position with a sterile dry dressing over the defect. Begin intravenous fluids to prevent dehydration.
    3. Place the infant in the prone position with a sterile moist dressing over the defect. Slowly begin oral gastric feeds to prevent the development of necrotizing enterocolitis.
    4. Place the child in the prone position with a sterile moist dressing over the defect. Begin intravenous fluids to prevent dehydration.

40. The parents of a 12-month-old with a neurogenic bladder ask the nurse if their child will always have to be catheterized. Select the nurse's best response.
1. "Your child will never feel when her bladder is full, so she will always have to be catheterized. Because she is female, she will always need assistance."
2. "As your child ages, she will likely be able to sense when her bladder is full and will be able to empty it on her own."
3. "Although your child will not be able to feel when her bladder is full, she can learn to urinate every 4 to 6 hours and therefore not require catheterizations."
4. "Your child will never be able to completely empty her bladder spontaneously, but there are other options to traditional catheterization. An opening can be made surgically through the abdomen, allowing a catheter to be placed into the opening."

41. Which does the nurse include in the postoperative plan of care for a child with myelomeningocele following ligament release?
1. Encourage the child to resume a regular diet, beginning slowly with bland foods that are easily digested, such as bananas.
2. Encourage the child to blow balloons to increase deep breathing and avoid postoperative pneumonia.
3. Assist the child to change positions to avoid skin breakdown.
4. Provide education on dietary requirements to prevent obesity and skin breakdown.

42. A 6-month-old infant was just diagnosed with craniosynostosis. The infant's father asks the nurse for more information about reconstructive surgery. Select the nurse's best response.
1. "The surgery is done for cosmetic reasons and is without many complications."
2. "The surgery is important to allow the brain to grow properly. Although most children do well, serious complications can occur, so your child will be closely observed in the intensive care unit."
3. "The surgery is important to allow the brain to grow properly. Most surgeons wait until the child is 18 months old to minimize potential complications."
4. "The surgery is mainly done for cosmetic reasons, and most surgeons wait until the child is 3 years old because the head has finished growing at that time."

43. A 6-month-old male has been diagnosed with positional brachycephaly. The nurse is providing teaching about the use of a helmet for his therapy. Which statement indicates that the parents understand the education? **Select all that apply.**
1. "We will keep the helmet on him when he is awake and remove it only for bathing and sleeping."
2. "He will start wearing the helmet when he is closer to 9 months because he will be more upright and mobile."
3. "He will wear the helmet 23 hours every day."
4. "Most children need to wear the helmet for 6 to 12 months."
5. "Most children gain some improvement."

44. The nurse tells a family of a child with cerebral palsy (CP) that since the 1960s the incidence of CP has:
1. Increased.
2. Decreased.
3. Remained the same.
4. Has decreased because of early misdiagnosis.

45. Which child is at increased risk for cerebral palsy (CP)?
1. An infant born at 34 weeks with an Apgar score of 6 at 5 minutes.
2. A 17-day-old infant with group B *Streptococcus* meningitis.
3. A 24-month-old child who has experienced a febrile seizure.
4. A 5-year-old with a closed-head injury after falling off a bike.

46. Which child requires continued follow-up because of behaviors suspicious of cerebral palsy (CP)?
    1. A 1-month-old who demonstrates the startle reflex when a loud noise is heard.
    2. A 6-month-old who always reaches for toys with the right hand.
    3. A 14-month-old who has not begun to walk.
    4. A 2-year-old who has not yet achieved bladder control during waking hours.

47. The parents of a child with meningitis and multiple seizures ask if the child will likely develop cerebral palsy (CP). Select the nurse's best response.
    1. "When your child is stable, she'll undergo computed tomography (CT) and magnetic resolution imaging (MRI). The physicians will be able to let you know if she has CP."
    2. "Most children do not develop CP at this late age."
    3. "Your child will be closely monitored after discharge, and a developmental specialist will be able to make the diagnosis."
    4. "Most children who have had complications following meningitis develop some amount of CP."

48. The nurse is caring for a 2-month-old infant who is at risk for cerebral palsy (CP) due to extreme low birth weight and prematurity. His parents ask why a speech therapist is involved in his care. Select the nurse's best response.
    1. "Your baby is likely to have speech problems because of his early birth. Involving the speech therapist now will ensure vocalization at a developmentally appropriate age."
    2. "The speech therapist will help with tongue and jaw movements to assist with babbling."
    3. "The speech therapist will help with tongue and jaw movements to assist with feeding."
    4. "Many members of the health-care team are involved in your child's care so that we will know if there are any unmet needs."

49. The nurse prepares baclofen for a child with cerebral palsy (CP) who just had her hamstrings surgically released. The child's parents ask what the medication is for. Select the nurse's best response.
    1. "It is a medication that will help decrease the pain from her surgery."
    2. "It is a medication that will prevent her from having seizures."
    3. "It is a medication that will help control her spasms."
    4. "It is a medication that will help with bladder control."

50. A child with cerebral palsy (CP) has been fitted for braces and is beginning physical therapy to assist with ambulation. The parents ask why he needs the braces when he was crawling without any assistive devices. Select the nurse's best response.
    1. "The CP has progressed, and he now needs more assistance to ambulate."
    2. "As your child grows, different muscle groups may need more assistance."
    3. "Most children with CP need braces to help with ambulation."
    4. "We have found that when children with CP use braces, they are less likely to fall."

51. The parents of a 12-month-old with cerebral palsy (CP) ask the nurse if they should teach their child sign language because he has not begun to vocalize. The nurse bases the response on the knowledge that sign language:
    1. May be a very beneficial way to help children with CP communicate.
    2. May cause confusion and further delay vocalization.
    3. Is difficult to learn for most children with CP.
    4. Is beneficial to learn, but it would be best to wait until the child is older.

52. The parents of a child with cerebral palsy (CP) are learning how to feed their child and avoid aspiration. The nurse would question which of the following when reviewing the teaching plan?
    1. Place the food on the tip of the tongue.
    2. Place the child in an upright position during feedings.
    3. Feed the child soft and blended foods.
    4. Feed the child slowly.

53. The nurse is caring for a child with cerebral palsy (CP) whose weight is in the fifth percentile and who has been hospitalized for aspiration pneumonia. His parents are anxious and state that they do not want a G-tube placed. Which would be the nurse's best response?
    1. "A G-tube will help your son gain weight and reduce his risk for future hospitalizations due to pneumonia."
    2. "G-tubes are very easy to care for and will make feeding time easier for your family."
    3. "Are you concerned that you will not be able to care for his G-tube?"
    4. "Tell me your thoughts about G-tubes."

54. The parent of an infant diagnosed with a neuroblastoma asks the nurse what the prognosis is. The nurse's best response is:
    1. Excellent, because a neuroblastoma is always cured.
    2. Excellent, because infants with a neuroblastoma have the best prognosis.
    3. Poor, because infants with a neuroblastoma rarely survive.
    4. Variable, depending on the site of origin.

55. Which should be included in the plan of care for a child who has a neuroblastoma with metastasis to the bone marrow and pancytopenia?
    1. Administer red blood cells.
    2. Limit school attendance to less than 4 hours daily.
    3. Administer warfarin (Coumadin).
    4. Encourage a diet high in fresh fruits and vegetables.

56. The parent of a child with neuroblastoma asks the nurse what the typical signs and symptoms are at first. Select the nurse's best answer.
    1. "Most children complain of abdominal fullness and difficulty urinating."
    2. "Many children in the early stages of a neuroblastoma have joint pain and walk with a limp."
    3. "The signs and symptoms vary depending on where the tumor is located, but typical symptoms include weight loss, abdominal distention, and fatigue."
    4. "The signs and symptoms are fairly consistent regardless of the location of the tumor. They include fatigue, hunger, weight gain, and abdominal fullness."

57. Which child would likely have experienced a delay in the diagnosis of a brain tumor?
    1. A 3-month-old, because signs and symptoms would not have been readily apparent.
    2. A 5-month-old, because signs and symptoms would not have been readily suspected.
    3. School-age child, because signs and symptoms could have been misinterpreted.
    4. Adolescent, because signs and symptoms could have been ignored and denied.

58. A child has been diagnosed with a midline brain tumor. In addition to showing signs of increased intracranial pressure (ICP), she has been voiding large amounts of very dilute urine. Which medication does the nurse expect to administer?
    1. Mannitol (Osmitrol).
    2. Vasopressin.
    3. Furosemide (Lasix).
    4. Dopamine (Intropin).

59. The nurse is caring for a child receiving radiation therapy for a brain tumor. The parents ask if their child will likely have any learning disabilities. Select the nurse's best answer.
   1. "All children who receive radiation have some amount of learning disability. As long as they receive extra tutoring, they usually do well in school."
   2. "Because your child is so young, she will likely do well and have no problems in the future."
   3. "Response varies with each child, but younger children who receive radiation tend to have some amount of learning disability later in life."
   4. "Response varies with each child, but younger children who receive radiation tend to have fewer problems later in life than older children."

60. A child involved in a motor vehicle accident (MVA) is currently on a backboard with a cervical collar in place. The child is diagnosed with a cervical fracture. Which would the nurse expect to find in the child's plan of care?
   1. Remove the cervical collar, keep the backboard in place, and administer high-dose methylprednisolone (Medrol).
   2. Continue with all forms of spinal stabilization and administer high-dose methylprednisolone (Medrol) and ranitidine (Zantac).
   3. Remove the backboard and cervical collar and prepare for halo traction placement.
   4. Remove the cervical collar and backboard, place the child on spinal precautions, and administer high-dose methylprednisolone (Medrol) and ranitidine (Zantac).

61. Which has the potential to alter a child's level of consciousness? **Select all that apply.**
   1. Metabolic disorders.
   2. Trauma.
   3. Hypoxic episode.
   4. Dehydration.
   5. Endocrine disorders.

ANSWERS AND RATIONALES

The correct answer number and rationale for why it is the correct answer are given in **boldface blue type**. Rationales for why the other possible answer options are incorrect also are given, but they are not in boldface type.

1. 1. "Coma" describes a state of consciousness in which the child is not responsive to any stimulation, including painful stimulation.
   2. "Delirium" describes a state of consciousness in which the child is extremely confused and anxious.
   3. **"Obtunded" describes a state of consciousness in which the child has a limited response to the environment and can be aroused by verbal or tactile stimulation.**
   4. "Confusion" describes a state of consciousness in which the child is not oriented to person, place, and time.

   TEST-TAKING HINT: The test taker needs to be familiar with terms describing states of consciousness.

2. 1. Most 3-year-olds are not capable of naming the president.
   2. **Asking the 3-year-old to identify her parents and state her name is a developmentally appropriate way to assess orientation.**
   3. Many 3-year-olds are not familiar with their phone number or may not be able to share this information during a stressful time, such as hospitalization.
   4. Many 3-year-olds do not know the current month.

   TEST-TAKING HINT: The test taker needs to be familiar with the concept of consciousness and applying normal developmental-specific age-groups.

3. 1. School-age children feel more comfortable when parents are present and are more likely to cooperate with a neurological assessment.
   2. **Parents should be encouraged to remain with their child for mutual comfort.**
   3. Describing a policy is not sufficient and does not give the parents enough information.
   4. School-age children feel more comfortable when parents are present and are more likely to cooperate with a neurological assessment.

TEST-TAKING HINT: The test taker needs to be familiar with growth and development of children and applying theories to specific clinical situations.

4. 1. The child is demonstrating a reflex called posturing. The parent should not be given any false hope that the child is responding at a higher level than is truly occurring.
   2. The posturing reflex often indicates irritability, and the child should not continue to receive stimulation.
   3. Posturing is a reflex, not a seizure.
   4. **Posturing is a reflex that often indicates that the child is receiving too much stimulation.**

   TEST-TAKING HINT: The test taker needs to be familiar with caring for the comatose child and what causes posturing.

5. 3, 5.
   1. The anterior fontanel is usually raised and bulging in infants with increased ICP.
   2. The infant is not able to comprehend blurred vision or make any statements.
   3. **A high-pitched cry is often indicative of increased ICP in infants.**
   4. The infant with increased ICP usually has a poor appetite and does not feed well.
   5. **The infant may be sleeping more than usual because of increased ICP.**

   TEST-TAKING HINT: The test taker needs to be familiar with hydrocephalus and how increased ICP is manifested in infants. Answer 2 can be eliminated because an infant cannot specifically verbalize.

6. 2, 3.
   1. Diagnostic tests include MRI scan, CT scan, ultrasound, and myelography. These tests give much more needed information than do skull x-rays.
   2. **Daily head circumference measurements are done to assess for hydrocephalus.**
   3. **Diagnostic tests include MRI scan, CT scan, ultrasound, and myelography.**
   4. Vital signs should be taken at least every 4 hours.
   5. Infants with repaired myelomeningocele are kept prone to prevent pressure on the surgical site.

   TEST-TAKING HINT: The test taker needs to be familiar with postoperative care for infants with myelomeningocele.

7. 1. These are symptoms of a shunt malfunction and should be evaluated immediately.
   2. Although these symptoms may be associated with the start of a girl's menstrual cycle, they are symptoms of a shunt malfunction and require immediate evaluation.
   3. A shunt can malfunction at any point and should be evaluated when signs of increased ICP are evident.
   4. **These are symptoms of a shunt malfunction and should be evaluated immediately.**

   TEST-TAKING HINT: The test taker should recognize these symptoms as signs of a shunt malfunction and can eliminate answers 1, 2, and 3 because they do not address the situation as an emergency.

8. 1. A semi-Fowler position in an infant seat may allow the ventricles to drain too rapidly in the immediate postoperative period.
   2. **Flat in the crib is the position usually used initially, with the angle gradually increasing as the child tolerates.**
   3. The Trendelenburg position is not used immediately after ventriculoperitoneal shunt placement because it would increase ICP.
   4. The head elevated to 90 degrees will allow the ventricle of the brain to drain too quickly.

   TEST-TAKING HINT: The test taker should note the word "initially" and consider why the position would be immediately beneficial. Answer 3 can be eliminated because that position could increase ICP.

9. 1. The CSF in viral meningitis is usually clear.
   2. **The CSF in bacterial meningitis is usually cloudy.**
   3. The CSF in healthy children is usually clear.
   4. Sepsis is an infection of the bloodstream.

   TEST-TAKING HINT: The test taker can eliminate answer 4 because an infection of the bloodstream would not be detected in the CSF.

10. 1. Administration of intravenous antibiotics should not be started until after all cultures have been obtained.
    2. Administration of maintenance IV fluids can wait until after the cultures have been obtained.
    3. Placement of a Foley catheter is not a priority procedure.
    4. **Cultures of spinal fluid and blood should be obtained, followed by administration of intravenous antibiotics.**

TEST-TAKING HINT: The test taker needs to think about priority of care. Answer 3 can be immediately eliminated because it is not a priority. Answer 4 should be considered a priority because antibiotics should not be started before the samples have been obtained and sent for culturing.

11. 1. **Brudzinski sign occurs when the child responds to a flexed neck with an involuntary flexion of the hips and/or knees.**
    2. Cushing triad is a sign of increased ICP and is manifested with an increase in systolic blood pressure, decreased heart rate, and irregular respirations.
    3. Kernig sign occurs when there is resistance or pain in response to raising the child's flexed leg.
    4. Nuchal rigidity occurs when there is a resistance to neck flexion.

   TEST-TAKING HINT: The test taker should be familiar with terms used to describe meningeal irritation.

12. 1. The child with bacterial meningitis should be placed in a private room isolated from all other patients. Bacterial meningitis is caused by many pathogens, and patients should be isolated from each other.
    2. The child with bacterial meningitis should be placed in a private room isolated from all other patients. Bacterial meningitis is caused by many pathogens, and patients should be isolated from each other.
    3. **A quiet private room with minimal stimulation is ideal because the child with meningitis should be in a quiet environment to avoid cerebral irritation.**
    4. A bright room with developmental activities may cause irritation and increase ICP.

   TEST-TAKING HINT: The test taker should consider what contributes to cerebral irritation and should not be influenced by the developmental requirements of a healthy child.

13. 1. Isolation precautions must be maintained for at least the first 24 hours of intravenous antibiotic therapy.
    2. **Intravenous fluids at 1½ times regular maintenance could cause fluid overload and lead to increased ICP.**
    3. Neurological checks are usually made at least every hour.
    4. Acetaminophen (Tylenol) is usually administered when the child has a fever, as increased temperature can lead to increased ICP.

TEST-TAKING HINT: The test taker should consider the answers and eliminate those that may increase ICP. Intravenous fluids are often given at less than maintenance unless the child is hemodynamically unstable.

14. 1. Although encephalitis is usually caused by a viral infection, the child is usually admitted for close observation.
2. Intravenous antibiotics are not given to the child with viral encephalitis.
3. **The young child with encephalitis should be admitted to a PICU where close observation and monitoring are available. The child should be observed for signs of increased ICP and for cardiac and respiratory compromise.**
4. The child would not be discharged because observation for complications is necessary. As a general rule, younger children tend to have more complications and require a PICU admission.

TEST-TAKING HINT: The test taker should be familiar with the diagnosis and treatment of encephalitis. The test taker should not be influenced by the word "viral" but should realize that the sequelae of encephalitis require close monitoring in an ICU environment.

15. 1. Having a child immunized helps prevent viral illnesses from occurring, thereby decreasing the likelihood of Reye syndrome.
2. The administration of aspirin or products containing aspirin has been associated with the development of Reye syndrome.
3. **The administration of aspirin or products containing aspirin has been associated with the development of Reye syndrome. A headache can be the first sign of a viral illness followed by other symptoms. It is best not to use aspirin or aspirin-containing products in children.**
4. Children with Reye syndrome are always admitted to the hospital because there is a strong possibility for complications and rapid deterioration.

TEST-TAKING HINT: The test taker should be aware that aspirin administration in children with viral infections has been linked to Reye syndrome.

16. 1. Decorticate posturing is seen with a less advanced stage of Reye syndrome and likely indicates that the child's condition is improving.
2. The child's condition is improving; therefore, cardiac and respiratory failure is less likely.

3. **Progressing from decerebrate to decorticate posturing usually indicates an improvement in the child's condition.**
4. Decorticate posturing is associated with inflammation above the brain stem, whereas decerebrate posturing is associated with inflammation in the brain stem.

TEST-TAKING HINT: The test taker needs to be familiar with posturing reflexes and their significance.

17. 1. A common manifestation is increased ICP, which is treated with an osmotic diuretic. Furosemide (Lasix) is a loop diuretic.
2. A common manifestation is hypoglycemia. Insulin does not treat hypoglycemia, but decreases the blood sugar instead.
3. **A common manifestation is hypoglycemia, which is treated with the administration of intravenous glucose.**
4. Morphine is a narcotic used for pain relief. It should be used with caution because it can lead to respiratory depression.

TEST-TAKING HINT: The test taker needs to be aware that increased ICP is a very common manifestation of Reye syndrome and should therefore eliminate any answers that do not treat increased ICP. The test taker can also eliminate answers 2 and 4 because they do not treat hypoglycemia, which is another common manifestation of Reye syndrome.

18. 1. **The child experiencing a seizure usually requires more oxygen because the seizure increases the body's metabolic rate and demand for oxygen. The seizure may also affect the child's airway, causing the child to be hypoxic. It is always appropriate to give the child blow-by oxygen immediately. The nurse should remain with the child and call for additional help.**
2. It is important to reassure the parents, but giving the child oxygen and calling for additional support is the priority of care.
3. It is not necessary to call a code unless the child experiences a cardiac or respiratory arrest. Research indicates that encouraging parents to remain with the child in emergency situations benefits both the child and family.
4. It is important to monitor and observe the child during a seizure, but it is very difficult to obtain a blood pressure from a seizing child. The priority of care involves administering oxygen and calling for additional help.

TEST-TAKING HINT: The test taker needs to prioritize care and choose answer 1 because it will help maintain the airway. Answer 3 could immediately be eliminated because the child is having a seizure, not a cardiac arrest.

19. 1. **Absence seizures occur frequently and last less than 30 seconds. The child experiences a brief loss of consciousness during which she may have a change in activity. These children rarely fall, but they may drop an object. The condition is often confused with daydreaming.**
    2. Akinetic seizures occur when the young child experiences a brief loss of consciousness and postural tone and falls to the ground. The child quickly regains consciousness.
    3. A non-epileptic seizure is a seizure that occurs secondary to another disorder, such as a fever or increased ICP.
    4. A simple spasm seizure is not a diagnosis.

    TEST-TAKING HINT: "Daydreaming" is the classic description of an absence seizure.

20. 1. **An atonic seizure is characterized by a loss of muscular tone, whereby the child may fall to the ground.**
    2. It is important to evaluate the child for life stressors, but suspected seizure activity needs immediate evaluation.
    3. An absence seizure is characterized by a change in activity whereby the child appears to be daydreaming or staring straight ahead. The child usually continues basic simple movements but loses an awareness of surroundings.
    4. The preschool years are a not a time of rapid growth. Many children in this age-group appear clumsy, but suspected seizure activity needs immediate evaluation.

    TEST-TAKING HINT: The test taker should recognize the description as seizure activity and, therefore, could immediately eliminate answers 3 and 4.

21. 1. **High fat and low carbohydrates are the components of the ketogenic diet.**
    2. High fat and low carbohydrates are the components of the ketogenic diet.
    3. High fat and low carbohydrates are the components of the ketogenic diet.
    4. High fat and low carbohydrates are the components of the ketogenic diet.

    TEST-TAKING HINT: The test taker needs to be familiar with the components of a ketogenic diet.

22. 1. It is very difficult and time consuming to establish an intravenous line in a child who is experiencing a generalized seizure. Rectal diazepam (Valium) is first administered in an attempt to stop the seizure long enough to establish a line, and then medication is administered intravenously.
    2. **Rectal diazepam (Valium) is first administered in an attempt to stop the seizure long enough to establish an IV, and then IV medication is administered.**
    3. Although the child may become hypoglycemic due to increased metabolic demands, stopping the seizure with rectal diazepam (Valium) is the first priority. Medication is not placed in the mouth of a child experiencing a generalized seizure because it increases the risk of injury and aspiration.
    4. Stopping the seizure with rectal diazepam (Valium) takes priority. Nothing should be administered orally to a patient who is unconscious.

    TEST-TAKING HINT: The test taker needs to consider the current situation and the level of difficulty in establishing intravenous access in a child experiencing a generalized seizure.

23. 1. Children who experience a febrile seizure are likely to experience another febrile seizure.
    2. **Most children over the age of 5 years do not have febrile seizures.**
    3. Antipyretics are administered to prevent the child's temperature from rising too rapidly.
    4. Most children are not prescribed anticonvulsant medication after experiencing a febrile seizure.

    TEST-TAKING HINT: There is an increased risk in siblings, but the 7-year-old child is above the usual age of febrile seizures.

24. 1. Although many children with epilepsy require more than one medication to achieve seizure control, it is recommended that only one medication be started at a time so that the child's reaction to the specific medication can be observed.
    2. **One medication is the preferred way to achieve seizure control. The child is monitored for side effects and drug levels.**
    3. Rectal gels are used to stop a seizure once it has begun; they are not used to prevent seizures.

4. The route of choice for the prevention of seizures is oral. There is no reason to assume that compliance will be an issue prior to beginning anticonvulsant therapy.

TEST-TAKING HINT: The test taker should eliminate answer 4 because IV medications are not included in the initial home medication regimen.

25. 1. Swimming does not need to be avoided as long as there is someone else present to call for help in the event of an emergency.
    2. **The rhythmic reflection of other car lights can trigger a seizure in some children.**
    3. There is no reason to avoid strenuous activity.
    4. It is important for adolescents to be with their peers in order to reach developmental milestones.

TEST-TAKING HINT: The test taker should consider the answers that can lead to a seizure. Answer 2 is the only answer that includes a common trigger.

26. 1. Nothing should be placed in the child's mouth because he is at risk for aspiration. Rescue Valium is usually administered rectally.
    2. **The nurse should remain with the child and observe the seizure. The child should be protected from his environment, and clothing should be loosened.**
    3. A tongue blade should never be placed in the child's mouth because it can cause injury or increase the risk of aspiration.
    4. The nurse should remain with the child and call for help. A child can be injured if carried during a seizure.

TEST-TAKING HINT: The test taker should eliminate answers 1 and 3 because nothing should ever be placed in the mouth of a child having a seizure.

27. 1. The child who has a closed-head injury has decreased perfusion to the brain and increased metabolic needs that lead to ischemia and brain damage.
    2. The child who has a closed-head injury has decreased perfusion to the brain and increased metabolic needs that lead to ischemia and brain damage.
    3. The child who has a closed-head injury has decreased perfusion to the brain and increased metabolic needs that lead to ischemia and brain damage.
    4. **Decreased perfusion of the brain and increased metabolic needs of the brain.**

TEST-TAKING HINT: The test taker needs to be familiar with the mechanics of a head injury.

28. 1. It is not a priority of care to find out if anyone else was injured.
    2. Although open-ended questions are important, the nurse needs specific information, and the anxious parent may need to be guided during triage assessment.
    3. **Asking specific questions will give the nurse the information needed to determine the level of care for the child.**
    4. Although it is important to provide safety education, this information should be given in a nonjudgmental manner at a point when the parent and child are less stressed.

TEST-TAKING HINT: The test taker needs to consider the role of a triage nurse to obtain specific information quickly. Answer 4 can be eliminated because it implies judgment and does not help the current situation.

29. 1. **Cushing triad is characterized by a decrease in heart rate, an increase in blood pressure, and changes in respirations. The triad is associated with severely increased ICP. Mannitol is an osmotic diuretic that helps decrease the increased ICP.**
    2. The child's vital signs need to be monitored, but a fluid bolus will increase the circulating volume and lead to an increase in the child's ICP. Fluid boluses are necessary in cases of shock but must be administered carefully and the child closely observed.
    3. An antihypertensive will not help decrease the ICP.
    4. The child will benefit from supplemental oxygen, but it will not help decrease the ICP.

TEST-TAKING HINT: The test taker should recognize the signs of Cushing triad. If not recognized, the child's condition should at least be seen as deteriorating and emergent. Answers 2 and 4 can be eliminated because they are only partially correct.

30. 1. Even if the child is unresponsive, the child can still feel pain.
    2. If pain medication is administered cautiously, the child can still be monitored and signs of improvement will be evident.
    3. **Pain medication promotes comfort and ultimately decreases ICP.**
    4. Pain medication decreases the demand for oxygen.

TEST-TAKING HINT: The test taker needs to consider the presence and significance of pain in the unresponsive child. Answer 1 can be immediately eliminated because the unresponsive child does feel pain.

31. 1. **A cooling blanket will help cool the child quickly and at a controlled temperature.**
    2. Acetaminophen (Tylenol) should be administered after the cooling blanket has been applied. Tylenol is an effective medication, but a cooling blanket will begin to be effective before the medication is absorbed.
    3. Acetaminophen (Tylenol) should be administered after the cooling blanket has been applied. Tylenol is an effective medication, but a cooling blanket will begin to be effective before the medication is absorbed.
    4. Ice packs will cause the child to shiver, which will increase oxygen consumption and possibly increase ICP. Shivering can also cause the child to experience a rebound increase in temperature.

TEST-TAKING HINT: The test taker should consider the cause of the increased temperature and how to cool the child quickly. Answer 4 should be eliminated because ice packs are no longer recommended to treat increased temperatures.

32. 1. Although peers play an important role in the adolescent's development, this particular patient is at risk for increased ICP and should have decreased stimulation.
    2. Loud talking may cause the child's ICP to increase.
    3. A bright, lively environment may lead to increased ICP.
    4. **A dark, quiet environment and minimal stimulation will decrease oxygen consumption and ICP.**

TEST-TAKING HINT: The test taker should consider the causes of ICP and select answers that will not increase ICP. Answers 1, 2, and 3 cause an increase in ICP and should be eliminated.

33. 1. **A computed tomography (CT) scan of the head will reveal trauma. Dilating the eyes is performed to check for retinal hemorrhages that are seen in an infant who has experienced shaken baby syndrome (SBS).**
    2. An EEG is not usually done as a priority test in an infant displaying symptoms of SBS.

3. X-rays of the head will show fractures, but CT and pupil examinations are the priority for this child.
4. X-rays of all long bones may be performed to rule out any old or new fractures, but CT and pupil examinations are the priority for this child.

TEST-TAKING HINT: The test taker should consider child abuse (SBS), because the story does not match the injury. The pupils are always dilated to rule out SBS.

34. 1. An open anterior fontanel allows for swelling, therefore decreasing the risk of injury.
    2. **Insufficient musculoskeletal support and a disproportionate head size place the infant at risk because the head cannot be supported during a shaking episode.**
    3. Superficial veins and arteries do not place the infant at a higher risk for injury.
    4. Although the myelination is immature, the immature musculoskeletal support places the infant at risk.

TEST-TAKING HINT: Answer 3 should be eliminated because superficial vessels do not lead to SBS.

35. 1. Meningocele is a sac that contains a portion of the meninges and cerebrospinal fluid.
    2. **A myelomeningocele is a sac that contains a portion of the meninges, the CSF, and the nerve roots.**
    3. Spina bifida occulta is the mildest form of spina bifida in which one or more vertebrae are malformed. The child usually has no symptoms, and in most cases, no one knows there is a spinal defect.
    4. Anencephaly is a neural tube defect in which the bones of the skull and head do not form correctly. Infants are missing large parts of their brain and skull.

TEST-TAKING HINT: The test taker would need to know the definition of myelomeningocele to answer this question.

36. 1. **Because a meningocele does not contain any nerve endings, most children experience no neurological problems after surgical correction.**
    2. Corrective surgery is done as soon as possible to minimize the risk of infection.
    3. Because a meningocele does not contain any nerve endings, most children experience no neurological problems after surgical correction.

4. Because a meningocele does not contain any nerve endings, most children experience no neurological problems after surgical correction.

TEST-TAKING HINT: The test taker should consider the risks of infection and immediately eliminate answer 2 because the surgery is not postponed but performed as soon as possible.

37. 1. Although it is important to measure the head circumference of all babies, children with myelomeningocele are at increased risk for hydrocephalus, which can be manifested with an increase in head circumference.
   2. **Children with myelomeningocele are at increased risk for hydrocephalus, which can be manifested with an increase in head circumference.**
   3. Although a defect in the spine can be a portal of entry for infection, children with myelomeningocele often have hydrocephalus as well.
   4. Children with myelomeningocele are not at risk for microcephaly.

TEST-TAKING HINT: The test taker should consider the diagnosis and choose a response that best fits the current diagnosis.

38. **2, 3.**
   1. Some children with myelomeningocele experience learning disabilities, but it is not the most common complication.
   2. **Urinary tract infections are the most common complication of myelomeningocele. Nearly all children with myelomeningocele have a neurogenic bladder that leads to incomplete emptying of the bladder and subsequent urinary tract infections. Frequent catheterization also increases the risk of urinary tract infection.**
   3. **About 90% to 95% of children with myelomeningocele experience hydrocephalus.**
   4. Children with myelomeningocele are at risk for skin breakdown and decubitus ulcers, but they are not the most common complications.
   5. Nutrition issues can occur, but are not the most common complication.
   6. Attention deficit disorders can occur, but are not the most common complications.

TEST-TAKING HINT: The test taker needs to be familiar with the complications of myelomeningocele. Neurogenic bladder and hydrocephalus are the most common complications, so the test taker should be led to select answers 2 and 3.

39. 1. Placing the child in the prone position is correct. A dry dressing may adhere to the defect, causing irritation.
   2. A dry dressing may adhere to the defect, causing irritation.
   3. Oral gastric feedings are not usually started unless there is going to be a delay in surgery. The defect is usually corrected within 24 hours to avoid infection.
   4. **The child is placed in the prone position to avoid any pressure on the defect. A sterile moist dressing is placed over the defect to keep it as clean as possible. Intravenous fluids are begun to prevent dehydration.**

TEST-TAKING HINT: The test taker can eliminate answer 2 because a dry dressing could cause irritation and stick to the sac.

40. 1. The child with a neurogenic bladder will never be able to spontaneously empty it completely. Most children learn to self-catheterize at a young age.
   2. The child with a neurogenic bladder will never be able to spontaneously empty it completely.
   3. Placing the child with a neurogenic bladder on a bladder training program is not helpful, because the child will never be able to spontaneously empty it completely.
   4. **A vesicostomy is an example of an option for children with myelomeningocele in which alternatives to traditional catheterizations are created.**

TEST-TAKING HINT: The test taker should recognize that the neurogenic bladder in a child with myelomeningocele is irreversible, and answers 2 and 3 should be eliminated.

41. 1. Children with myelomeningocele are prone to latex allergies and therefore should not eat bananas.
   2. Children with myelomeningocele are prone to latex allergies and therefore should not be exposed to balloons.
   3. **Preventing skin breakdown is important in the child with myelomeningocele because pressure points are not felt easily.**

4. It is always important to provide education on dietary needs, but it is not the priority in the immediate postoperative period.

TEST-TAKING HINT: The test taker should consider that children with myelomeningocele are prone to latex allergies and therefore should eliminate answers 1 and 2.

42. 1. Although there is a cosmetic benefit, the surgery is done to reconstruct the skull to allow the brain to grow properly. There are potential complications associated with this surgery, such as increased ICP.
    2. **The surgery is done to reconstruct the skull to allow the brain to grow properly. Because there are potential complications associated with this surgery, such as increased ICP, the child is usually closely observed in the PICU.**
    3. The surgery is not usually postponed but instead done in early infancy.
    4. The surgery is not usually postponed because it will allow for brain growth.

TEST-TAKING HINT: The test taker should consider the importance of allowing room for brain growth. Answers 3 and 4 can be eliminated because the surgery is performed in early infancy.

43. **3, 5.**
    1. The infant needs to wear the helmet 23 hours daily. It is removed for bathing but not sleeping.
    2. The helmet is most effective when the child is younger because the bones in the skull are more malleable. The child is less likely to need the helmet when upright and mobile because there is less pressure in one area.
    3. **The helmet is worn 23 hours every day and removed only for bathing.**
    4. Most children wear the helmet for 3 months.
    5. **Most children gain some improvement from a helmet.**

TEST-TAKING HINT: The test taker should recognize that the helmet is worn 23 hours daily and can eliminate answer 1.

44. 1. **The incidence of CP has increased, partly as a result of the increased survival rate of extreme low-birth-weight and premature infants.**
    2. The incidence of CP has increased since the 1960s.
    3. The incidence of CP has increased since the 1960s.
    4. There is no evidence to suggest that CP has been diagnosed erroneously.

TEST-TAKING HINT: The test taker should consider the causes of CP and be led to answer 1 because technology has increased the survival rate of low-birth-weight and premature infants. The test taker should resist the temptation to select answer 2 because it has not decreased as have many disorders.

45. 1. There is an increased incidence of CP when the infant has an Apgar score of 3 or less at 5 minutes.
    2. **Any infection of the central nervous system increases the infant's risk of CP.**
    3. A febrile seizure does not increase the risk of CP.
    4. Although head trauma can increase the risk of CP, the school-age child is not likely to develop CP from falling off a bike.

TEST-TAKING HINT: The test taker should consider the risks for CP. Answers 3 and 4 should be eliminated because these symptoms are least likely to lead to CP.

46. 1. The startle reflex is expected in an infant 1-month-old.
    2. **The clinical characteristic of hemiplegia can be manifested by the early preference of one hand. This may be an early sign of CP.**
    3. Although many children walk before the age of 14 months, it is not considered a motor delay not to have achieved this milestone at this point.
    4. Many 2-year-olds have not achieved bladder control.

TEST-TAKING HINT: The test taker should be familiar with normal developmental milestones and eliminate answers 1, 3, and 4 because they are all developmentally appropriate.

47. 1. CP is diagnosed based on clinical characteristics and developmental findings. It is not diagnosed with any type of radiological examination.
    2. Although most cases of CP occur in the neonatal period, some children can develop CP at a later age.
    3. **The child will be given a chance to recover and will be monitored closely before a diagnosis is made.**
    4. Although many children develop CP after having complications of meningitis, many do not. Although the parents should not be given false hope, they should not be led to lose hope for a complete recovery.

TEST-TAKING HINT: The test taker should be led to answer 3 because it explains the process and does not state that the child definitely will or will not develop CP.

48. 1. The nurse cannot assume that the child will have speech difficulties. Speech therapy does not guarantee vocalization at a developmentally appropriate age.
    2. Although speech therapy will assist with babbling at a later age, its primary purpose is to assist with feeding.
    3. **It is important to involve speech therapy to strengthen tongue and jaw movements to assist with feeding. The infant who is at risk for CP may have weakened and uncoordinated tongue and jaw movements.**
    4. Members of a multidisciplinary team become involved in a child's care based on specific needs, not hospital routine.

TEST-TAKING HINT: The test taker should immediately eliminate answer 4 because it does not consider the child's individual needs.

49. 1. Baclofen is not given for postoperative pain control.
    2. Baclofen is not given for seizures.
    3. **Baclofen is given to help control the spasms associated with CP.**
    4. Baclofen is not given for bladder control.

TEST-TAKING HINT: The test taker needs to be familiar with the medication baclofen.

50. 1. CP is a nonprogressive disorder.
    2. **CP can manifest in different ways as the child grows. It does not progress, but its clinical manifestations may change.**
    3. Children with CP have different abilities and needs. CP can result in mild to severe motor deficits; therefore, one treatment regimen cannot be used or recommended for all children.
    4. Although braces may assist some children with ambulation, they will not be useful in all cases.

TEST-TAKING HINT: The test taker can eliminate answers 3 and 4 because generalizations cannot be made regarding CP. Each child has different abilities and disabilities.

51. 1. **Sign language may help the child with CP communicate and ultimately decrease frustration. Children with CP may have difficulty verbalizing because of weak tongue and jaw muscles. They may be able to have sufficient motor skills to communicate with their hands.**
    2. Sign language does not cause confusion and may help reinforce vocabulary and vocalization.
    3. CP is manifested differently in all children; therefore, generalizations cannot be made.
    4. The earlier sign language is taught, the more it will be beneficial.

TEST-TAKING HINT: The test taker can immediately eliminate answer 3 because it makes a generalization. All forms of language are beneficial and well tolerated by children, especially young children.

52. 1. **The food should be placed far back in the mouth to avoid tongue thrust.**
    2. The child should be placed in an upright position.
    3. Soft and blended foods minimize the risk of aspiration.
    4. Allowing the child time to feed minimizes the risk of aspiration.

TEST-TAKING HINT: The test taker should consider which methods will decrease the risk of aspiration. Answers 2, 3, and 4 all decrease the risk of choking and should be eliminated.

53. 1. Sharing information may not be helpful if the family is not ready to listen.
    2. Sharing information may not be helpful if the family is not ready to listen.
    3. The family may have other concerns that would be communicated through an open-ended question.
    4. **An open-ended question will encourage family members to share what they know and potentially clear up any misconceptions.**

TEST-TAKING HINT: The test taker should consider the principles of therapeutic communication. Answer 4 is an open-ended question that will not be perceived as judgmental and should elicit the most information.

54. 1. Neuroblastoma is not always cured and can be fatal depending on the stage at diagnosis, site of origin, and the age of the child.
    2. **Infants younger than 1 year have the best prognosis.**
    3. Infants younger than 1 year have the best prognosis.
    4. Although the prognosis varies with the site of origin, infants have the most favorable outcome.

TEST-TAKING HINT: The question requires the test taker to be familiar with the prognosis of neuroblastoma.

55. 1. **Red blood cells will be needed to increase the red blood cell count.**
    2. The child should not be around groups of people because of the potential of exposure to infection.
    3. Blood thinners are not given to the child with a decreased platelet count.
    4. Fresh fruits and vegetables should be avoided because they may contain microorganisms that can lead to infection in the child with a low white blood cell count.

    TEST-TAKING HINT: The test taker should consider all components of pancytopenia and select the answer that will not harm the child. Answers 2 and 4 should be immediately eliminated because they both increase the risk of infection.

56. 1. Although abdominal fullness is often seen, difficulty urinating is not a common symptom.
    2. Bone manifestations are a sign of bone metastasis, which is not seen in the early stages of neuroblastoma.
    3. **The signs and symptoms vary depending on where the tumor is located, but typical symptoms include weight loss, abdominal distention, and fatigue.**
    4. The signs and symptoms vary according to the location of the tumor. Generally, hunger and weight gain are not seen.

    TEST-TAKING HINT: The test taker should eliminate answer 2 because bone metastases are a late sign, and the test taker is looking for initial signs.

57. 1. **In infants, signs and symptoms may not be readily apparent because the open fontanel allows for expansion.**
    2. Although brain tumors are not suspected in infants, a delay in diagnosis is most likely because of the open fontanel, allowing some expansion to go unnoticed.
    3. Signs and symptoms may be misinterpreted, but increased ICP will become apparent.
    4. Signs and symptoms may be denied, but increased ICP will become apparent.

    TEST-TAKING HINT: The test taker should consider growth and development in answering this question. The anterior fontanel allows for brain expansion, therefore delaying the discovery of signs and symptoms of a brain tumor.

58. 1. The child is experiencing diabetes insipidus, a common occurrence in children with midline brain tumors. Mannitol (Osmitrol) is an osmotic diuretic that will not treat diabetes insipidus.
    2. **The child is experiencing diabetes insipidus, a common occurrence in children with midline brain tumors. Vasopressin is a hormone that is used to help the body retain water.**
    3. The child is experiencing diabetes insipidus, a common occurrence in children with midline brain tumors. Furosemide (Lasix) is a diuretic that will not treat diabetes insipidus.
    4. The child is experiencing diabetes insipidus, a common occurrence in children with midline brain tumors. Dopamine (Intropin) is a beta-adrenergic agonist that is not used to treat diabetes insipidus.

    TEST-TAKING HINT: The test taker should be familiar with diabetes insipidus. The question describes its symptoms. Diabetes insipidus commonly occurs in children with midline brain tumors. The test taker can eliminate answers 1 and 3 because they increase diuresis, which needs to be avoided.

59. 1. Not all children who receive radiation experience learning disabilities.
    2. Younger children tend to experience more learning difficulties than do older children.
    3. **Although variable, younger children tend to experience more learning difficulties than do older children.**
    4. Although variable, younger children tend to experience more learning difficulties than do older children.

    TEST-TAKING HINT: The test taker should be familiar with radiation therapy. The test taker should be led to answers 3 and 4 because they both state that difficulties are variable.

60. 1. The cervical collar should not be removed. In addition to the methylprednisolone (Medrol), ranitidine (Zantac) should be administered to prevent gastric ulcer formation.
    2. **All forms of spinal stabilization should be continued while methylprednisolone (Medrol) and ranitidine (Zantac) are administered.**
    3. The backboard and cervical collar should not be removed until after the halo traction has been applied.
    4. The cervical collar should not be removed.

    TEST-TAKING HINT: The test taker should be familiar with spinal cord injuries. The test taker should eliminate any answer stating the cervical collar be removed, such as 1, 3, and 4.

61. 1, 2, 3, 4, 5.
    1. Many metabolic disorders are associated with hypoglycemia. The hypoglycemic child experiences a decreased level of consciousness because the brain does not have stores of glucose.
    2. Trauma can lead to generalized brain swelling with resultant increased ICP.
    3. Hypoxemia leads to a decreased level of consciousness because the brain is intolerant to the lack of oxygen.
    4. Dehydration can lead to inadequate perfusion to the brain, which can result in a decreased level of consciousness.
    5. Endocrine disorders often result in a decreased level of consciousness because they can lead to hypoglycemia, which is poorly tolerated by the brain.

    TEST-TAKING HINT: Metabolic disorders, trauma, hypoxic episodes, dehydration, and endocrine disorders are examples of disorders that can alter a child's level of consciousness by either increasing ICP or decreasing the perfusion of blood to the brain.

14

Leadership and Management

KEYWORDS

The following words include English vocabulary, nursing/medical terminology, concepts, principles, or information relevant to content specifically addressed in the chapter or associated with topics presented in it. English dictionaries, your nursing textbooks, and medical dictionaries such as *Taber's Cyclopedic Medical Dictionary* are resources that can be used to expand your knowledge and understanding of these words and related information.

Advocacy

Assent

Confidentiality

Delegation

Ethical principles

Followership

Informed consent

Leadership

Malpractice

Management

Mentor

Nurse practice act

Priority

Risk management

Scope of practice

ABBREVIATIONS

Activities of daily living (ADLs)

Against medical advice (AMA)

Cardiopulmonary resuscitation (CPR)

Emergency department (ED)

Gastrointestinal (GI)

Glycosylated hemoglobin (HbA1c)

Health Insurance Portability and
 Accountability Act (HIPAA)

Health maintenance organization (HMO)

Licensed practical nurse (LPN)

Licensed vocational nurse (LVN)

Peripherally inserted central catheter
 (PICC)

Prothrombin time (PT)

QUESTIONS

1. An adolescent is hospitalized for treatment of gunshot wounds acquired in a gang conflict. The teen often shouts at the nurses and uses vulgar language. Which activity is the best example of client advocacy?
   1. Accepting the rude behavior without comment.
   2. Avoiding entering the room except for scheduled treatments.
   3. Meeting all demands in order to achieve peace.
   4. Asking the teen to describe any fears about current treatment.

2. An adolescent is seen in the ED and diagnosed with a bowel obstruction. Despite the nurse's best attempt to explain the reason for a nasogastric (NG) tube, the teen refuses to let the nurse insert the tube. The parent's approach is also ineffective. Which would be most appropriate for the nurse to do first?
   1. Obtain an order for sedation, physically restrain the client, and insert the tube.
   2. Page the physician and document the client's refusal to accept the nasogastric tube.
   3. Explain the against-medical-advice (AMA) form to the adolescent and parent.
   4. Notify the hospital's client advocate to meet with the adolescent and parent.

3. An infant returned from GI surgery 4 hours ago. The parent refuses pain medication for the baby and states, "The baby is crying because of hunger. Can I offer a bottle?" How should the nurse best advocate for the infant?
   1. Review the results of the observational pain scale with the parent and explain why the infant must have nothing by mouth.
   2. Use nonpharmacological measures first to see if the pain rating of 8 (out of 10) decreases.
   3. Ask the parent to use the observational pain tool to measure the infant's pain.
   4. Call the physician to obtain an order to feed the infant.

4. At lunch, several nurses are discussing how difficult it is to care for an adolescent who constantly complains of pain unrelieved by morphine via a patient-controlled analgesia (PCA) pump. One nurse comments, "The teen is addicted to drugs. What do you expect?!" Which is the best response to this statement?
   1. "The teen should be moved to an adult unit, where the teen will be told what to do."
   2. "We should make sure that the teen has a nursing student to give the staff some relief."
   3. "Perhaps we should call a team conference to review the pain complaints and treatment."
   4. "I think we should speak with the physician about changing to non-narcotic pain medications."

5. A case manager works in an outpatient clinic that administers palivizumab (Synagis) to premature infants at high risk for respiratory syncytial virus (RSV). Which outcome is most significant as an indication of effective treatment?
   1. Prevention of hospitalization.
   2. Optimal weight gain.
   3. Promotion of parent-infant bonding.
   4. Early detection and treatment of congenital defects.

6. A case manager is called to arrange for medical equipment and medications at discharge for a child with multiple social problems. Which problem is likely to have the greatest impact on discharge planning?
   1. The child and family are homeless.
   2. The child is not covered by insurance.
   3. The family cannot pay for medications.
   4. The child does not have a primary care provider.

7. Which outcome would indicate effective case management for a child with moderate to severe asthma?
   1. The child attends school regularly with few absences for the year.
   2. The child has an asthma action plan.
   3. The family fills prescriptions for prophylactic inhaled steroids.
   4. The child does not utilize the peak flowmeter when cared for at home.

8. Which of the following is a component of family-centered care?
   1. Reinforce all parenting practices.
   2. Accept all cultural practices and rituals.
   3. Guarantee that financial needs are met.
   4. Recognize family strengths.

9. Nurses are aware that current trends affecting health-care consumers include which of the following? Consumers:
   1. Generally are less informed about health-care issues than previous generations.
   2. Are comfortable with health insurance benefits, services, and conditions.
   3. Are more trusting and less demanding of health-care organizations and staff.
   4. Expect to be more involved in decisions about health-care options.

10. A child and family are addressed by the nurse during admission to the pediatric unit. Which statement is the best example of a proactive service orientation?
    1. "Do you have any special questions or concerns that I can address?"
    2. "It is important that you keep the crib side rails up at all times you are not at the bedside."
    3. "We ask that you restrict visitors to two persons at the bedside because of space limitations."
    4. "Because your child is on contact precautions, your child will have to remain in the room."

11. A seriously ill child is treated in the intensive care unit. Which aspect of care is the easiest for family members to evaluate and most important for consumer satisfaction?
    1. The compliance with standards.
    2. The efficiency of the medical equipment used in care.
    3. The relationship with the nurse and other staff.
    4. The accuracy of completion of medical orders.

12. An interdisciplinary team is assembled to review protocols for management of central intravenous lines. Which staff should be represented on the team?
    1. Experienced RNs and pharmacists.
    2. RNs, physicians, and pharmacists.
    3. RNs, LPNs/LVNs, and physicians.
    4. Charge nurses and staff physicians.

13. The staff nurse is discharging an infant with a tracheostomy and gastrostomy to be cared for at home. The case manager has arranged for home health supplies and services. Whose discussion would be of most direct benefit to ensure individualized care in the home?
    1. Case manager and community pediatrician.
    2. Case manager and home health company supervisor.
    3. Staff RN and medical supply company.
    4. Hospital staff nurse and home health nurse.

14. An experienced nurse notes that a child is developing a rash shortly after the first dose of an intravenous antibiotic. Which team member should be called first?
    1. Physician.
    2. Pharmacist.
    3. Charge nurse.
    4. Unit manager.

15. It is a busy day on the pediatric unit, and the nurses are short-staffed. A school-age child is scheduled to undergo an invasive radiological procedure. Which staff member would be most appropriate to meet the child's support needs by accompanying the child to the radiology department?
1. The staff nurse with the least busy assignment.
2. The staff nurse assigned to this child.
3. A volunteer grandparent who is on the unit.
4. The child life–worker for the unit.

16. Which activity, encouraged by the management, would be most effective in helping a new nurse manager develop transformational leadership abilities in a rapidly changing practice setting?
1. Select a mentor and a professional support group.
2. Focus on activities that avoid change and involve minimal risk.
3. Reward or correct followers to maintain current levels of practice.
4. Use your own judgment when making decisions, with little input from staff.

17. Which activity best falls within the scope of management rather than leadership?
1. Planning the staffing schedule for a 2-month period.
2. Empowering the staff to meet client-care goals for the year.
3. Encouraging staff to utilize reflective practice and self-awareness.
4. Inspiring staff to develop a shared vision of quality client care.

18. Tasks of followership that would be expected of a new nursing graduate include which of the following?
1. Collaborates with others, honors standards, demonstrates individual accountability.
2. Envisions organizational goals, affirms values, represents the group.
3. Motivates others, develops standards, eliminates barriers to care.
4. Evaluates system processes, recommends ways to improve the system.

19. The pediatric unit is reevaluating the procedure used by staff to suction tracheostomies. Which activity demonstrates followership activities appropriate to a recent nursing graduate?
1. Rewrite the hospital policy and procedure for tracheostomy suctioning.
2. Work with information technology to plan new computer screens for charting.
3. Provide input on the feasibility and effectiveness of the new procedure.
4. Hold in-service presentations to educate staff on the techniques and rationale for the new procedure.

20. The nurse receives a telephone call from a staff member who works on another unit. The member is inquiring about the test results of a friend's child, who is hospitalized on the nurse's unit. Which response is appropriate? **Select all that apply.**
1. Summarize the test results, because they are within the normal range.
2. Move to a private phone to prevent being overheard before sharing the information.
3. Decline to give out information.
4. Direct the staff member to the test results in the hospital electronic medical record.
5. Suggest the staff member ask the child's parent about test results.

21. A pediatric hospital nurse receives a telephone call from an individual who is the parent of a child assigned to the nurse's care. Which action by the nurse is most correct?
1. Verify the privacy code assigned to the child before giving any information.
2. Decline to give out information over the telephone because no ID can be shown.
3. Update the parent on the child's condition because no family members are in the room.
4. Take the parent's name and telephone number and give it to the other parent when visiting.

22. A nursing student records notes about a pediatric client's condition in preparation for a clinical experience. Which information is considered individually identifiable health-care information and cannot be attached to the notes?
    1. Date of birth.
    2. Medical diagnosis.
    3. Nursing diagnosis.
    4. Diagnostic test results.

23. If an employee has medical testing at a facility where that employee works, what is the appropriate way to access the test results?
    1. Complete the authorization form and receive a copy of the results.
    2. Get a fellow employee who works in that department to access the results.
    3. Call a friend who has access to the records and ask for a copy of the test results.
    4. Check the computer system for the test results.

24. For a school-age child who has Kawasaki disease and is taking aspirin, which laboratory value should be reported to the physician?
    1. Blood urea nitrogen 18 mg/dL.
    2. Hematocrit 42%.
    3. Potassium 3.8 mEq/L.
    4. PT 14.6 sec.

25. During a home visit to an 8-month-old infant in congestive heart failure on digoxin (Lanoxin), the nurse obtains assessment information. Which assessment indicates that the nurse needs to consult the physician?
    1. The infant's apical pulse is 70 at rest.
    2. After crying, the infant's heart rate is 170.
    3. Respirations are 40 per minute at rest.
    4. Capillary refill is <3 sec.

26. A premature infant with chronic lung disease is going home with oxygen, tracheostomy suction, and gastrostomy feedings. Which discharge planning activity will be most effective in promoting continuity of care?
    1. Send the parents to meet staff at the nursing agency that will be providing care in the home.
    2. Plan a team conference at the hospital before discharge to include parents and hospital and home health staff.
    3. Ask the parents to meet with the hospital respiratory therapy staff to discuss adapting the home environment to meet equipment needs.
    4. Teach parents how to care for the infant by utilizing hospital equipment and protocols.

27. Which client can benefit most by a primary nursing approach in which one nurse cares for the child whenever on duty and coordinates other staff care?
    1. A child admitted for a diagnostic workup of mononucleosis.
    2. A child who had surgery 1 day ago for appendicitis.
    3. An infant treated with phototherapy for hyperbilirubinemia.
    4. A toddler with leukemia, admitted for chemotherapy.

28. When caring for an infant admitted for pyloric stenosis surgery, which tasks would be appropriate for the RN to delegate to a nursing assistant? **Select all that apply.**
    1. Physical assessment on admission.
    2. Vital signs every 4 hours.
    3. Discharge teaching for parents.
    4. Bed, bath, and change of linens.
    5. Daily weights.

29. The nurse is managing care of a school-age child with new-onset type 1 diabetes. Which tasks must be performed only by the RN and cannot be delegated to an LPN/LVN or nursing assistant? **Select all that apply.**
    1. Teaching parents how to give subcutaneous injections of insulin.
    2. Performing blood glucose monitoring before meals and bedtime.
    3. Evaluating the child's response to insulin doses.
    4. Determining the educational goals for the day.
    5. Teaching the child signs for hypoglycemia and hyperglycemia.

30. Assigning the right task to the right person is a principle of nursing delegation and assignment. Which scenario best meets this principle?
    1. A 4-month-old with Down syndrome is assigned to a nurse whose own child died of heart disease due to Down syndrome 6 months ago.
    2. A child with a central intravenous line that occluded on the previous shift is assigned to a new LPN/LVN.
    3. A child newly diagnosed with acute leukemia is assigned to an experienced pediatric oncology nurse who floated to the general pediatric unit.
    4. A child with new-onset type 1 diabetes is assigned to an RN who has four other complex-care clients.

31. An experienced pediatric nurse relocates to a new city and state. In the new position, the nurse questions which skills and tasks can be performed by unlicensed nursing personnel. To obtain answers to this question, which resource is considered primary?
    1. Hospital policies and procedures manual.
    2. State's nurses' association.
    3. Educational program for nursing assistants.
    4. State's nurse practice act.

32. When caring for a client in pain, which activity is appropriate to delegate to unlicensed nursing personnel?
    1. Coaching the client during painful procedures.
    2. Assessment using a self-report pain scale.
    3. Evaluating pain after giving medication.
    4. Bathing the client and hygiene measures.

33. After receiving the change-of-shift report, the nurse prioritizes care for the day. Which child should the nurse assess first?
    1. A 1-month-old admitted 1 day ago with fever and possible sepsis.
    2. A 14-month-old with a tracheostomy admitted for respiratory syncytial virus (RSV) bronchiolitis.
    3. An 18-month-old with acute viral meningitis.
    4. A 7-year-old 1 day after an appendectomy.

34. After a school bus accident, four elementary school children are delivered by ambulance to the emergency department (ED). Which child should be directed to the physician first by the triage nurse?
    1. The child who is crying uncontrollably and tries to move off the stretcher.
    2. The child with severe abdominal pain; who is anxious and responsive; and whose blood pressure is 100/60, heart rate is 120, and respiratory rate is 28.
    3. The child with severe pain and distorted alignment of the right lower leg, indicating a possible fracture.
    4. The child who is unresponsive, with fixed and dilated pupils; blood pressure is 58/44, heart rate is 60, and RR is 10.

35. The nurse is providing care for an adolescent with complex needs after surgical correction of a severe bowel obstruction. On entering the room, the nurse prioritizes care and decides to complete which task first?
    1. Change the central intravenous line dressing, which is loose and gaping.
    2. Empty the ileostomy bag, which is moderately full of liquid stool.
    3. Change the gauze dressing around the Jackson Pratt drain.
    4. Check for correct positioning of the nasogastric (NG) tube in the stomach.

36. An adolescent is received in the PICU after scoliosis surgery. Using Maslow's Hierarchy of Needs as a guide, which problem takes priority?
   1. Hypotension related to analgesia.
   2. Fear of being left alone by parents.
   3. Frustration with postoperative immobility.
   4. Concern with the extensive skin incision.

37. A child is receiving continuous morphine by patient-controlled analgesia (PCA) pump (basal and bolus) to control pain. Which side effect is the nurse's greatest concern?
   1. Sedation.
   2. Respiratory depression.
   3. Nausea and vomiting.
   4. Constipation.

38. Which question represents an ethical issue in nursing practice that cannot be resolved through clinical research?
   1. How does the incidence of medication errors on the pediatric unit compare with the incidence of errors on the neonatal unit?
   2. Does the use of local anesthesia during circumcision make a difference in infants' pain scores, as measured on the face, legs, activity, cry, consolability (FLACC) scale?
   3. Is the emergency department nurse obligated to report suspicion of child abuse if signs of abuse are noted in the assessment?
   4. Which method of irrigating central venous lines results in less line obstruction and infection?

39. Shortly before a child's elective surgery, the parent tells the nurse, "I am having second thoughts about my child undergoing this surgery." The nurse respects the parent's concern and calls the surgeon. What ethical/moral principle is represented by this situation?
   1. Autonomy.
   2. Equality.
   3. Fidelity.
   4. Justice.

40. During a clinic visit, a child's mother tells the nurse, "I'm afraid of what my husband will do." Following an ethical decision-making process, the nurse's first step is to:
   1. Direct the mother to a center for abused women.
   2. Provide the phone number of the domestic violence hotline.
   3. Clarify what the mother means by her statement.
   4. Ask the mother, "Why does your husband feel this way?"

41. Which situation would be appropriate to refer to the hospital ethics committee?
   1. The physician recommends that a young child in the end stages of terminal cancer be taken off the ventilator. The parents, who are divorced and have joint custody of the child, have different views about whether to discontinue the ventilator.
   2. A child in end-stage renal failure is placed on the renal transplant list. The parents are asked to sign permission for surgery after a cadaver kidney is located. One parent is out of town and gives telephone consent.
   3. After initial therapies have failed, a child with leukemia is evaluated for a new cancer protocol. The child, aged 8 years, gives assent for the new treatment, and his parents give consent as well.
   4. Parents are shocked when their child is diagnosed with a malignant bone tumor. The orthopedic surgeon discusses the options of limb amputation and a limb-salvage procedure. The parents are asked to consider each option.

42. Organizational policies on the security of computer data mandate that system users keep which piece of user information confidential?
    1. Name.
    2. ID.
    3. Password.
    4. Credentials.

43. The nurse is charting on the computer at the nursing station when a parent exits a nearby room and asks for help because the child has vomited. Which immediate action is best?
    1. Immediately assist the parent.
    2. Put the computer in "suspend mode" so that the screen is blank and then assist the parent.
    3. Finish recording information and exit out of the computer before assisting the parent.
    4. Continue charting and call another team member to assist the parent.

44. If a staff member has the right to access the computer system, the member has a right to view which health records?
    1. Personal.
    2. Immediate family members.
    3. Clients assigned to their care.
    4. Clients' family members.

45. Individually identifiable health information may not be:
    1. Faxed.
    2. Mailed.
    3. Copied.
    4. Sold.

46. Which client is able to give informed consent for a surgical procedure in many U.S. states?
    1. A 13-year-old abused male.
    2. A 15-year-old pregnant female.
    3. A 16-year-old cancer patient.
    4. A 17-year-old college freshman.

47. Which of the following situations would be considered a failure to obtain informed consent?
    1. Parents who speak Spanish receive information about their child's surgery from the surgeon using a telephone language-line Spanish translator.
    2. Bilingual parents sign the consent form for a lumbar puncture. Later, they tell a Spanish-speaking nurse, "We do not understand why they are doing this test."
    3. The physician addresses the benefits of a procedure with a child's parents but gets called away. Later, the physician returns to finish the discussion before parents sign the consent.
    4. Only one parent of a child is present in the hospital to sign the surgical consent. The other parent is out of town on business.

48. Staff members working with school-age children believe it is important for each child to understand and agree to medical treatment, especially when treatment is part of research protocols. This process is:
    1. Assent.
    2. Informed consent.
    3. Confidentiality.
    4. Emancipation.

49. When explaining the procedure to the parent of a child undergoing surgery, the provider must give which of the following information as part of informed consent? **Select all that apply.**
    1. Date and time the specific procedure will be performed.
    2. Alternative therapies.
    3. Benefits that are likely to result from the procedure.
    4. Names and titles of all staff members who will be in the operating room.
    5. The statement that the client and family may withdraw consent at any time.

50. When making assignments for the oncoming shift on the pediatric unit, the charge nurse assigns a float RN from another unit to care for an infant with complex needs. What is the legal responsibility of the charge nurse in this situation?
    1. Assurance of scope of practice.
    2. Duty to orient, educate, and evaluate.
    3. Client's rights and responsibilities.
    4. Determination of nurse/client ratios.

51. After the parent leaves the side rail down, a hospitalized toddler falls from the crib and suffers a skull fracture. Earlier that day, the nurse had discussed the importance of side rails with that parent and recorded the discussion in the nursing notes. Which element of malpractice is missing in this case?
    1. Relationship with the client.
    2. Breach of duty of care.
    3. Injury.
    4. Damage.

52. The nurse should check the agency's policy and procedure manual as the primary legal authority for which of the following?
    1. Whether an RN can initiate a blood transfusion.
    2. Sharing of client-sensitive information.
    3. Legal protection when providing CPR to a non-client.
    4. Procedure for flushing a central venous line.

53. Which situation might be considered assault and battery of a child?
    1. The nurse sticks a hysterical infant five times in an attempt to start a PICC line, although the parent verbally refuses to allow the procedure to continue after the third try.
    2. A 2-year-old screams while being restrained for a dressing change of a complex burn wound.
    3. A nurse attempts to administer an oral antibiotic to a young child, who then spits the entire dose of medication out on the sheet.
    4. A postoperative school-age child refuses when told to get out of bed and walk in the hall four times a day.

54. The nurse makes an error by giving the wrong medication to a client. An incident report is completed per hospital policy. What information should the nurse chart in the medical record? **Select all that apply.**
    1. Description of the specific occurrence.
    2. What treatment was given.
    3. Completion of the incident report.
    4. Date, time, and name of person completing the incident report.
    5. Nothing.

55. Which event should be reported to a risk management committee by documentation?
1. A nurse administered a double therapeutic dose of medication based on an incorrect physician order.
2. A client's heparin lock became clotted between intermittent medication doses.
3. A toddler dislodged the intravenous catheter, resulting in an occluded intravenous line.
4. An uncooperative child spit out an undeterminable amount of oral medication despite the nurse's best effort.

56. Which event represents a departure from safe practice as defined by risk management?
1. A nurse double-checks an insulin dose with a nursing assistant before administration to the client.
2. The physician writes an illegible order, then draws a line through it, initials it, and prints the same information above the line.
3. The nurse repeats a verbal order back to the physician and asks for verification of accuracy.
4. A nurse asks another RN to double-check a dose of morphine before administering the drug via intravenous push.

57. The diabetes clinic conducts a disease management program for children with type 1 diabetes. Which test is the most valid indicator of compliance with the diabetes regimen?
1. Fasting blood glucose level.
2. Fingerstick glucose for 24 hours.
3. Urine ketone strip.
4. HbA1c assay.

58. A charge nurse overhears a staff nurse make an erroneous statement to a parent in the hallway. What should the charge nurse do first?
1. Discuss the correct information with the parent.
2. Discuss the observation with the manager of the unit.
3. Write a description of the incident and share it with the staff nurse.
4. Ask the staff nurse to describe the situation in private.

59. Which situation should be referred by the pediatric nursing staff to the nurse manager?
1. Several staff members plan to get together to celebrate the end of a successful year working on the unit.
2. Staff members complain about the cafeteria food and want a broader menu.
3. Clients with occluded saline locks are repeatedly being transferred from the emergency department to the pediatric unit.
4. Nursing staff members who have joined the union are in disagreement with union policies.

60. A 9-year-old child on the pediatric unit is immobilized in a spica cast. When the parents are absent, the child presses the call light constantly. Which action would be most appropriate to meet the child's needs?
1. Consult with the charge nurse to obtain a 24-hour sitter for the child.
2. Speak with the parents and ask them not to leave the bedside.
3. Refer to the child-life worker for bedside play activities.
4. Obtain a social service referral to meet emotional needs.

61. A young child hospitalized with asthma is ready for discharge. A home nebulizer is ordered by the physician. In order to obtain the nebulizer, a referral should be made to which staff member?
1. Case manager.
2. Nurse manager.
3. Materials management staff.
4. Child-life staff.

The correct answer number and rationale for why it is the correct answer are given in **boldface blue type.** Rationales for why the other possible answer options are incorrect also are given, but they are not in boldface type.

1. 1. Acceptance of the teen's humanity does not mean acceptance of inappropriate or rude behavior. The nurse also has rights and should communicate to the teen how the behavior is being interpreted.
   2. Avoidance of the teen is likely to further alienate and isolate the teen, increasing fears and concerns.
   3. Meeting all demands may not be appropriate in this situation. Nursing staff members need to negotiate, clarify, and explain which behaviors are acceptable, without reinforcing negative behavior.
   4. **All clients have the right to be informed and to participate in care decisions. Assessment of needs is the first step in providing culturally congruent care and education.**

TEST-TAKING HINT: Client advocacy is based on protecting the basic rights of clients in the health-care system. Understanding the disease process and its treatment is one of these rights. As in all aspects of care, assessment of the client's questions and fears is the beginning of client education.

2. 1. This approach involves little advocacy for the client, because it bypasses rather than supports self-determination.
   2. This approach would be used only after other methods to communicate with the client have been attempted.
   3. This is the least effective approach, because if the adolescent leaves against medical advice, no care will be received.
   4. **Because of the client's age, the teen should be treated as an adult. The nurse best promotes self-determination by making additional attempts to elicit any fears and concerns that are preventing effective care. The client advocate may be able to gain this information.**

TEST-TAKING HINT: Client advocacy includes promoting the rights of the client, in this case the right to self-determination and informed consent. Utilizing the client advocate in this situation is an effective way to further determine why the client is refusing care.

3. 1. **As the advocate for the infant and the parent, the nurse has the responsibility to educate the parent about the infant's condition after surgery, the rationale for having nothing by mouth, and the assessment and treatment of pain. By being informed, the parent can make educated assessments and decisions, collaborating with the nurse to meet the infant's needs.**
   2. A pain rating of 8 indicates severe pain and the need for pharmacological and nonpharmacological pain control measures.
   3. Although the parent should be educated about the pain tool, the parent should not be accountable to use the tool to measure the infant's pain.
   4. If the infant had major GI surgery, it would be contraindicated to feed the infant immediately postoperatively.

TEST-TAKING HINT: Advocacy helps to ensure that pain and other postoperative needs are met by nursing staff. Because parents have the legal authority to consent for their child's treatment, it is critical that they be fully informed and understand the child's postoperative status and rationale for treatment.

4. 1. Passing responsibility for care to another unit where staff do not know the teen is unlikely to resolve problems with care.
   2. Recruiting a student, who is less experienced in the care of complex pain clients, is unlikely to resolve problems with care.
   3. **As a client advocate, the nurse is responsible for recognizing when current approaches are ineffective and for working with other staff members to develop effective care. Planning a team conference is one way to brainstorm new approaches.**
   4. If morphine does not relieve the pain, this answer is unlikely to be effective.

TEST-TAKING HINT: As a client advocate, the nurse promotes the rights of this client to optimum treatment and pain relief. Because pain is a complex phenomenon, a multidisciplinary approach is often helpful to come up with new and more effective approaches.

5. 1. **Palivizumab (Synagis) is an antibody administered monthly to premature and other high-risk infants during respiratory syncytial virus (RSV) season. The goal is prevention of serious RSV bronchiolitis requiring hospitalization.**
2. Although weight gain is an important health outcome for growing premature infants, it is not the focus of a clinic for RSV prophylaxis.
3. Promotion of parent-infant bonding is a goal for nurses working with infants; however, this is not the focus of a clinic for RSV prevention.
4. Early detection and treatment of congenital problems are important for the health of premature infants, but they are not the focus of a clinic for RSV prevention.

TEST-TAKING HINT: Because of the expense and special authorization needed from third-party payers, palivizumab (Synagis) is often administered in specialty clinics. Case managers work with clients to coordinate care, promote cost savings, use resources efficiently, and improve client outcomes.

6. 1. **Homelessness is likely to have the greatest impact on discharge planning because all other aspects of care revolve around this issue.**
2. The social worker can assist the family in applying for medical aid because of their low income.
3. Discharge medications can often be secured through the assistance of the social worker and hospital pharmacy.
4. The child can be referred to a clinic that works with indigent clients for follow-up and continued care.

TEST-TAKING HINT: Homelessness affects all other issues and requires social services in both the community and hospital.

7. 1. **Regular school attendance is a positive outcome of case management because asthma can result in frequent absences from school.**
2. The asthma action plan is important for the client to have so that the parents, school nurse, and others know what to do if the client has an asthma exacerbation. The better determinant of compliance is school attendance.
3. This situation is considered a negative outcome, because children with moderate or severe asthma need inhaled steroids to decrease lung inflammation.
4. This situation is a negative outcome. Peak flowmeters should be used to monitor lung function and guide treatment decisions.

TEST-TAKING HINT: The goal of case management in asthma is improved health outcomes, including prevention of exacerbations of illness. School attendance, prevention of hospital admissions, regular checkups, early diagnosis of illness, and compliance with medications are indicators of effective case management.

8. 1. Parenting practices are respected as long as children's needs are met; however, this may not be true of all parenting practices. Parent education and negotiation may be required.
2. There may be times that cultural practices directly conflict with medical treatments; therefore, acceptance is based on compatibility.
3. Although financial support for families is included in family-centered care guidelines, there is no guarantee that all financial needs will be met.
4. **Recognizing and building on family strengths is an important component of family-centered care.**

TEST-TAKING HINT: All pediatric health-care organizations include family-centered care as part of their client rights documents. Family-centered care includes recognizing the family as the constant in the child's life, creating parent-professional collaboration, encouraging parent-to-parent support, and building on family strengths.

9. 1. Today's health-care consumer is better educated, often from searching the Internet, and expects to receive more information from providers.
2. In contrast, many clients are dissatisfied or confused about benefits under their health insurance plans.
3. To the contrary, data show that clients are more demanding and aggressive in situations involving health care.
4. **Data show that current health-care consumers expect to participate more in decisions about medical treatment.**

TEST-TAKING HINT: Consider the effect of societal trends, such as Internet access, advertising and marketing, increased rights of women and minorities, changes in insurance and HMOs, and increasing diversity.

10. 1. **This is a proactive statement with a "ready to help" attitude.**

2. This statement provides information about crib safety.

3. This statement provides information about visiting policies.

4. This statement provides information about isolation policies.

TEST-TAKING HINT: A service orientation focuses on customer satisfaction. Proactive statements with a "ready to help" attitude include such phrases as "How may I help you?" "I'd be happy to …" "It's my pleasure to …"

11. 1. Consumers are frequently unable to judge this aspect of care.

2. This is not a known aspect of care for most family members.

3. **Consumers always have the ability to evaluate the quality of the relationship with the person delivering the service.**

4. Family members as consumers seldom have the information to judge this aspect of care.

TEST-TAKING HINT: Although consumers are frequently unable to judge or evaluate the quality of interventions, they always have the ability to evaluate the quality of the relationship with the person delivering the service. Most consumer complaints revolve around problems with staff, such as feeling ignored or disrespected or being treated poorly.

12. 1. The team should be composed of these staff members; however, this answer omits physicians, who write the orders for the central intravenous line.

2. **Because all three of these disciplines are involved in care of central intravenous lines, this answer is the most complete.**

3. In many locations, LPNs/LVNs are not authorized to care for central intravenous lines and would not be involved in this care. Furthermore, this answer omits pharmacists, who are concerned with medication administration through these lines.

4. Involving only persons at the leadership level may lead to omission of valuable input from staff RNs, resident physicians, and other disciplines such as pharmacy.

TEST-TAKING HINT: Involving all team members who have responsibilities related to this activity helps to ensure that all important factors are considered. When members of all involved disciplines participate in decision making, they are more likely to agree to any changes made.

13. 1. These team members have oversight for assessing, planning, and evaluating care of the child but do not provide direct nursing care in the hospital or home.

2. Both of these team members are in managerial roles, which are essential for providing resources, but may not guarantee an individualized approach to care.

3. Planning for home-care supplies is an important function but not as broad as that provided by other team members.

4. **If the goal is individualized care, the best team members to discuss this child's care are the two staff members with the most direct caretaking responsibilities—the hospital staff nurse and the home health nurse.**

TEST-TAKING HINT: The key to deciding among staff members is the phrase "individualized care." Which two team members will be in most direct contact with the child and family? These staff members are most likely to know the individual characteristics of the child and family members.

14. 1. **Development of an allergic reaction, which is most likely happening in this situation, requires prompt treatment to prevent complications such as anaphylaxis. The physician should be called first so that prompt treatment can be ordered.**

2. The pharmacist cannot change the drug without a physician's order.

3. Although the charge nurse should be informed in a timely manner, the nurse has the responsibility to communicate directly with the physician when an allergic reaction is suspected.

4. This incident may or may not require communication to the unit manager.

TEST-TAKING HINT: Problem-solving requires knowledge of clearly delegated roles and duties. Only the physician has the authority to prescribe an antihistamine in this situation. Furthermore, the nurse has the legal responsibility to notify the physician of any complication, such as a rash.

15. 1. The child does not know that nurses have other client assignments and may not feel supported. Additionally, this arrangement takes the staff nurse away from assigned clients.

2. In a short-staffed situation, it may be impossible to take a nurse off the floor for even a short radiological procedure. Care of other assigned clients may be compromised.

3. A volunteer may not be able to support the child adequately in an unfamiliar situation and may have difficulty coping with the stress of an intrusive procedure.

4. **Helping children cope with intrusive or frightening procedures is part of the job description of the child life–worker. This answer has the added advantage of maintaining staff nurse numbers on the unit.**

TEST-TAKING HINT: **The best answer considers the staffing needs of the unit as well as the individual support needs of the child. In answers 1 and 2, staffing may be compromised by sending a nurse off the unit. In answer 3, the volunteer may not be able to support the child adequately. Because support during intrusive procedures is a common function of the child life–worker, answer 4 is most likely to provide the child with maximum support without reducing nursing staffing.**

16. 1. **A mentor can model new behavior and coach the new nurse manager while providing support during new experiences.**
2. The novice nurse leader-manager must be willing to change, grow, and take risks.
3. Transformational leadership involves inspiring new visions rather than maintaining the status quo.
4. A good leader gathers input from all levels of staff when making decisions.

TEST-TAKING HINT: **Transformational leadership is best in changing environments. This leadership style involves creativity, change, risk, shared vision, and attention to the importance of people. The challenges of developing these leadership abilities are best met by the novice leader-manager who has the support of a mentor who can serve as a coach, teacher, and resource person.**

17. 1. **Managers coordinate and utilize resources. Planning for staffing is an example of both coordination and utilization of staff.**
2. Empowerment of staff best fits within the scope of leadership.
3. Encouraging self-reflection is a motivational activity included in leadership theories.

4. Leaders help to transform organizations through motivation and inspiration of employees.

TEST-TAKING HINT: **"Management" is defined as a process of coordinating activities and utilizing resources to achieve goals. Actions tend to be more specific, such as preparing the staffing schedule. "Leadership" is a broader concept, involving staff empowerment, system redesign, ethics, and increased motivation.**

18. 1. **These followership activities are appropriate for a newly graduated nurse.**
2. These activities are leadership and management tasks, appropriate for the experienced practitioner.
3. These tasks fall within the scope of leadership and management.
4. These tasks require experience in an organization and are appropriate for leaders and managers.

TEST-TAKING HINT: **Bleich's tasks of leadership, management, and followership are included in the examples above. The new nursing graduate would be expected to demonstrate good followership before taking on leadership and management tasks.**

19. 1. Writing policies and procedures is an advanced activity, performed by nurse managers.
2. Designing systems for charting is an advanced task, requiring experienced staff.
3. **Testing a new procedure falls within the scope of a new practitioner and is an appropriate followership activity.**
4. Staff educators are experienced staff members whose responsibility is to plan in-service education.

TEST-TAKING HINT: **Because the new graduate focuses on followership tasks, the key to answering this question is to determine whether actions fall within the scope of leadership, management, or followership. Testing out a new procedure is most clearly a followership task.**

20. **3, 5.**
1. Providing information to a staff member who is not involved in the client's care is a violation of privacy and must be avoided.
2. It is a violation of privacy to share information with others without client/family permission.

3. **The pediatric nurse cannot legally share this information, but the parent can choose to do so. This response does not violate client/family right to privacy.**

4. It is a clear violation of privacy to access electronic medical records without a need to know this information to provide care. Because the staff member is not involved in the child's care, that person cannot legally access the child's medical information.

5. **The pediatric nurse cannot legally share this information, but the parent can choose to do so. This response does not violate the client/family right to privacy.**

TEST-TAKING HINT: Sharing clinical information is guided by the "need to know" in order to care for a client. In this case, the staff member works on another unit and is not caring for the friend's child. "Need to know" does not exist here.

21. 1. **The nurse is correct to verify the privacy code, which is given only to the child's legal guardians, before relating medical information over the telephone.**

2. The nurse is correct to deny information to individuals who do not have the privacy code.

3. Failure to verify the caller's right to receive information is a violation of the client's right to privacy and confidentiality.

4. The nurse is incorrect to deny information if the caller can provide proper ID.

TEST-TAKING HINT: Institutions can reduce violation of a client's privacy and confidentiality by allowing access to client data only by individuals who are legally allowed to receive it. Most hospitals maintain privacy of data by assigning a privacy code, which is given to immediate family members, or maintaining a list of persons who are allowed information. Verification of a caller's right to receive information should be made by the nurse before giving out information over the telephone.

22. 1. **Date of birth is information that can be used to identify an individual and should not be attached to students' notes.**

2. The medical diagnosis is not considered individually identifiable information.

3. A nursing diagnosis is not considered individually identifiable information.

4. Diagnostic test results are not considered individually identifiable information.

TEST-TAKING HINT: Information that can be used to identify an individual includes name, birth date, Social Security number, and medical record number. Attaching this information to health-care data violates client confidentiality and privacy.

23. 1. **Employees who seek access to their own medical records must follow the same procedures as any other client treated by the health-care facility.**

2. This action violates federal laws regarding protected health information because the employee does not have a "need to know" to provide care.

3. This action constitutes a privacy violation because the friend does not have a "need to know" to provide care.

4. Clinical information systems should be accessed only as necessary to provide client care. This does not include access to personal records.

TEST-TAKING HINT: Federal guidelines require that all clients access their personal medical records following the same procedures. The standard for accessing client information is a "need to know" for the performance of the job.

24. 1. This value is in the normal range. Normal blood urea nitrogen is 10–20 mg/dL. For a client on aspirin, an elevated blood urea nitrogen value might be a result of chronic GI bleeding.

2. This value is in the normal range. Normal hematocrit values are 37–47 (females) and 42–52 (males). Hematocrit values decrease if bleeding occurs.

3. This value is in the normal range. Normal potassium values are 3.5–5.0 mEq/L. The nurse monitors for a decrease in potassium.

4. **This value indicates an increase in PT and should be reported to the physician. Normal range is 11–12.5 seconds. Prolonged bleeding time can be a side effect of aspirin.**

TEST-TAKING HINT: Two variables must be considered when answering this question: Which laboratory values are abnormal and what changes are likely to be seen with aspirin due to the side effect of bleeding?

25. 1. **Bradycardia (heart rate below 90–110 bpm in infants) is a common sign of digoxin toxicity. The provider should be notified.**

2. Increased heart rate after crying is a normal finding in an infant.

3. This is a normal RR in an infant. Tachypnea, a complication in congestive heart failure, is usually defined as an RR greater than 60–80 breaths per minute.

4. This is a normal capillary refill (<2–3 sec). Delayed capillary refill is a sign of complications in congestive heart failure.

TEST-TAKING HINT: Digoxin (Lanoxin) is a potentially dangerous drug because of the narrow margin of safety between therapeutic and toxic doses. Accidental overdose is possible because such small doses are given to infants (usually less than 1 mL).

26. 1. This activity is appropriate but does less than other answers to promote continuity of care because it omits hospital staff.
    2. **By including parents, hospital staff, and home-care staff, a joint team conference is the best option to promote continuity of care.**
    3. Adaptation of the home environment is important in the discharge process, but it is not focused on the goal of continuity of care.
    4. Teaching parents how to care for the child in the hospital is an important first step to home care, but it does less than other options to meet the goal of continuity of care.

TEST-TAKING HINT: The question focuses on effective promotion of continuity of care. Although other answers are important in planning for home care, only answer 2 involves all family and staff members, promoting continuity between hospital and home.

27. 1. Primary nursing is less important in this situation. This child is likely to have a short hospital stay, without readmission.
    2. Appendicitis, without complications, usually results in early discharge or a short hospital stay. Continuity of staff is less important.
    3. The hospital treatment of hyperbilirubinemia is likely to be very short because this condition can also be treated in the home. Primary nursing is less important.
    4. **This child is likely to be admitted for repeated hospitalizations and over a longer period of time than other clients. Having a close relationship with one or a few nurses can lead to increased satisfaction for all.**

TEST-TAKING HINT: The advantage of primary nursing is continuity in the relationship between the child/family and the nurse. A more individualized approach can be provided, leading to more holistic care. This approach is most valuable for clients with repeat hospitalizations and longer stay.

28. 2, 4, 5.
    1. RNs should perform all admission assessments. By law, this function cannot be delegated.
    2. **Determination of vital signs is within the scope of practice of the nursing assistant and is an appropriate task for the RN to delegate.**
    3. RNs perform all client teaching. Therefore, it is not appropriate to delegate this task to a nursing assistant.
    4. **ADLs are appropriate for the RN to delegate to a nursing assistant.**
    5. **Daily weights are appropriate for the RN to delegate to a nursing assistant.**

TEST-TAKING HINT: The test taker must know which tasks can be assigned to nursing assistive personnel. Baseline assessments and client teaching are never delegated and must be completed by the RN. Vital signs and ADLs are within the scope of practice of a nursing assistant and may be delegated.

29. 1, 3, 4, 5.
    1. **All education must be completed by the RN and cannot be delegated. This includes insulin administration.**
    2. Blood glucose monitoring is within the scope of practice of an LPN/LVN and nursing assistant and can be delegated by the RN.
    3. **Evaluation of a client's responses to treatments and medications must be completed by the RN and cannot be delegated.**
    4. **Determining the plan of care, including educational goals, must be completed by the RN. This task is not within the scope of practice of the LPN/LVN or nursing assistant.**
    5. **Teaching the child about hypoglycemia and hyperglycemia is the responsibility of the RN and cannot be delegated.**

TEST-TAKING HINT: Determining the plan of care and client teaching are functions that are only within the scope of practice of the RN and cannot be delegated to an LPN/LVN or nursing assistant.

30. 1. This might not be the best match between client and nurse if the emotions of the nurse who recently lost a child are still overwhelming.
  2. A newly graduated LPN/LVN might not be intravenous certified and would probably have little experience with central intravenous line malfunctions. Some states exclude LPNs/LVNs from working with central intravenous lines.
  3. **Even though the pediatric oncology nurse has floated to the pediatric unit, this client's care involves routine skills and knowledge used in the nurse's oncology practice. This makes this assignment the best example of "right task to right person."**
  4. Extensive teaching is involved for a child with new-onset diabetes. The nurse with a very busy assignment is not likely to have the time required for teaching.

  TEST-TAKING HINT: The "right task" is one that can be safely and effectively assigned to the nursing staff person who has the knowledge and skills required. In answers 1 and 4, the nurse may be distracted by interpersonal or environmental factors. In answer 2, the newly graduated LPN/LVN may not have the skills. Answer 3 is the best answer because the oncology nurse is likely to have the needed knowledge and skills.

31. 1. The hospital's policies and procedures must be based on the state's nurse practice act and is a secondary resource.
  2. The nurses' association in each state focuses on the welfare of nurses, not the legal scope of practice.
  3. Educational programs for nursing assistants must take scope of practice into consideration, but they are not the legally defining bodies.
  4. **Each state establishes legal guidelines for health-care professionals in various roles. These guidelines are in the state's nurse practice act, which is the ultimate legal document.**

  TEST-TAKING HINT: The word "primary" is the key to answering this question. Each state has its own definition of scope of practice for different nursing roles. These are legal definitions, passed by the state legislature, and are therefore the primary sources of information.

32. 1. Rules of management dictate that the RN does not delegate the function of client teaching.
  2. Rules of management dictate that the RN does not delegate the function of assessment.
  3. Rules of management dictate that the RN does not delegate the function of evaluation.
  4. **The nursing assistant may help the client in hygiene matters, including bathing.**

  TEST-TAKING HINT: When answering delegation questions, follow the rules of nursing management. The RN does not delegate assessment, teaching, or evaluation to unlicensed personnel such as nursing assistants.

33. 1. Fever is likely to be the most acute problem of this infant, but it is not life threatening.
  2. **Following the ABCs (airway, breathing, circulation), this baby has the greatest potential for a life-threatening complication if the tracheostomy becomes obstructed by mucus.**
  3. Although fever and discomfort may need prompt attention, neither one is life threatening.
  4. Pain is the critical assessment area for this child, but it is not life threatening.

  TEST-TAKING HINT: The question is asking the nurse to prioritize care based on physiological parameters. The toddler in answer 2 presents the greatest possibility for an acute life-threatening complication— respiratory obstruction. Although other clients are acutely ill, their conditions are more stable and unlikely to be life threatening.

34. 1. This child is experiencing a psychological crisis. The child is alert and mobile, behavior that indicates there are no severe physical injuries.
  2. **Presentation indicates possible abdominal injury and internal bleeding in early shock. With immediate attention, the injuries may be treatable; therefore, this child should be seen first.**
  3. Relief of pain is this child's immediate priority, which is not life threatening.
  4. Although this child is the sickest, presentation indicates irreversible brain injury; therefore, this child would not be the first priority for treatment.

  TEST-TAKING HINT: Physiological injuries always take priority over psychological issues, eliminating answer 1. If a client cannot be saved, the client does not need to be seen first, eliminating answer 4. Of the two remaining answers, the child in answer 2 is the more unstable and should be treated first.

35. 1. **The best method for preventing contamination of the central intravenous line site is to complete this procedure first. This lessens the likelihood of spreading microorganisms from the GI tract to the central line. The possible complication of sepsis is most life threatening.**
2. Accurate measurement of output and maintaining patency of the ileostomy bag are lower priority than preventing sepsis of the central intravenous line.
3. Maintaining patency of the Jackson Pratt drain and dressing is lower priority than is maintaining asepsis of the central intravenous line.
4. Correct positioning of the nasogastric tube is lower priority than prevention of sepsis.

TEST-TAKING HINT: Determine which principle of care supersedes the others. In this case, maintaining sterility of the central intravenous line takes precedence over accuracy of output, patency of an abdominal dressing, or nasogastric tube position.

36. 1. **Physiological needs take priority over other needs; therefore, hypotension is the priority need.**
2. Fear of being alone falls within the "security" category, which is lower than physiological needs.
3. Frustration with immobility falls within the "self-esteem" category, which is lower than physiological needs.
4. Body image concerns fall within the category of "self-esteem," which is lower than physiological needs

TEST-TAKING HINT: Maslow's Hierarchy of Needs begins with physiological needs and proceeds to safety and security, love and belonging, self-esteem, and self-actualization. Hypotension is the only clear physiological need listed.

37. 1. Sedation is to be expected and is not the greatest concern.
2. **Airway and breathing complications are the most serious side effects.**
3. As long as the nurse is careful to prevent aspiration, nausea and vomiting are less serious side effects.
4. Constipation is a more long-term and less serious side effect.

TEST-TAKING HINT: Prioritizing following the ABCs (airway, breathing, circulation) indicates that respiratory depression is the most dangerous side effect of treatment.

38. 1. This question can be answered by collecting data on medication errors on each unit and comparing the data.
2. This research question can be answered by comparing pain scores for infants with and without local anesthesia.
3. **This is a legal/ethical issue that is guided by state mandates and the nurse's values of altruism and justice.**
4. This question involves a nursing treatment (irrigation) and client outcomes (line obstruction and infection) that can be determined through action and data collection.

TEST-TAKING HINT: This question involves ethical principles such as altruism (doing good for another), human dignity (each individual has intrinsic worth), and justice (treat persons equally).

39. 1. **Autonomy is the right to make one's own decisions, in this case, the right of the parent to make decisions about the child's surgery. As legal guardian, the parent has the right to choose or not choose for the child to undergo an elective procedure.**
2. Equality is the value for uniformity or evenness between cases or clients. This is not directly related to the situation.
3. Fidelity means keeping promises or agreements. While important in any nurse-parent interaction, it is not the focus of this situation.
4. Justice is the moral principle of fairness. Although this is a universal principle of care, it is not the main issue in this situation.

TEST-TAKING HINT: By knowing the meaning of each principle or value, the test taker can select the correct one.

40. 1. This answer is based on the assumption that the couple's relationship involves abuse; however, this has yet to be established.
2. Only after the nurse clarifies that the mother is experiencing violence will this answer be appropriate.
3. **Clearly identifying the problem, as suggested in this answer, is the first step in the ethical decision-making process.**
4. This statement is an example of the consideration of causative factors; however, the problem has not been clearly identified yet.

TEST-TAKING HINT: Ethical decision making follows steps that closely resemble the nursing process: Identify the problem, consider causative factors, explore answers for action, develop a plan, implement the action, and evaluate the results.

41. 1. **This situation involves differences of opinion among persons who have a legal responsibility to make decisions for the child. Consultation by the multidisciplinary members of the ethics committee may help caregivers reach an agreement.**
2. Routine care and consent are involved in this situation. No ethical dilemma is apparent.
3. Chemotherapy protocols require parental consent and, when appropriate, child assent before implementing. In this situation, all are in agreement about care; therefore, no ethical dilemma is involved.
4. Parents in this situation are given information and asked to make decisions about two possible courses of treatment. Although each course has advantages and disadvantages, both are acceptable for treating the diagnosis. Unless parents disagree on what course to pursue, there is no ethical dilemma.

TEST-TAKING HINT: Ethics committees provide a forum for discussing different views, especially when caregivers, clients, or providers differ in their preferences for treatment. A situation most likely to be reviewed by a committee is one involving differences of opinion about what should be done for a child.

42. 1. The user name can often be linked to the system user's real name and is not considered confidential.
2. The user ID can often be linked to the system user's real name and is not considered confidential.
3. **A password uniquely identifies a user and provides access to data appropriate to the user. System users must maintain confidentiality of their password.**
4. The credentials of the system user are not considered confidential.

TEST-TAKING HINT: System users must never share their passwords. When the nurse signs on to a system, data and information that are entered can be traced to that nurse's password. The nurse is accountable for all actions linked to that password.

43. 1. Although this action gives immediate attention to the client, it violates confidentiality of client information by leaving the computer screen open.
2. **Changing the computer to suspend mode requires only a few seconds. This answer is the best choice, because confidentiality is maintained and the client receives prompt attention.**
3. The amount of information left to be recorded is unknown, and completing charting may delay the assistance needed by the parent.
4. How soon will another staff member be able to assist the client? Because this information is unknown, meeting client needs may be delayed.

TEST-TAKING HINT: Two issues are involved: meeting client needs in a timely manner and maintaining confidentiality of client information. This clinical situation does not appear to be a true emergency. Therefore, confidentiality takes priority and should be maintained by closing the computer screen before leaving the computer unattended.

44. 1. Although staff members may have access to their own records, HIPAA regulations disallow personal access that bypasses institutional policies and procedures.
2. As in answer 1, this access is disallowed under HIPAA regulations.
3. **The right to access information is based on the need to know this information to provide client care. Staff must have access to records of assigned clients in order to provide care.**
4. As in answers 1 and 2, this access is disallowed under HIPAA regulations.

TEST-TAKING HINT: In order to maintain clients' rights and confidentiality of health-care information, HIPAA regulations spell out the standard for accessing client information—a need to know for the performance of the job.

45. 1. Individually identifiable health information, such as client name or ID number, may be shared via fax with other health-care personnel who have a need to know the information to provide care.
2. As in answer 1, this information may be mailed to others who have a need to know to provide proper care.
3. Following the "need to know" rule, individually identifiable information may be copied, as long as confidentiality is maintained.
4. **Selling information such as lists of names and addresses is disallowed by law, because the purpose of sharing the information is not the provision of care.**

TEST-TAKING HINT: The key to sharing or utilizing health information that can be traced to an individual client is the "need to know" to provide individual health care. Confidentiality must be maintained, and providers may not benefit financially by selling such information.

46. 1. Abuse alone is not a basis for emancipation.
    2. **Pregnant minors are considered emancipated minors in many U.S. states and are able to give informed consent.**
    3. A diagnosis of cancer is not a basis for emancipation.
    4. Attending college is not a basis for emancipation.

    TEST-TAKING HINT: Emancipated minors are individuals younger than 18 years of age who are able to give valid informed consent. State statutes mandate who can be considered emancipated. Examples include pregnant females and adolescents treated for substance abuse or communicable disease.

47. 1. Use of a competent translator does not violate the method of obtaining informed consent.
    2. **This situation violates the principle of informed consent. Despite signing the written consent form, the parents state a lack of understanding of the procedure.**
    3. As long as full information is revealed to parents, the timing of information can vary. This situation does not violate the principle of informed consent.
    4. It is acceptable for either parent to sign the consent, if both have custody of the child. This practice does not violate the principle of informed consent.

    TEST-TAKING HINT: The primary care provider is responsible for informing the legal guardian of a pediatric client about a procedure and its potential benefits and risks. Criteria that must be satisfied for informed consent are the following: The person giving consent must understand the procedure, expected outcomes, risks or side effects, and alternate treatments; and a person who is considered legally capable, such as a legal guardian or parent, must give consent.

48. 1. **Assent is the process by which children give their consent for medical treatment. Assent does not have the same legal implications as informed consent, which is given by parents or legal representatives.**

2. Children younger than 18 years cannot give legal informed consent unless they are emancipated minors. Parents serve as children's legal representatives and give informed consent.
3. Confidentiality is one component of the consent process, but it is not a term used to designate the consent process.
4. Emancipation is a different process from consent for treatment. Emancipated minors may include pregnant adolescents and minors seeking treatment for substance abuse or communicable diseases.

TEST-TAKING HINT: The test taker must understand the legal implications of informed consent. Informed consent is based on legal capacity, voluntary action, and comprehension. Unless a child is an emancipated minor, he or she does not have the legal capacity to give informed consent. However, a child younger than 18 years may be able to comprehend the implications of treatment and give voluntary assent.

49. 2, 3, 5.
    1. Although this is helpful information for a client, it is not required on the informed consent form.
    2. **Alternative treatments are part of the informed consent process.**
    3. **Benefits likely to result from the procedure are part of the process of informed consent.**
    4. Only the names of the persons performing the procedure are required for informed consent.
    5. **The statement that the client and family may withdraw consent at any time is required for informed consent.**

    TEST-TAKING HINT: Information required for informed consent includes an explanation of the procedure, risks involved, benefits likely to result, options other than the procedure, name of the person(s) performing the procedure, and statement that the client and family may withdraw consent at any time.

50. 1. "Scope of practice" refers to the legally permissible boundaries of practice and is applicable to all RNs. In this situation, it is the float nurse's lack of familiarity with care, rather than scope of practice, that influences the legal responsibility of the charge nurse.
    2. **The charge nurse has a duty to orient the float nurse to the pediatric unit, educate the nurse on any unfamiliar procedures, and evaluate the float nurse's competency to provide care.**

3. The client's right to competent care can be maintained as long as the assignment of the float nurse is implemented to meet care standards.

4. In this situation, the established nurse/client ratio may be maintained and is not the primary issue raised by floating a nurse from another unit.

TEST-TAKING HINT: Floating nurses from one clinical unit to another to fill a staffing vacancy can be an effective strategy, if floating guidelines are met. The charge nurse is responsible for ensuring that the floating nurse has the required competencies for working on the unit and is supported in carrying out the assigned care. This legal responsibility includes the supervisory duty to orient, educate, and evaluate the floating staff.

51. 1. The nurse has a relationship with the client because the nurse has been assigned to care for the child in the hospital. This element is present.

2. **Breach of duty of care is missing in this case, because the nurse met the standard of care. The nurse educated the parent on the importance of side rail safety before the incident occurred.**

3. The element of injury is present in this case, because the child suffered a skull fracture.

4. The child sustained damage in this case, as evidenced by the skull fracture.

TEST-TAKING HINT: In order for malpractice to be proved, four elements must be present: The nurse has a relationship with the client by being assigned to care for the client; the nurse failed to observe a standard of care in the specific situation; the client sustained harm, injury, or damage; and the harm must have occurred as a direct result of the nurse's failure to act in accordance with the standard of care.

52. 1. Each state's nurse practice act defines the scope of nursing practice, such as what level of practitioner can initiate a blood transfusion.

2. The national HIPAA is in place to ensure that providers protect the privacy and security of health information.

3. Each state has a Good Samaritan act to protect health-care workers who give assistance in emergency situations.

4. **The local agency's policy manual would describe acceptable procedures for performing specific skills such as flushing a central venous line. These procedures serve as the legal standard of care.**

TEST-TAKING HINT: The nurse needs to know major laws that govern practice, at both state and national levels. Where these laws exist, they serve as the primary legal authority for care. Examples include nurse practice acts, Good Samaritan acts, HIPAA, the Patient Self-Determination Act, and child and elder abuse reporting. The legal basis for most specific technical procedures can be found in agencies' policy and procedure manuals.

53. 1. **The parent's refusal to allow the nurse to continue constitutes a revocation of informed consent; therefore, the nurse is acting without permission. In addition, the nurse should consult the agency policy and procedure manual regarding the number of attempts allowed in this procedure.**

2. Normal toddler behavior is being exhibited here. This response might occur despite use of analgesics, parental presence, and other coping measures.

3. Many young children have difficulty taking oral medication, and this situation falls within normal parameters.

4. Initial refusal of a painful activity is typical behavior for a school-age child, but it can often be overcome by motivational and diversional measures.

TEST-TAKING HINT: Battery is intentional physical contact that is wrongful in some way, such as causing embarrassment or injury or done without permission. In pediatrics, the parent gives consent for the child and must give permission for a procedure of this type.

54. 1, 2.
1. **After an error occurs, the nurse should document what occurred.**

2. **After an error, the nurse should document what was done to solve or treat the problem.**

3. The fact that an incident report was completed should not be documented in the client medical record.

4. No information regarding the incident report should be documented in the client medical record.

5. The facts concerning the medication error should be recorded, because of the effect on the client's health status.

TEST-TAKING HINT: An incident report helps an organization track client care–related problems. The facts of what occurred, the effect on the client, and the treatment given should be recorded.

55. 1. **Administration of a medication dose outside the therapeutic range is an execution error and should be reported as a critical incident. The nurse is held responsible for administering the wrong dose, just as the physician is responsible for ordering the wrong dose.**
2. This event is not considered to be a nursing error because it is not under the control of the nurse, if proper flushing protocol has been followed. Rather, it is a complication of intravenous therapy.
3. This event is a complication of intravenous therapy and is not a nursing error.
4. This event is an example of the challenges of giving oral medications to uncooperative children and is not considered a nursing error.

TEST-TAKING HINT: The goal of risk management is to promote quality client care and minimize adverse outcomes. Medication errors are monitored through incident reporting. Events that represent a departure from safe practice, with or without resulting harm to the client, should be reported.

56. 1. **This answer is an example of a violation of the policy for administering a high-risk drug such as insulin. Policy dictates that another RN (not a nursing assistant) double-check the dose before administering.**
2. This is an example of a potential error that was corrected appropriately before it was completed.
3. This is an example of appropriate verification of orders.
4. This is an example of appropriate double-checking of a high-risk drug.

TEST-TAKING HINT: The goal of risk management is to create an awareness of potential risk factors and set up various mechanisms to control and/or eliminate risk. The protocol for high-risk medications, including insulin, is to check the dose with another RN before administering.

57. 1. Fasting blood glucose level may be used as a diagnostic test.
2. Fingerstick blood glucose values reflect compliance over the previous 1–2 days, making this test less valid as a long-term indicator of compliance. This test allows for short-term adjustment of the therapeutic regimen.

3. Urine ketones are measured to detect diabetic ketoacidosis.
4. **HbA1c reflects the average blood glucose level over 3 months, making it the most valid indicator.**

TEST-TAKING HINT: Blood glucose levels are the best indicators of compliance with insulin, diet, and exercise regimens in diabetes. Long-term measurements, such as HbA1c, are better indicators than short-term levels, such as fasting glucose or fingerstick glucose checks.

58. 1. The charge nurse needs to validate correct understanding of what was observed by speaking with the staff nurse before addressing the parent.
2. Until validation with the staff nurse, the charge nurse does not know whether a problem has occurred.
3. Verbal assessment and validation of the situation should occur before a written reprimand.
4. **Validation of information that was actually communicated to the parent should be the next step. This should come from the staff nurse in a private discussion.**

TEST-TAKING HINT: Before disciplinary action is taken in regard to any personnel situation, the charge nurse should give the staff member the opportunity to discuss the situation from the personal viewpoint.

59. 1. Social interactions among staff are not necessarily within the jurisdiction of the nurse manager.
2. The cafeteria is not a responsibility of nursing administration, and staff would better facilitate change by giving input directly to this department.
3. **This is a client-care issue that will take some investigation and correction on a unit-to-unit level. Pediatric unit and emergency department managers should be involved. This situation is most appropriate to refer to nurse managers.**
4. Union policies are separate from hospital administration and nursing management.

TEST-TAKING HINT: Focus on the role of the nurse manager and the activities under that role. Only answer 3 focuses on events that are within the job description of the nurse manager.

60. 1. Employing a sitter is not a cost-effective solution because the child is not in danger when adults are out of the room.
2. Parents need break times to deal with the stress of having a hospitalized child. It is unreasonable to expect them to stay at the bedside 24 hours a day.
3. **The role of the child-life worker is to help hospitalized children meet normal developmental needs. Referring to them is the most appropriate action.**
4. The behavior shown is normal and does not indicate unusual social or emotional needs. Therefore, a social service consult is not indicated.

TEST-TAKING HINT: The child has difficulty only on the occasions that parents are absent, indicating a need for attention from staff or the diversion of play activities. A child-life worker is the best staff person to meet these needs.

61. 1. **The role of case manager includes ordering medical equipment for discharge; therefore, this is an appropriate referral.**
2. Most nurse manager activities are broader in scope than discharge planning.
3. Materials management stocks hospital supplies but is usually not involved in discharge supplies.
4. Child-life staff members focus on emotional needs during hospitalization and would not be involved in this aspect of discharge planning.

TEST-TAKING HINT: The test taker must know the role of each staff member listed. Obtaining equipment for discharge is an important role of the case manager.

15

Comprehensive Exam

1. Which outcome is expected in a breastfed newborn?
   1. Voids spontaneously within 12 hours of life.
   2. Loses 10% of body weight in the first 5 days.
   3. Regains birth weight by the 14th day of life.
   4. Awakens spontaneously for all feedings.

2. The average newborn weighs 3400 g. The nurse will tell the parents that the baby weighs _____ lb.

3. The posture of a healthy term newborn is described as:
   1. Hypotonic.
   2. Asymmetric.
   3. Extended.
   4. Flexed.

4. The nurse is working in the newborn nursery and accidentally bumps the crib of one of the babies. This baby demonstrates a Moro reflex. The nurse sees this baby in which posture?
   1. Trunk extended upward and head lifted.
   2. When placed on abdomen, crawling movement occurs.
   3. A "fencing" posture.
   4. Extremities extended and abducted and fingers fanned.

5. The parent of a newborn wants to know what the newborn screening test does. What is the nurse's best response?
   1. "It detects a large number of congenital diseases."
   2. "It screens after birth for some inherited and congenital conditions."
   3. "Parents choose which diseases to screen for."
   4. "It screens for congenital diseases that insurance companies cover."

6. A family is adopting a child from a foreign country. What suggestions can be given to the parents for incorporating the child into the family? **Select all that apply.**
   1. Learn as much about the child as possible before adoption.
   2. Expect conflict and determine how to work through it with the child.
   3. Do not discuss the biological parents with the child.
   4. Discuss your expectations with the child.
   5. Try to maintain a part of the child's original family name.

7. When the parents of a 5-year-old tell the child they are divorcing, the parents need to be aware of which behaviors that the child may demonstrate? **Select all that apply.**
   1. Increased self-esteem, bragging.
   2. Changes in sleep and appetite.
   3. Feelings of abandonment.
   4. Develops dictatorial attitude.
   5. Verbalizes feelings about divorce-related changes.

8. The mother of a 6-month-old is going back to work. The nurse should make which of the following suggestions for ways to evaluate day-care options? **Select all that apply.**
   1. Size of day-care center.
   2. Strict health and safety requirements.
   3. Caretakers who are loving and kind.
   4. Challenging activities for all the children.
   5. Child-care ratios that maximize staff use.
   6. Small class size.

9. Match each genetic term with its definition and function.
   1. Congenital
   2. FISH analysis
   3. Genome
   4. Malformation
   5. Phenotype
   6. Syndrome

   A. Morphogenic defect of an organ
   B. Recognized pattern of malformation
   C. Present at birth
   D. Clinically exhibited characteristic
   E. Fluorescent in situ hybridization
   F. Complete genetic information of organism

10. Parents are concerned that Turner syndrome is suspected in their newborn. Which physical characteristics led to this suspicion? **Select all that apply.**
    1. Cleft lip and palate.
    2. Weak, high-pitched cry.
    3. Webbed neck and lymphedema.
    4. Long arms and small genitalia.
    5. Coarctation of the aorta.

11. A pregnant teen is to have prenatal testing. She is afraid of needles and wants to know the least invasive way she can get the testing done. The nurse should suggest which testing procedure?
    1. Triple marker screen.
    2. Ultrasound examination.
    3. Amniocentesis.
    4. Chorionic villus sampling.

12. Parents are told by the genetic counselor that they have a 1 : 4 probability of having a second child with cystic fibrosis (CF). They already have one child who is affected. The parents state their risk is lower now than when they had the previous child. What should the nurse tell the parents about the 1 : 4 probability?
    1. Each pregnancy is an independent event.
    2. The probability of having another child with CF is twice as likely as it was when they had the first child.
    3. The probability of having a healthy child is twice as likely with this pregnancy.
    4. The probability of miscarrying is greater now than with the previous pregnancy.

13. A young woman tells a nurse she is pregnant and concerned that her boyfriend may be "slow" mentally. The nurse should do which activity first?
    1. Develop a pedigree.
    2. Take a family history.
    3. Inform the provider about the concern.
    4. Refer the client for genetic counseling.

14. A parent who is Jehovah's Witness has a child with leukemia and a very low RBC count. The nurse should recognize that the family faces which dilemma?
    1. Numerous dietary kosher laws exist.
    2. A belief that only Allah cures illness.
    3. Desire for anointing of the sick.
    4. Opposition to transfusions and vaccines.

15. The nurse is working in a clinic, and the next client is an infant with deaf parents. In addition to providing an interpreter for the deaf, the nurse should incorporate what additional aid in communicating with the family?
    1. Talk just as with hearing families.
    2. Maintain good eye contact to let them read the nurse's lips.
    3. Explain procedures thoroughly.
    4. Recommend a trained hearing dog.

16. A teenager is legally blind. The teen is wearing thick glasses and is carrying some schoolbooks. Which question should the nurse ask the teen?
    1. "Just how blind are you?"
    2. "Can you see enough to read those books?"
    3. "Tell me what you can see in this room."
    4. "Is your vision worse than 20/200 in either of your eyes?"

17. The nurse is working in a school health clinic, and a child comes in complaining of "something in my eye." What should the nurse do first?
    1. Have the child wash hands.
    2. Refer the child to an ophthalmologist.
    3. Wash out the affected eye with tap water.
    4. Examine the eye for a foreign body.

18. A child assigned to the nurse's floor has a dysfluency. The nurse should recognize what symptoms?
    1. Stuttering.
    2. Substitution of one sound for another.
    3. Speaking in a monotone.
    4. Hypernasal speech.

19. Parents confide to the nurse that their child, who is 35 months old, does not talk and spends hours sitting on the floor watching the ceiling fan go around. They are concerned their child may have autism. The nurse should ask the parents which question?
    1. "Does your child have brothers or sisters?"
    2. "Does your child seek you out for comfort and love?"
    3. "Do you have trouble getting babysitters for your child?"
    4. "Does your child receive speech therapy?"

20. The nurse in the emergency department is caring for an 8-month-old who suffered a concussion from an automobile accident. The infant was in the car seat at the time. The nurse should assess the infant for which symptoms?
    1. Sweating, irritability, and pallor.
    2. Plethora and hyperthermia.
    3. Crying with fear.
    4. Negative Babinski reflex.

21. A parent tells the nurse that the 3-month-old infant is fussy, spits up constantly, and has a lot of gas, and there is a family history of allergies. These symptoms are related to which diagnosis?
    1. Failure to thrive.
    2. Sensitive to cow's milk.
    3. Phenylketonuria.
    4. Pancreatic insufficiency.

22. The nurse on the previous shift charted that a newborn demonstrated cutis marmorata. The nurse now caring for the baby should check which vital sign?
    1. Blood pressure.
    2. Respirations.
    3. Skin color.
    4. Temperature.

23. The nurse is caring for a newborn with Erb palsy and a phrenic nerve paralysis. The most effective way to promote respiratory effort is for the nurse to position the newborn in what way?
    1. Supine.
    2. On the affected side.
    3. On the unaffected side.
    4. Prone.

24. A 2-day-old baby is being readied for discharge but looks jaundiced. The nurse reviews the baby's birth records and notes that the baby has A blood type, and the mother has O blood type. The nurse should check which blood test?
    1. Hepatitis B titer.
    2. Total bilirubin.
    3. Complete blood count.
    4. Sedimentation rate.

25. An infant at 12 hours of age has a positive Coombs test result and a bilirubin level of 18 mg/dL. The provider has ordered an exchange transfusion for the infant. As the transfusion is proceeding, the nurse should watch for which sign?
    1. Increasing jaundice.
    2. Lethargy.
    3. Temperature instability.
    4. Irritability.

26. A baby is brought into the clinic for follow-up review of phenylketonuria. The baby is 9 months old and weighs 22 lb. If the recommendation is to limit the phenylalanine in the diet to 25 mg/kg/day, this infant should have no more than _____ of phenylalanine/day.

27. The nurse working in the newborn nursery has to draw a heel-stick blood sample before an infant's discharge. What can the nurse do to decrease the pain the infant feels from this procedure? **Select all that apply.**
    1. Wrap the heel in a warm, damp cloth.
    2. Use EMLA before doing the stick.
    3. Swaddle the infant.
    4. Have the infant do non-nutritive sucking.
    5. Do the stick while the infant is asleep.

28. The nurse's unit is using the POPS pain scale for measuring pain in infants. The nurse knows this tool is which of the following?
    1. Pain Assessment Tool for infants 27 weeks to term gestation.
    2. The Neonatal Infant Pain Scale for infants 3 to 12 months.
    3. Premature Infant Pain Profile for infants 32 weeks to term gestation.
    4. Post-Operative Pain Score for infants 1 to 7 months.

29. The nurse tells a parent which of the following data can be provided by a polysomnogram? **Select all that apply.**
    1. Heart rate and respirations.
    2. Brain waves.
    3. Eye and body movements.
    4. Cyanosis or plethora.
    5. End-tidal carbon dioxide.

30. Parents tell the nurse that their 18-month-old is always curious about the environment and is learning new words every day. The toddler is entering a phase of rapid _____ development.

31. Parents are concerned that their toddler refuses to sleep in the new toddler bed and wonder what to do. The nurse explains that the child is using "global organization." What does the nurse mean by this term?
   1. The preoperational phase of developing cognitive thought starts around 3 years old.
   2. The child is self-centered and does not want to learn.
   3. The child sees changing to a toddler bed as changing the whole process of sleeping and going to bed.
   4. The toddler may have a phobia to the bed.

32. Parents express concern that their 5-year-old has started having more temper tantrums. The parents want to know if this is normal for this age. What should the nurse ask the parents about the tantrums? **Select all that apply.**
   1. "Do you notice and praise your child when your child does something right?"
   2. "Are the tantrums related to one specific aspect of life?"
   3. "Are the tantrums causing any harm to self or others?"
   4. "Have you consulted the Internet for any suggestions?"
   5. "How do you handle your child during a tantrum?"

33. Parents are told they should start taking their toddler to the dentist. They are concerned the dentist will be too rough with their child. The nurse suggests the parents do which of the following before the dental visit? **Select all that apply.**
   1. Tell the child it will not hurt.
   2. Warn that they will have the dentist give a needle in case of bad behavior.
   3. Tell the child they will go along to the dentist so that they can model comfortable, safe behavior.
   4. Offer the child a treat for good behavior.
   5. The dentist will look in their child's mouth and count the teeth.

34. A 17-month-old is brought into the clinic, and the nurse notes the toddler has tooth decay on the maxillary upper incisors. Which tactic(s) would the nurse suggest to wean the toddler from the bottle? **Select all that apply.**
   1. Hide the bottle and tell the toddler that it is not needed anymore.
   2. Put only tap water in the bottle.
   3. Give the bottle only at night.
   4. Give the toddler a pacifier and take the bottle away.
   5. Do not give any bottles before bed.

35. Parents are frustrated with toilet-training their 2-year-old. Both parents work full-time and claim they do not have time to spend on toilet-training. How will the nurse respond to the parents' concern? **Select all that apply.**
   1. "You will have to invest some time if the child is to be toilet-trained."
   2. "A child needs to be both physically and psychologically ready to learn the skills needed to be continent."
   3. "Do you think your child is stubborn?"
   4. "Have the child sit on the toilet until the child voids."
   5. "If the child can stay dry for two hours, then he might be ready to toilet train."

36. Parents are interested in switching their child from a booster seat to a regular seat belt. The child is 7 years old and weighs 51 lb. What can the nurse tell the parents about switching the child to a seat belt? **Select all that apply.**
    1. The safest place to ride in the car is in the front seat.
    2. The child needs to weigh 60 lb and be 8 years old to qualify legally for a seat belt.
    3. The seat belt should be worn low on the hips.
    4. Use a shoulder belt only if it does not cross the child's neck.
    5. Tether straps are optional.

37. The nurse goes to the kindergarten classroom to evaluate a rash. A 5-year-old has patches of itchy vesicles on the chest and face. The teacher tells the nurse the child had a runny nose a couple of days ago. The nurse suspects that the rash is caused by which virus?
    1. Fifth disease (parvovirus B-19).
    2. Roseola (herpesvirus type 6).
    3. Scarlet fever (group A beta-hemolytic *Streptococcus*).
    4. Chickenpox (varicella zoster).

38. The clinic is doing a lead screening program for children in a low-income community. The nurse working in the program wants to tell the parents the reasons to have their children screened for lead poisoning. **Select all that apply.**
    1. Young children absorb 10% of the lead to which they are exposed.
    2. Homes built between 1900 and 1950 may contain lead-based paint.
    3. The blood level of lead should be below 12.8 mcg/dL.
    4. Lead can affect any part of the body, but the brain and kidneys are at greatest risk.
    5. Foods such as fruit, candy, and antacids contain lead.

39. A 9-year-old boy is brought to the clinic for a physical. The child's weight is 95 lb (95th percentile), and his height is 4 feet 4 inches (50th percentile). Blood pressure is 118/75. Reading the blood pressure graph in the following figure, the boy is in the _____ percentile for systolic and in the _____ percentile for diastolic readings for his age.

Blood Pressure Levels for Boys by Age and Height Percentile

Age (year)	HP Percentile	Systolic BP (mmHg) ← Percentile of Height →							Diastolic BP (mmHg) ← Percentile of Height →						
		5th	10th	25th	50th	75th	80th	95th	5th	10th	25th	50th	75th	80th	95th
1	50th	60	61	63	65	87	88	89	34	35	36	37	35	39	39
	90th	94	95	97	99	100	102	103	40	50	51	52	53	53	54
	95th	98	99	101	103	104	106	106	54	54	55	54	57	58	58
	99th	105	106	108	110	112	113	114	61	62	63	64	65	66	66
2	50th	84	85	87	88	88	92	92	39	40	41	42	43	44	44
	90th	97	89	100	102	102	106	106	54	55	56	57	58	58	59
	95th	101	102	104	105	105	109	110	59	59	60	61	62	63	63
	99th	109	110	111	113	113	117	117	66	67	63	69	70	71	71
3	50th	86	87	89	91	91	94	95	44	44	45	48	47	46	48
	90th	100	101	103	105	105	108	109	59	59	60	61	62	63	63
	95th	104	105	107	109	109	112	113	63	63	64	65	66	67	67
	99th	111	112	114	116	116	110	120	71	71	72	73	74	76	76
4	50th	88	89	91	93	93	96	97	47	48	49	50	51	51	52
	90th	107	103	105	107	107	110	111	62	63	64	65	66	66	67
	95th	106	107	109	111	111	114	115	66	67	68	69	70	71	71
	99th	113	114	116	118	118	121	122	74	76	76	77	78	78	79
5	50th	90	91	93	95	85	98	98	50	51	52	53	54	55	55
	90th	104	105	106	108	108	111	112	65	66	67	68	69	60	70
	95th	106	109	110	112	112	115	116	69	70	71	72	73	74	74
	99th	115	116	118	120	120	123	123	77	78	79	80	81	81	82
6	50th	91	92	94	95	98	99	100	53	53	54	55	56	57	57
	90th	105	106	109	110	110	113	113	66	68	69	70	71	72	72
	95th	109	110	112	114	114	117	117	72	72	73	74	75	76	76
	99th	116	117	119	121	121	125	125	80	80	81	82	83	84	84
7	50th	93	94	95	97	97	100	101	55	55	66	57	58	69	59
	90th	106	107	109	111	111	114	115	70	70	71	72	73	74	74
	95th	110	111	113	115	115	118	119	74	74	75	76	77	78	78
	99th	117	118	120	122	122	125	126	82	82	83	84	85	86	86
8	50th	94	95	97	99	99	102	102	56	57	63	60	60	60	61
	90th	107	109	110	112	112	115	116	71	72	72	73	74	76	76
	95th	111	117	114	116	116	119	120	76	76	77	78	79	79	80
	99th	119	120	122	123	123	127	127	83	84	83	86	87	87	88
9	50th	95	96	88	100	100	103	104	57	58	60	60	61	61	62
	90th	109	110	112	114	114	117	118	72	73	74	75	76	76	77
	95th	113	114	116	116	116	121	121	76	77	78	79	80	81	81
	99th	120	121	123	125	125	128	129	81	85	88	87	88	88	89
10	50th	97	98	100	102	102	105	106	50	59	60	61	61	62	63
	90th	111	112	114	115	115	119	119	73	73	74	75	76	77	78
	95th	115	116	117	119	119	122	123	77	78	79	80	81	81	82
	99th	122	123	125	127	127	130	130	85	86	86	88	88	89	90

40. The nurse is working in a school health clinic, and a teen mentions that her older sister just had a baby born with a myelomeningocele. The teen is wondering if there is anything she can do to prevent this from happening to her baby when she decides to have children. Which is the best response?

1. Take a multivitamin with folic acid daily.
2. Eat more fruits and vegetables daily.
3. Have breakfast every morning.
4. There is nothing that can be done to decrease the risk.

41. A 16-year-old comes into the clinic for a physical examination. The teen weighs 180 lb and is 5 feet 5 inches tall. According to the following figure, the teen's body mass index (BMI) is _____.

Body Mass Index Table

	Normal						Overweight					Obese										Extreme Obese															
BMI	19	20	21	22	23	24	25	26	27	28	29	30	31	32	33	34	35	36	37	38	39	40	41	42	43	44	45	46	47	48	49	50	51	52	53	54
Height (inches)												Body Weight (pounds)																								
58	91	96	100	106	110	115	112	124	129	134	138	143	145	153	155	162	167	172	177	181	186	191	196	201	205	210	215	220	224	229	234	239	244	248	253	258
59	94	99	104	109	114	119	124	128	133	138	143	148	153	158	163	168	173	178	183	188	193	196	203	208	212	217	222	227	232	237	242	247	252	257	262	267
60	97	102	107	112	118	123	128	133	138	143	148	153	155	163	168	174	179	184	189	194	199	204	209	215	220	225	230	235	240	245	250	255	261	266	271	276
61	100	106	111	116	122	127	132	137	143	148	153	158	164	169	174	180	185	190	195	201	206	211	217	222	227	232	238	243	248	254	259	264	269	275	280	286
62	104	109	115	120	129	131	136	142	147	153	158	164	169	175	180	186	191	196	202	207	213	218	224	229	235	240	246	251	256	262	267	273	278	284	289	295
63	107	113	118	124	130	135	141	148	152	158	163	169	175	180	186	191	197	203	205	214	220	225	231	237	242	248	254	259	266	270	278	282	287	293	299	304
64	110	116	122	128	134	140	145	151	157	163	169	174	180	186	192	197	204	209	215	221	227	232	238	244	250	256	262	267	273	279	285	291	296	302	308	314
65	114	120	126	132	136	144	150	156	162	168	174	180	186	192	198	204	210	216	222	228	234	240	246	252	258	264	270	276	282	288	294	300	306	312	318	324
66	118	124	130	136	142	148	155	161	167	173	179	186	192	198	204	210	216	223	229	235	241	247	253	260	266	272	278	284	291	297	303	309	315	322	328	334
67	121	127	134	140	146	153	159	166	172	178	185	191	198	204	211	217	223	230	236	242	249	255	261	268	274	280	287	293	299	306	312	319	325	331	338	344
68	125	131	138	144	151	158	164	171	177	184	190	197	203	210	216	223	230	236	243	249	256	252	269	276	282	289	295	302	308	315	322	328	335	341	348	354
69	128	135	142	147	155	162	169	176	182	189	196	203	209	216	223	230	236	243	250	257	263	270	277	284	291	297	304	311	318	324	331	338	345	351	358	365
70	132	139	146	153	160	167	174	181	188	195	202	209	216	222	229	236	243	250	257	264	271	278	285	292	299	306	313	320	327	334	341	348	355	362	369	376
71	138	143	150	157	165	172	179	186	193	200	208	215	222	229	236	243	250	257	266	272	279	286	293	301	308	315	322	329	338	343	351	358	366	372	379	386
72	140	147	154	162	169	177	184	191	199	206	213	221	228	235	242	250	258	265	272	279	287	294	302	309	316	324	331	338	346	353	361	368	375	383	390	397
73	144	151	159	166	174	182	189	197	204	212	219	227	235	242	250	257	265	272	280	288	295	302	310	318	325	333	340	348	355	363	371	378	386	393	401	408
74	148	155	163	171	179	186	194	202	210	218	225	233	241	249	256	264	272	280	287	295	303	311	319	326	331	342	350	358	365	373	381	389	396	404	412	420
75	152	160	168	176	184	192	200	208	216	224	232	240	248	256	264	272	279	287	295	303	311	319	327	335	343	351	359	367	375	383	391	399	407	415	423	431
76	155	164	172	180	189	197	205	213	221	230	238	246	254	263	271	279	287	295	304	312	320	328	336	344	353	361	369	377	386	394	402	410	418	426	435	443

42. A 12-year-old girl with a thoracic myelomeningocele has had numerous urinary tract infections and has difficulty doing her clean intermittent self-catheterization. She and her parents are seeking an alternative way to empty her bladder. The surgeon has offered to do a Mitrofanoff procedure. The surgeon will use the _____ to create a continent conduit between the bladder and the abdominal wall.

43. The parent of a school-age child who is a paraplegic and uses a wheelchair states that the child is allergic to latex. Which is the most important intervention for this child?
1. Giving antihistamines and steroids after procedures.
2. Prevention of contact with latex products.
3. Doing a radioallergosorbent test before each procedure.
4. Using only latex-free gloves when doing procedures.

44. An infant with a lumbar myelomeningocele is admitted to the unit with an Arnold-Chiari malformation. The infant has which other diagnosis?
1. Hydrocephalus.
2. Anencephaly.
3. Tethering of the spinal cord.
4. Perinatal hemorrhage.

45. Which would the nurse assess in a 4-week-old infant who has developmental dysplasia of the hip and is wearing a Pavlik harness?
1. Diaper dermatitis.
2. Talipes equinovarus.
3. Leg shortening and limited abduction.
4. Pain.

46. Which is the primary goal for a newborn with a cleft of the soft palate?
1. Prevent ear infections.
2. Help the mother bond with the baby.
3. Repair the cleft palate.
4. Establish feeding and sucking.

47. When an infant is born with a herniation of the abdominal wall with intestine present and the peritoneal sac absent, it is called _____.

48. What are the two organizations in the United States that make and govern the recommendations for immunization policies and procedures?
    1. National Advisory Committee on Immunization and American Medical Association.
    2. U.S. Public Health Service Centers for Disease Control and American Academy of Pediatrics.
    3. National Immunization Program and Pediatric Infectious Disease Association.
    4. National Institutes of Health and Minister of National Health and Welfare.

49. A nurse is working in a well-child clinic administering immunizations to preschoolers. Which procedure will minimize local reactions to the injections?
    1. Apply EMLA cream 1 hour before.
    2. Change the needle on the syringe after drawing up the biological drug.
    3. Inject into the vastus lateralis or ventrogluteal muscle.
    4. Use distraction such as telling the child to hold their breath.

50. A fixed splitting of the S_2 heart sound is heard in an otherwise healthy child. This is a diagnostic sign of which cardiac defect?
    1. Mitral regurgitation.
    2. Atrial septal defect.
    3. Functional murmur.
    4. Pericardial friction rub.

51. An innocent murmur has which characteristics? **Select all that apply.**
    1. Short induration.
    2. S_2 murmur.
    3. Loudest in the pulmonic area.
    4. Fixed and can be heard in many positions.
    5. Grade III or less.

52. A child is giggling and laughing, and the nurse gently places one hand on the child's front and the other on the back of the chest. The sounds can be felt through the skin. This finding is called _____.

53. A child returns from surgery, having had tonsils and adenoids removed. When the parents are getting ready for discharge, the nurse gives which of the following instructions about home care? **Select all that apply.**
    1. Some secretions may be blood-tinged for a few days.
    2. Run a cool-mist vaporizer in the bedroom.
    3. Pain relief should be provided every 4 hours.
    4. The child can resume a normal diet.
    5. The child should blow the nose and cough every 4 hours.

54. A 2-year-old is brought to the emergency department for fever and ear pain. The parent reports the child has had many ear infections and that polyethylene tubes have been recommended, but the parent cannot afford surgery. The child is diagnosed with bilateral otitis media. The toddler is carrying a baby bottle full of juice, and the parent is carrying a pack of cigarettes. Which preventive measures could be taught to the parent to decrease the incidence of ear infections? **Select all that apply.**
    1. Wean the toddler from the bottle.
    2. Give the toddler a decongestant before bedtime.
    3. Encourage the parent to smoke outside the house.
    4. Counsel the parent to change his shirt and wash his hands after smoking.
    5. Have the child's hearing checked.

55. For the past 2 nights, an 18-month-old who attends day care has been having a barking, hoarse-sounding cough that comes in spasms with very noisy respirations. The parent is concerned that the child has picked up an infection at day care. The day-care staff indicates the child does not cough during the day, has no fever, and is eating and drinking well. This description is most likely which condition?
    1. Laryngotracheobronchitis.
    2. Bacterial tracheitis.
    3. Asthma.
    4. Acute spasmodic laryngitis.

56. An 11-month-old was born at 28 weeks' gestation and required 2 weeks of ventilation. The baby is currently well and is being seen in the clinic. The physician recommends that the baby receive preventive therapy for respiratory syncytial virus (RSV) for the next 5 months since winter is approaching. Which medication will be ordered?
    1. Respiratory syncytial virus immune globulin (RespiGam).
    2. Ribavirin.
    3. Palivizumab (Synagis).
    4. Pneumococcal vaccine.

57. Three preschool children and their foreign-born parents come to a homeless shelter. The family has been homeless for 3 months. The children appear somewhat unkempt but nourished. One of the children has several enlarged cervical lymph nodes and is running a low-grade fever. Which chronic infectious illness should be suspected in the child?
    1. Chlamydial pneumonia.
    2. Tuberculosis.
    3. Pertussis (whooping cough).
    4. Asthma.

58. Which is assessed to diagnose pediculosis capitis? **Select all that apply.**
    1. Crawling insects.
    2. White flakes in the hair.
    3. Nits attached close to scalp.
    4. Inflammatory papules.
    5. Dark brown hair.

59. A child in a classroom is disruptive with loud talking, has a short attention span, and has difficulty organizing work. Which is the most likely diagnosis for this child?
    1. Enuresis.
    2. Sexual abuse.
    3. Learning disability.
    4. Attention deficit-hyperactivity disorder.

60. A child is taking haloperidol (Haldol) for schizophrenia, and the family has been instructed to watch for extrapyramidal side effects. Which are characteristic of these side effects?
    1. Abnormal movements and twitches.
    2. Inappropriate behaviors.
    3. Excessive aggressiveness.
    4. Thoughts of suicide.

61. A sports physical examination is being performed on a 12-year-old male. He is evaluated as a Tanner stage II. Which physical characteristic would the nurse expect? **Select all that apply.**
    1. Enlarging penis.
    2. Height spurt.
    3. Gynecomastia.
    4. Deepening voice.
    5. Enlarging scrotum.

62. A 15-year-old girl who is an avid basketball player comes to the clinic for menstrual irregularities. She skips meals and has lost some weight. She mentions that she has menstrual periods every 2 weeks. Women who have menstrual periods more often than every 21 days are _____.

63. Which is the nurse's best approach to teach high school students about smoking prevention?
    1. Discuss health consequences of smoking.
    2. Use scare tactics and point out the negative effects of smoking.
    3. Offer alternatives to smoking such as chewing gum or doing activities that distract.
    4. Have the adolescents talk with their parents about smoking.

64. A child with moderate asthma is wheezing and coughing. Which test should the nurse perform before the health-care provider (HCP) sees the child? **Select all that apply.**
    1. Skin testing for allergens.
    2. PCO_2 levels.
    3. Biox level.
    4. Metered dose inhaler.
    5. Peak flow.

65. Which should the nurse teach the child and parents about montelukast (Singulair) ordered for moderate persistent asthma? **Select all that apply.**
    1. This is an add-on medication to the child's regular medications.
    2. It can be given when the child needs it.
    3. It is not to be used to treat acute episodes.
    4. The parents will need to give up smoking.
    5. The child will require chest physiotherapy in conjunction with the medication.

66. The nurse is caring for a child dying from leukemia. The parents want to know how comfortable the nurse is in giving doses of pain medication that are larger than customary. Which ethical principle of care are the parents asking about?
    1. Double effect.
    2. Justice
    3. Honesty.
    4. Beneficence.

67. The parents of a 19-year-old ask the nurse what they should do in terms of long-term care placement for their severely disabled child. Which is the nurse's best response?
    1. "How much care do you want?"
    2. "Do you have other children who could take your child into their home?"
    3. "Do you have a detailed plan of care?"
    4. "Are you working with an agency or social worker about this matter?"

68. Parents of a 2-year-old with Down syndrome are told the child should be screened for atlantoaxial instability. The nurse tells the parents that which of the following are symptoms of this instability?
    1. Mental retardation.
    2. Neck pain and torticollis.
    3. Vision and hearing loss.
    4. Early onset of puberty.

69. Which are early signs and symptoms of hydrocephalus in infants?
    1. Confusion, headache, diplopia.
    2. Rapid head growth, poor feeding, confusion.
    3. Papilledema, irritability, headache.
    4. Full fontanels, poor feeding, rapid head growth.

70. A newborn with suspected hydrocephalus is transferred to the intensive care unit for further evaluation and treatment. The infant's nurse knows which of the following?
1. To use sedation as needed to keep the baby from crying or being fussy.
2. To keep the crib in a flat and neutral position.
3. To expect the infant to sleep more than an infant without hydrocephalus.
4. To not use any scalp veins for intravenous infusions.

71. Which is immediate postoperative care for shunt placement in an infant diagnosed with hydrocephalus?
1. Wet-to-dry dressing changes at both the shunt insertion site and the abdominal incision site.
2. Measure the child's head at least once a day.
3. Position the infant's head off the shunt site for the first 2 postoperative days.
4. Complete vital signs and neurological checks every 4 hours.

72. In preparing the patient and family for hospital discharge, which of the following signs and symptoms of shunt malfunction and infection should the nurse include in the teaching plan? **Select all that apply.**
1. Emesis, lethargy.
2. A change in neurological behavior.
3. Fever, irritability.
4. Diarrhea or constipation.
5. Redness along the shunt system.

73. The parents of an infant with hydrocephalus ask about future activities in which their child can participate in school and as an adolescent. The nurse should tell the parents which of the following is appropriate?
1. A helmet should be worn during any activity that could lead to head injury.
2. Only non-contact sports should be pursued, such as swimming or tennis.
3. Because of the risk of shunt system infection, swimming is not a sports option.
4. The child should wear a MedicAlert bracelet; then there is no need to be concerned about the shunt.

74. While assisting with a lumbar puncture procedure on an infant or small child, the nurse should do which of the following?
1. Have the patient in a clean diaper to avoid contamination of the site.
2. Monitor the patient's cardiorespiratory status at all times.
3. Position the patient in the prone position with the head to the left.
4. Start an intravenous line to facilitate use of conscious sedation.

75. A 10-month-old has fallen out of the high chair and is brought to the emergency department (ED). Place the following components of the nurse's assessment into order of priority.
1. Airway _____
2. Bleeding _____
3. Appetite _____
4. Breathing _____
5. Circulation _____
6. Level of consciousness _____

76. Which are associated with Guillain-Barré? **Select all that apply.**
1. Always fatal after 18 to 24 months.
2. Progresses cephalocaudally.
3. Complications are associated with immobility.
4. Respiratory support is a nursing priority.
5. Tube feedings or total parental nutrition may become necessary.

77. An adolescent is complaining of knees swelling and hurting, hands and feet being cold all the time, frequent headaches, and a red rash on the cheeks and nose. Which does the nurse suspect?
    1. Multiple sclerosis.
    2. Normal adolescent concerns.
    3. Myasthenia gravis.
    4. Systemic lupus erythematosus.

78. Which does the nurse include in discharge teaching for a 15-year-old with systemic lupus erythematosus? **Select all that apply.**
    1. High-protein diet.
    2. Low salt intake.
    3. Exposure to the sun.
    4. Killed-virus vaccines.
    5. Systemic corticosteroids.
    6. Antimalarials.

79. A 12-year-old cut a hand while climbing a barbed-wire fence. What should the nurse discuss with the parents regarding need for tetanus vaccine? **Select all that apply.**
    1. No tetanus vaccine is necessary; it is too soon since the child's scheduled Tdap was given.
    2. Tetanus is a potentially fatal disease.
    3. Puncture wounds are less susceptible to tetanus.
    4. There will be mild soreness at the injection site.
    5. Tdap should be administered.
    6. Td should be administered.

80. A parent calls the nurse for dosing information for Pepto-Bismol and aspirin for children who are 8 and 9 years old and are ill. Which does the nurse advise? **Select all that apply.**
    1. 15 mL of Pepto-Bismol after every diarrhea stool.
    2. 81 mg baby aspirin every 4 hours.
    3. No medications are necessary.
    4. Pepto-Bismol contains aspirin.
    5. Diet as tolerated.
    6. Reye syndrome is associated with aspirin use.

81. Which is/are the most common, nonlethal complication(s) occurring from meningitis?
    1. Cranial nerve deficits.
    2. Epilepsy.
    3. Bleeding intracranially.
    4. Cerebral palsy.

82. Which should the nurse teach the parent of a child with suspected meningitis?
    1. Antibiotics are not initiated until the cerebrospinal fluid cultures are definitive for specificity to prevent resistance.
    2. Antibiotics are useless against viral infections, so they are not used for meningitis.
    3. Antibiotics should be started before the cerebrospinal fluid cultures are definitive; culture results may take up to 3 days.
    4. Antibiotic initiation is based on the age, signs, and symptoms of the child, not on the causative agent.

83. During the nurse's assessment, a child begins to have a generalized tonic-clonic seizure. The drug of choice and method of administration the nurse expects the health-care provider (HCP) to order are which of the following?
    1. Lorazepam and diazepam, combined in an intravenous solution of D₅W.
    2. Lorazepam given intravenously or diazepam given directly into a vein.
    3. Phenobarbital administered in an intravenous solution of D₅W, 0.45 normal saline.
    4. Phenytoin in a dextrose solution given intravenously over 1 hour.

84. Parents of a child with generalized seizures ask the nurse for information to give their child's teachers. Which of the following should be included?
    1. A soft-padded spoon should be kept nearby to put between the child's teeth at the onset of a seizure.
    2. Roll the child onto the abdomen, with the head to the left, so any contents can flow from the mouth.
    3. If a seizure lasts longer than 5 minutes, an ambulance should be called.
    4. As the child grows, medication dosages may need to be adjusted to control seizure activity.

85. Which best describes the type of seizure displayed in the accompanying figure?
    1. Tonic-clonic.
    2. Absence.
    3. Atonic.
    4. Akinetic.
    5. Myoclonic.
    6. Infantile spasm.

86. Which best describes the type of seizure displayed in the accompanying figure?
    1. Infantile spasm.
    2. Febrile seizure.
    3. Simple partial seizure with motor signs.
    4. Simple partial seizure with sensory signs.
    5. Atonic partial seizure.

87. A 14-year-old sustained a grade III concussion while playing football. Which statement made by the parents indicates that further education is needed?
    1. "Our child will not be able to play football until recovery is complete."
    2. "Our child needs to get back to school quickly because there are midterms next week."
    3. "Our child's headaches may continue for the next 6 months; we should call the physician if the headaches get worse."
    4. "If our child suffers another concussion before recovery is complete, brain injury will be compounded."

88. The nurse is doing discharge teaching for a 3-month-old with a new shunt placed for hydrocephalus. Which are signs and symptoms of hydrocephalus that the parents may see if the shunt malfunctions? **Select all that apply.**
    1. Vomiting.
    2. Irritability.
    3. Poor feeding.
    4. Headache.
    5. Sunken fontanel.
    6. Seizures.
    7. Inability to wake up infant.
    8. Hyperactivity.

89. When introducing solid foods into an infant's diet, it is important to introduce one food at a time in order to rule out _____.

90. The injection site of choice for a 6-month-old receiving immunizations is the _____.

91. Infants should ride in a _____ car seat until 2 years of age.

92. According to Piaget, the school-age child is in the _____ stage of cognitive development.

93. According to Freud, the most significant achievement of toddlers is
_____.

94. Seizures that originate in one hemisphere are called _____.

95. The term _____ is commonly defined as stiffness of the neck.

96. Which applies to brain tumors? **Select all that apply.**
    1. Brain tumors are the most common malignancy in the United States.
    2. Although an exact cause is unknown, an association has been linked to paints and radiation.
    3. All children with brain tumors present with very similar manifestations.
    4. Brain tumors in children usually occur below the cerebellum.
    5. Symptoms of brain tumors always appear rapidly.

97. Which applies to cerebral palsy? **Select all that apply.**
    1. It is the most common chronic disorder of childhood.
    2. Hyperbilirubinemia increases the risk of cerebral palsy.
    3. It is a progressive chronic disorder.
    4. Most children do not experience any learning disabilities.
    5. There is a familial tendency seen in children with cerebral palsy.

98. Which applies to encephalitis? **Select all that apply.**
    1. Usually caused by a bacterial infection.
    2. A chronic disease.
    3. Most commonly seen after a varicella infection in the newborn population.
    4. Newborns diagnosed with encephalitis often have extensive neurological problems.
    5. Can be seen with meningitis.

99. Which approach gives the most support to parents grieving over a terminally ill newborn?
    1. State, "You are both still young and will be able to have more children."
    2. Avoid the parents; let them ask you questions.
    3. Offer rationalizations for the child's terminal illness.
    4. State, "You are still feeling all the pain of your child's illness."

The correct answer number and rationale for why it is the correct answer are given in **boldface blue type.** Rationales for why the other possible answer options are incorrect also are given, but they are not in boldface type.

1. 1. Newborns may not void spontaneously in the first 12 hours of life, but they void within the first 24 hours of life.
   2. Most, but not all, babies lose approximately 10% of their body weight in the first 3 to 4 days of life.
   3. **Breastfed infants should regain their birth weight by the 14th day of life.**
   4. Many babies do not initially awaken spontaneously for nursing; initially, the mother may need to offer the baby the breast every 2 to 3 hours.

   TEST-TAKING HINT: Breastfed infants usually start to gain weight once their mother's milk comes in at about day 3 or 4 of life. Be aware of words such as "all" or "never" because in health care very few things are "all" or "never."

2. 7.5.
   Change 3400 g to kg, and then multiply by 2.2 lb/kg. Divide 3400 g by 1000 g/kg = 3.4 kg. Multiply 3.4 kg by 2.2 lb/kg = 7.48 lb. Round up to 7.5 lb.

   TEST-TAKING HINT: The test taker must know the correct formulas and equivalencies to use.

3. 1. Hypotonia is of concern because a floppy, limp infant may have suffered a birth insult or has a genetic condition such as Down syndrome.
   2. Babies have a symmetric appearance and do not develop hand preference (asymmetry) until 18 to 24 months.
   3. A full-term, healthy newborn initially has a flexed posture because it has been curled up in the uterus.
   4. **A full-term, healthy newborn initially has a flexed posture because it has been curled up in the uterus.**

   TEST-TAKING HINT: The nurse should expect to see an infant who has tone and strength, although not in its fully developed state.

4. 1. The Landau reflex occurs when the infant is suspended prone; the infant will raise the head and extend the trunk upward.

2. Clonus is elicited by a brisk dorsiflexion of the foot that elicits oscillating movements of the ankles and knees.
   3. This reflex is the asymmetric tonic neck. When an infant's head turns to one side, the arm and leg on the same side extend, and the opposite arm and leg flex.
   4. **The Moro reflex is another name for the startle reflex.**

   TEST-TAKING HINT: The asymmetric tonic neck reflex is a specific posture that is assumed by the newborn when the head is turned or moved quickly.

5. 1. Newborn screening tests screen for a large number of congenital diseases.
   2. **It screens for some inherited and congenital conditions after birth.**
   3. Individual states determine which diseases are screened for, not the parents.
   4. Insurance companies do not determine which newborn screening tests are conducted.

   TEST-TAKING HINT: The parents want to know the purpose of the test.

6. 1, 2, 4, 5.
   1. **Learn as much as possible about the child.**
   2. **Expect to have some conflict with cultural differences and age.**
   3. Children who are adopted when they are older than 2 years of age know their biological families and have feelings about their adoption. It is best to discuss this openly with the child.
   4. **Setting clear behavioral expectations for the child will aid in the assimilation into the family.**
   5. **It is always good to retain some part of the child's original name, such as a middle name, to maintain the link with the previous family and culture.**

   TEST-TAKING HINT: When children are adopted at an older age, they have memories of their previous family, and these will need to be incorporated into rearing the child.

7. 2, 3, 5.
   1. Young children who are experiencing a divorce have poor self-esteem and blame themselves for the separation.
   2. **They exhibit loss of appetite and poor sleep patterns.**

3. **Preschool and young school-age children feel the parent who is leaving the family is abandoning them. They also develop increased anxiety.**
4. Older rather than young school-age children may become dictatorial and aggressive and show a decline in school performance.
5. **The 5-year-old can verbalize feelings about divorce and the changes that are going to take place within the family.**

TEST-TAKING HINT: The young school-age child is in the Piaget stage of ego formation.

8. **2, 3, 6.**
   1. Larger day care facilities do not necessarily have qualified staff and age-appropriate activities for the child or infant.
   2. **In choosing a day care, it is important for parents to see that the health and safety requirements of the law are maintained.**
   3. **Each child gets the attention that is required for maintaining a healthy, happy child. Caretakers should be loving and supportive of the children and parents.**
   4. Activities should be age-appropriate for the child.
   5. Child-care ratios, as well as class size, should be small, and staff should not feel they have more work to do than they can manage.
   6. **Child-care ratios, as well as class size, should be small, and staff should not feel they have more work to do than they can manage.**

TEST-TAKING HINT: The infant is only 6 months old.

9. **1, C; 2, E; 3, F; 4, A; 5, D; 6, B.**

TEST-TAKING HINT: First match the word with the definition you know, then look for matches that are less familiar.

10. **3, 5.**
    1. Cleft lip and palate occur in many syndromes such as trisomy 13 and VATER, but they are not associated with Turner syndrome.
    2. A weak, high-pitched cry is seen in babies with cri du chat syndrome.
    3. **A low-set posterior hairline, webbing of the neck, and lymphedema of the hands and feet are characteristic of Turner syndrome.**
    4. Small genitalia and long, thin arms and legs are seen with Klinefelter syndrome; this is seen only in males.
    5. **Coarctation of the aorta or bicuspid atrial valve pose the most serious risks for children with Turner syndrome.**

TEST-TAKING HINT: Turner syndrome is a sex chromosome anomaly that is missing one complete X chromosome. It is the only known monosomy defect that produces a viable fetus.

11. 1. The triple marker screen, amniocentesis, and chorionic villus sampling require either a venipuncture or uterine puncture.
    2. **The ultrasound is appropriate for a noninvasive procedure. It would detect multiple gestations and structural abnormalities, but it would not detect biochemical abnormalities.**
    3. The triple marker screen, amniocentesis, and chorionic villus sampling require either a venipuncture or uterine puncture.
    4. The triple marker screen, amniocentesis, and chorionic villus sampling require either a venipuncture or uterine puncture.

TEST-TAKING HINT: The only test that does not require a blood sample is the ultrasound. Biochemical testing, however, should be encouraged because it will provide valuable information about the pregnancy.

12. 1. **In a probability equation, each pregnancy is an independent event.**
    2. The probability of having a child with cystic fibrosis is 1 chance in 4, whether the first or the fourth baby.
    3. The probability of having a child with cystic fibrosis is 1 chance in 4, whether the first or the fourth baby.
    4. The probability of a miscarriage does not increase with this pregnancy.

TEST-TAKING HINT: "Probability" is a risk assessment term and denotes that a risk is present for the family.

13. 1. It is appropriate to develop a pedigree once the provider has discussed this issue with the patient.
    2. It is appropriate to take a family history once the provider has discussed this issue with the patient.
    3. **Working as a team with the provider and sharing this information enables the provider to make appropriate decisions.**
    4. It is appropriate to make a referral for genetic counseling once the provider has discussed this issue with the patient.

TEST-TAKING HINT: The young woman is questioning whether mental retardation can be inherited. The provider will need to discuss what her understanding of that concept is.

14. 1. Some Jewish sects, not Jehovah's Witnesses, believe in numerous dietary kosher laws that they must follow.
2. Muslims, not Jehovah's Witnesses, believe that Allah cures but sometimes works through humans to provide treatment.
3. Catholics, not Jehovah's Witnesses, encourage anointing of the sick.
4. **Jehovah's Witnesses are opposed to transfusions, and many are opposed to albumin, globulin, and factor replacement. Generally, they are not opposed to non-blood plasma expanders.**

TEST-TAKING HINT: The child's complete blood count is low, and the child will require blood or a blood volume expander.

15. 1. People tend to "do other things" while talking. The family does not hear well, so this will be inappropriate.
2. **When communicating with parents who are hearing-impaired, maintain good eye contact and allow them to read lips.**
3. It is best to talk in short but concrete ideas. For teaching complex material, drawings and charts should be used. Enunciate clearly and talk slowly.
4. The visit requires that the family be able to understand what is being said by the provider. A trained hearing dog is not part of this priority.

TEST-TAKING HINT: The parents are deaf. Scheduling an interpreter for the hearing-impaired will benefit the family in understanding the entire message. In helping the family benefit from the visit, also utilize the senses of sight, touch, and smell to communicate.

16. 1. The term "legally blind" means a person has a central visual acuity of 20/200 or less in the better eye using corrective lens.
2. This statement asks the teenager to tell if there is enough vision to read books, which may not be the case.
3. **Having the teenager explain what can be seen will assist in learning the teen's visual capabilities. Asking the teenager to explain initiates rapport and builds trust.**
4. This statement asks the teenager to tell you if there is enough vision to read books, which may not be the case.

TEST-TAKING HINT: This is a teenager with a chronic disability; therapeutic communication is always appropriate to use in interactions.

17. 1. Although washing the child's hands needs to occur, this is not the first priority.
2. Many eye injuries require immediate care with follow-up by an ophthalmologist.
3. Irrigating the eye, unless there is a chemical injury, may further irritate the eye problem. With chemical injuries, time is of the essence in diluting the chemical. This injury is stated to be a foreign body.
4. **Examine the eye and check for a foreign body before attempting to treat the injury or determining the plan of action.**

TEST-TAKING HINT: The first step in the nursing process is to assess the problem.

18. 1. **Dysfluency is speech with abnormal rhythms, such as repetitions in sounds or words. A stutter is described as tense repetitions of sounds or complete blockages of sounds.**
2. Children who substitute or omit consonants have articulation errors.
3. A child who speaks in a monotone has a voice disorder. Hypernasal speech is prominent in children with palatal weakness and cleft palate repair.
4. Hypernasal speech is prominent in children with cleft repairs of the hard and soft palates.

TEST-TAKING HINT: The definition of "fluent speech" is understandable speech.

19. 1. It is important to discuss the findings that the parents have presented and not peripheral information that may or may not be necessary to their concern.
2. **Children with autistic-like features lack many social skills, such as seeking reciprocity and comfort from parents and maintaining eye contact when someone is speaking with them. They have an inability to develop peer relationships.**
3. It is important to discuss the findings that the parents have presented and not peripheral information that may or may not be necessary to their concern.
4. It is important to discuss the findings that the parents have presented and not peripheral information that may or may not be necessary to their concern.

TEST-TAKING HINT: Autism is a complex developmental disorder that presents with behavioral and intellectual deficits. Language acquisition is an indicator of cognitive development.

20. 1. **Post-concussion syndrome is a common finding in children who have suffered a head injury. Symptoms in the infant include pallor, sweating, irritability, and sleepiness. The symptoms begin within minutes to hours.**
2. Plethora and hyperthermia may indicate a number of problems, such as being overdressed, crying, and stress.
3. Crying with fear in an 8-month-old is an expected behavior at this time.
4. Babies have a positive Babinski reflex until they are walking, which means they have toe fanning; after that, it should be a negative finding.

TEST-TAKING HINT: Post-concussion syndrome is common in children younger than 1 year who have suffered a head injury.

21. 1. Babies who have failure to thrive can tolerate a cows' milk formula, but they need to have a diet modifier to increase calories, such as polycose powder or medium-chain triglycerides oil.
2. **The parent is describing symptoms of a cow's milk allergy and mentions there are many family members with allergies.**
3. Phenylketonuria is an inborn error of metabolism presenting with growth failure, failure to thrive, and frequent vomiting. The infants are placed on a low phenylalanine formula, such as Lofenalac.
4. Portagen formula is used to nourish babies with pancreatic insufficiency or intestinal resections. Frequently these children are diagnosed with cystic fibrosis and present with failure to thrive, steatorrhea, bulky stools, and abdominal pain.

TEST-TAKING HINT: Consider the symptoms and the history of allergies in other family members.

22. 1. This is an important vital sign to assess, but it is not specific to cutis marmorata.
2. This is an important vital sign to assess, but it is not specific to cutis marmorata.
3. This is an important vital sign to assess, but it is not specific to cutis marmorata.
4. **Cutis marmorata is transient mottling of the body when the infant is exposed to cold. It is important to check the baby's temperature. Cutis marmorata is a change in the color of the skin.**

TEST-TAKING HINT: This question involves a newborn with a somewhat common problem.

23. 1. Placing the infant supine will compromise the function of the unaffected lung.
2. **To optimize the baby's breathing, position the infant with the affected side down. In this way, the unaffected lung can expand fully. Infants are primarily thoracic breathers, so it is important to maximize use of the unaffected lung. The infant also has an Erb/brachial palsy, which further limits the function on the affected side.**
3. Placing the infant on the unaffected side will decrease the ability to expand the unaffected lung maximally and increase the work of breathing.
4. Placing the infant prone compromises the function of the unaffected lung.

TEST-TAKING HINT: A phrenic nerve paralysis results in diaphragmatic paralysis and paradoxical chest movements.

24. 1. The baby would not have a hepatitis B titer unless the mother was hepatitis B–positive.
2. **This baby has an ABO blood incompatibility, with the mother being O+ and the baby being A+. The total bilirubin is a value that combines the unconjugated and the conjugated bilirubin levels. The newborn would have an increase in the unconjugated bilirubin (lipid-soluble) as a result of the presence of antibodies to the mother's blood type.**
3. The complete blood count does not necessarily explain the jaundice.
4. The sedimentation rate indicates inflammation somewhere in the body.

TEST-TAKING HINT: The baby is 2 days old, the mother's blood is O+, and the baby's blood is A+. Mothers with O+ blood type have the antibodies to types A and B, regardless of whether they have had other children.

25. 1. The baby is already becoming increasingly jaundiced; if the bilirubin level is not controlled, there is the risk of kernicterus.
2. Lethargy is symptomatic of a number of risks that a newborn might encounter, such as sepsis, dehydration, and hypothermia.

3. The signs of a blood exchange transfusion reaction are focused on an unstable temperature. If the newborn becomes too cool, the infant could develop respiratory distress or bradycardia. If the baby's temperature becomes too high, there would be a dramatic change in blood pressure, with either hypertension or hypotension causing vascular collapse. If the baby becomes hyperthermic, the donor red blood cells could also be damaged, further increasing the jaundice.

4. Irritability would be symptomatic of a number of risks that a newborn might encounter, such as sepsis, dehydration, or hypothermia.

TEST-TAKING HINT: The question is asking for signs of a transfusion reaction in a newborn.

26. **250 mg.**
Convert the weight of 22 lb to kilograms. There are 2.2 lb per kilogram of body weight, so divide 22 lb by 2.2. The baby weighs 10 kg. By multiplying 10 kg by 25 mg/kg recommendation per day, the total intake of phenylalanine per day for this infant is 250 mg.

TEST-TAKING HINT: The test taker must know the correct formulas and equivalencies to use.

27. **1, 3, 4.**
    1. **Wrapping the foot in a warm washcloth increases the vasodilation and makes obtaining the sample easier.**
    2. Using EMLA cream on the heel before the stick has not been shown to decrease the pain response of the infant.
    3. **Swaddling appears very effective in decreasing neonatal pain.**
    4. **Non-nutritive sucking appears very effective in decreasing neonatal pain.**
    5. The baby will feel the pain whether asleep or awake.

TEST-TAKING HINT: The question is asking for nursing measures that will help decrease the pain with a heel stick.

28. 1. The Pain Assessment Tool would not likely be used on an inpatient unit other than a neonatal intensive care unit.
    2. The Neonatal Infant Pain Scale would not likely be used on an inpatient unit other than a neonatal intensive care unit.

3. The Premature Infant Pain Profile would not likely be used on an inpatient unit other than a neonatal intensive care unit.
4. **The acronym POPS stands for Post-Operative Pain Score.**

TEST-TAKING HINT: The test-taker needs to know about pain scales and when to use which one.

29. **1, 2, 3, 5.**
    1. **A polysomnogram can record heart rate and respirations.**
    2. **A polysomnogram can record brain waves.**
    3. **A polysomnogram can record eye movements and body movements.**
    4. Unless the child is being videotaped while asleep, the polysomnogram is not able to pick up cyanosis or plethora.
    5. **A polysomnogram can record end-tidal carbon dioxide.**

TEST-TAKING HINT: A polysomnogram is a complex diagnostic tool that records electrical and muscle movements.

30. **Cognitive.**
Piaget's late phase of sensorimotor development occurs between 12 and 24 months and is a time when cognitive development occurs rapidly. Reasoning skills are still very primitive. The main cognitive skill of early childhood is language acquisition.

TEST-TAKING HINT: Language acquisition is the main cognitive achievement of early childhood.

31. 1. Preoperational thought starts around 2 years of age and continues until late in the third year.
    2. Toddlers are self-centered but are curious and want to learn. They love to explore their environment and try new things.
    3. **Toddlers think in very broad terms; it is difficult for them to see that changing the bed will not change the entire process of sleeping. "Global organization" means that change in one part changes the whole process.**
    4. The toddler is globally afraid of changes but is not phobic about the bed.

TEST-TAKING HINT: Preoperational thought implies that the child does not think in logical patterns. "Global organization" means that changing one part and affecting the entire process.

32. 1, 2, 3, 5.
1. **Many children who have difficulty with temper tantrums are described by the family as "bad" or "difficult" in all aspects of their life. This description often carries over into all the activities and conversations that the family has with the child and degrades the positive aspects of the child's personality.**
2. **Tantrums are frequently associated with only one aspect of a child's life, and this should be identified quickly so that changes can be instituted in the approach to the problem.**
3. **Tantrums that result in harm to the child or to others should be dealt with quickly; professional help may be needed.**
4. The Internet is often a source of conflicting information, but families frequently seek help from it. Not all the information on the Internet is appropriate or correct.
5. **Discipline and inappropriate behavior management techniques may worsen the temper tantrums.**

TEST-TAKING HINT: Consider the child's age and what are appropriate and inappropriate behaviors for this age.

33. 3, 5.
1. It would be more appropriate for the parents to tell the child what "might" happen at the visit rather than say the visit will not hurt. Often, children perceive simple activities such as looking in the mouth or touching the skin as invasive and hurtful.
2. Telling the child that there are consequences for having fear of something new is inappropriate.
3. **Modeling appropriate behavior for the child by having the child go with a parent creates a positive preparation for visiting the dentist.**
4. Bribing a child to "be good" sets up a negative approach to teaching a child. The child will then want a treat for every visit to the dentist.
5. **The dentist will look in the child's mouth and count the teeth.**

TEST-TAKING HINT: The parents may be projecting their fear of the dentist on to the child.

34. 1, 2, 5.
1. **Hiding the bottle and offering a cup is a good way to start to wean a toddler.**
2. **Putting only drinking water in the bottle is a good way to start to wean a toddler.**

3. Nighttime bottles should be discontinued as soon as the child is able to drink fluids from the cup. Nighttime bottles allow the milk or formula to coat the teeth all night long, encouraging tooth decay.
4. Starting to use a pacifier with a toddler who should be weaned from the bottle by 11 to 12 months of age is inappropriate.
5. **Nighttime bottles should be discontinued as soon as the child is able to drink fluids from the cup. Nighttime bottles allow the milk or formula to coat the teeth all night long, encouraging tooth decay.**

TEST-TAKING HINT: Weaning should occur before the first birthday unless medically indicated. The bottle should be less appealing and less available to the child once the child is able to drink from a cup.

35. 2, 5.
1. The parents have indicated that neither one has the motivation or time to do the toilet-training.
2. **The child is 2 years old and may not be physically, emotionally, or psychologically ready to toilet-train.**
3. A toddler will say "no" to most questions; that does not make the child stubborn.
4. Having the child sit on the toilet for more than 2 or 3 minutes is inappropriate.
5. **One of the indicators for a child to be ready to train is if the toddler stays dry for 2 hours.**

TEST-TAKING HINT: Most children initiate toilet-training at 24 to 36 months on their own.

36. 2, 3, 4.
1. The safest place for a child to ride in a car is in the middle of the back seat.
2. **Legally, a child must weigh 60 lb and be 8 years old to ride in a seat belt without a booster.**
3. **The seat belt, whether in a booster or on a seat, should be worn low on the hips and not across the abdomen.**
4. **The shoulder strap, for safety purposes, should be across the chest and not across the face or neck.**
5. Tether straps help to secure the seat belt in position when using a car seat or booster seat and should not be optional.

TEST-TAKING HINT: The child's age and weight determine the seat belt/booster seat requirements.

37. 1. Fifth disease is caused by the parvovirus, and the rash is initially described as "slapped cheek," with this impression lasting 3 to 4 days.
2. Roseola is caused by herpesvirus type 6 and is usually seen in children from 6 months to 3 years of age.
3. Scarlet fever is a bacterial disease and has a rash that feels like sandpaper.
4. **The most likely diagnosis for this child is chickenpox, which is caused by the varicella zoster virus. This is seen in young children and is highly contagious to others in the classroom and at home. It initially presents with a high fever for 3 to 4 days.**

TEST-TAKING HINT: The pruritic nature of the rash and the distribution primarily on the trunk in clusters and patches give clues as to its cause.

38. **2, 4.**
1. Young children absorb most of the lead that enters their body.
2. **Homes built between 1900 and 1950 most likely contain lead-based paints.**
3. The acceptable blood level is 5.0 mcg/dL or less.
4. **Lead can affect any part of the body, but the brain, nervous system, kidneys, and blood are likely to be most affected.**
5. In Hispanic and Arabic cultures, some painted jars in which candy is stored are painted with lead paints. Some medicinals, such as azarcon, greta, payloon, surma, and lozeena, are sources of lead.

TEST-TAKING HINT: Low-income families are frequently at risk for lead exposure because they may live in older homes that are in disrepair. Often, families who have emigrated from other countries are unaware of risks such as lead toxicity in the community.

39. **95th/90th.**
The blood pressure table for boys aged 1 to 17 years is based on height for age. The vertical column represents the percentiles for a specific age. The horizontal columns represent the percentiles of blood pressure for a specific height. Locating the blood pressure percentile shows the systolic pressure to be in the 95th percentile and the diastolic pressure to be in the 90th percentile.

TEST-TAKING HINT: Find the 50th percentile vertical line for systolic pressure and follow it to age 9. Find the 50th percentile on the vertical line for diastolic pressure and follow it to age 9.

40. 1. **The American Academy of Pediatrics recommends a daily intake of 0.4 mg of folic acid daily for all women of childbearing age.**
2. Although eating fruits and vegetables is part of a healthy lifestyle, the young woman will not gain any additional folic acid in her diet through those foods.
3. Although eating breakfast is part of a healthy lifestyle, the young woman will not gain any additional folic acid in her diet.
4. The addition of folic acid at 0.4 mg daily to the diet will decrease the risk of having a baby with a neural tube defect by 50% to 70%.

TEST-TAKING HINT: The teen is looking for a suggestion for preventing neural tube defects.

41. **30.**
Change the height to inches. Locate the height of 65 inches on the vertical axis. Locate the weight of 180 lb on the horizontal axis on the same line as the height. Look up at the body mass index line at the top, and it indicates the BMI is 30. This classifies as obese.

TEST-TAKING HINT: Weight for a person's height is the determinate of a BMI.

42. **Appendix.**
The appendix is used to create the stoma between the bladder and the abdominal wall. The abdominal stoma allows the young woman to perform the clean intermittent catheterization comfortably with less dexterity required.

TEST-TAKING HINT: The family is looking for an alternate way to do clean intermittent catheterizations. The appendix is not a necessary piece of bowel, so it can be utilized easily for this procedure.

43. 1. Giving antihistamines and steroids before and after procedures will help to decrease the response to the exposure.
2. **The most important intervention for any person with latex allergy or sensitivity is to prevent contact with latex products.**
3. Once the radioallergosorbent test confirms that a person is allergic to latex, the test does not need to be repeated.

4. Using latex-free gloves is one way to decrease exposure to latex.

TEST-TAKING HINT: This is a known allergen in a child at risk for latex sensitivity or allergy.

44. 1. **Arnold-Chiari malformation is a herniation of the brainstem into the cervical spinal canal through the foramen magnum.**
2. Anencephaly is absence of the brain.
3. Tethering of the spinal cord occurs when the tissue surrounding the cord adheres to the underlying bony or tissue structure of the spinal canal.
4. Perinatal hemorrhage is one cause of hydrocephalus but is not a brain malformation.

TEST-TAKING HINT: Type 2 Arnold-Chiari malformation is frequently seen in infants and children with myelomeningocele.

45. 1. Diaper dermatitis should be assessed with the diaper change, but it is not specific to the risks of wearing a Pavlik harness.
2. Talipes equinovarus is congenital clubfeet and does not occur as a result of the harness.
3. **An infant wearing a Pavlik harness is at risk of leg shortening on the affected side and limited abduction. The straps on the harness may need adjustment and lengthening frequently.**
4. Pain of any kind warrants further assessment.

TEST-TAKING HINT: The child has hip dysplasia and is wearing a corrective (therapeutic) device, the Pavlik harness. It is important to check for problems or complications that are caused by the harness.

46. 1. Infants with clefts of the palate are at greater risk for ear infections once they are eating and sucking on a breast or bottle.
2. It is important to help the mother bond with the baby, but nursing or sucking on the bottle helps to create positive feelings between the baby and the mother.
3. The cleft palate is not repaired until the baby is closer to 9 to 15 months of age when speech begins.
4. **The primary goal of any newborn with a cleft palate is to establish feeding and sucking.**

TEST-TAKING HINT: Getting started with feeding and nursing is difficult for the newborn with a cleft palate.

47. **Gastroschisis.**
Gastroschisis is a herniation of the abdominal wall without a peritoneal sac and intestines outside the abdominal cavity.

TEST-TAKING HINT: The stem of the word, *gastroc-*, is "stomach," and *-schisis* is "a split." This is different from an omphalocele, which has the peritoneal sac present and intact.

48. 1. The National Advisory Committee on Immunizations is a subgroup of the U.S. Public Health Service. The American Medical Association makes recommendations on adult care.
2. **The two organizations in the United States that govern the recommendations on immunization practices are the Advisory Committee on Immunization Practices (ACIP) of the U.S. Public Health Service and the Committee on Infectious Diseases of the American Academy of Pediatrics.**
3. The National Immunization Program is a part of the U.S. Public Health Service. Pediatric Infectious Disease Committee makes recommendations on treatment of known infectious diseases in children.
4. Canada has its own advisory committee called the National Advisory Committee on Immunization under the Minister of the National Health and Welfare Department.

TEST-TAKING HINT: The U.S. Public Health Service is the umbrella organization for all national health issues. The American Academy of Pediatrics has been instrumental in combating infectious diseases in the United States and publishes the Red Book on recommendations for preventing and managing infectious diseases in children.

49. 1. EMLA cream does not decrease local reactions.
2. EMLA cream does not decrease local reactions, and changing the needle has not been shown to decrease local reactions.
3. **The vastus lateralis and the ventrogluteal muscles are recommended sites for a child of any age.**
4. Using distraction will minimize pain but not minimize local reactions.

TEST-TAKING HINT: The question is asking for a procedure that the nurse can perform to minimize local reactions.

50. 1. Mitral regurgitation is best heard between S_2 and the beginning of S_1. It is accentuated by exercise.

2. The S₂ sound is caused by the closure of the pulmonic and aortic valves. A fixed splitting of the S₂ sound is indicative of an atrial septal defect.

3. A functional murmur does not denote a cardiac defect but may indicate anemia or some other physiological abnormality.

4. The pericardial friction rub is a high-pitched grating sound that is indicative of pericarditis.

TEST-TAKING HINT: The S₁ sounds are caused by closure of the tricuspid and mitral valves. The question involves an S₂ sound and is indicative of closure of the semilunar valves.

51. **1, 3, 5.**
   1. **An innocent murmur does not have an anatomical or physiological abnormality; it is a sound of short duration, grade III or less, and is best heard in the pulmonic area of the chest (second intercostal space close to the sternum).**
   2. An S₂ murmur is considered pathological until proved otherwise.
   3. **An innocent murmur does not have an anatomical or physiological abnormality; it is a sound of short duration, grade III or less, and is best heard in the left pulmonic area of the chest (second intercostal space close to the sternum).**
   4. Murmurs that are innocent or functional vary in their intensity and the position in which they can be heard. Pathological murmurs are fixed and radiate throughout the chest.
   5. **An innocent murmur does not have an anatomical or physiological abnormality; it is a sound of short duration, grade III or less, and heard best in the pulmonic area of the chest (second intercostal space close to the sternum).**

TEST-TAKING HINT: This is an otherwise healthy child. The Erb point (second and third intercostal space, midclavicular area on the left) is a frequent site to locate innocent murmurs.

52. **Vocal fremitus.**
   The conduction of voice sounds through the chest and respiratory tract is called vocal fremitus. The decrease in fremitus indicates obstruction in the airways, as would occur with asthma or pneumothorax. The increase in fremitus occurs with pneumonia.

TEST-TAKING HINT: Fremitus is the conduction of voice sounds through the respiratory tract.

53. **1, 2, 3.**
   1. **The nurse should alert the parents to the fact that the child may have some blood-tinged secretions for a few days afterward.**
   2. **Using a cool mist vaporizer helps to decrease the viscosity of the secretions.**
   3. **Pain relief every 4 hours is indicated.**
   4. The child should not be eating foods that are rough or fibrous but rather should stay on a soft or liquid diet for a few days to allow healing.
   5. Blowing the nose and coughing are contraindicated because this may loosen the clot that has formed over the surgical site.

TEST-TAKING HINT: The care and comfort measures are those that enable the parents to relieve pain and have decreased stress and worry about the surgery.

54. **1, 3, 4.**
   1. **Most toddlers are weaned from the bottle at about 12 to 15 months. Children who continue to drink from a bottle while lying down have a higher incidence of colds and ear infections.**
   2. Giving the toddler a decongestant before bedtime is not recommended because the primary problem is obstruction of the eustachian tube due to intrinsic or extrinsic causes. Decongestants thicken and make passage of fluid out of the middle ear more difficult.
   3. **Smoking outside the house is recommended as a way to prevent exposure of secondhand smoke to children, but the smoke still clings to the parents' clothing and hands and continues to be a source of exposure.**
   4. **Smokers should change their shirts and wash hands before handling a child to help prevent exposure to smoke.**
   5. Following treatment for otitis media, it is important to have the child's hearing checked because drainage from the middle ear may persist beyond the days of treatment. It will not prevent recurrence of the otitis media.

TEST-TAKING HINT: The question is asking for a major preventive measure for otitis media.

55. 1. Laryngotracheobronchitis is seen in infants and young school-age children and is viral in origin with accompanying symptoms of brassy cough, low-grade fever, hoarseness, but otherwise well appearance.

2. Bacterial tracheitis is caused by *Staphylococcus* and is characterized by a croupy cough, purulent secretions, high fever, and a need for antibiotics.

3. Asthma is a chronic inflammatory disease of the airways. In susceptible children, inflammation causes cough, wheezing, and chest tightness.

4. **This is the history of a child with acute spasmodic laryngitis. Symptoms of inflammation are absent or mild. Some children are thought to be predisposed to this, with allergy or psychogenic factors as an underlying cause.**

TEST-TAKING HINT: The child is well during the day and asymptomatic for fever or loss of appetite.

56. 1. RespiGam is also a prophylactic for respiratory syncytial virus, but it is primarily an immunoglobulin G that provides neutralizing antibodies against subtypes A and B of the virus. It must be given intravenously monthly, which is more difficult in terms of administration.

2. Ribavirin is an antiviral agent and is given in a hospital for treatment of respiratory syncytial virus.

3. **The American Academy of Pediatrics recommends that infants born before 32 weeks' gestation and younger than 2 years who have chronic lung disease should receive palivizumab (Synagis) monthly as a prophylactic to prevent respiratory syncytial virus during the winter months.**

4. The pneumococcal vaccine could be given during these 5 months but would not protect the infant from respiratory syncytial virus.

TEST-TAKING HINT: The infant is premature, and the winter season is starting.

57. 1. Chlamydial pneumonia is a sexually transmitted disease that would not be expected unless sexual abuse had occurred.

2. **The chronic infectious illness for which this child is at risk is tuberculosis. The disease may present as asymptomatic or include fever, enlarged lymph nodes, anorexia, weight loss, night sweats, and, occasionally, hemoptysis. It is recommended that Mantoux skin tests be performed annually for at-risk populations such as the homeless, first generation immigrants, and residents of correctional facilities.**

3. Pertussis is an acute respiratory tract infection that lasts approximately 4 to 6 weeks.

4. Asthma is not contagious.

TEST-TAKING HINT: Tuberculosis is on the rise in homeless and immigrant populations, and the child is in both categories.

58. 1, 3, 4.
1. **The lice can be seen crawling about on the scalp.**

2. The nits can be described as "looking like dandruff," but it could also be dandruff or seborrhea that is seen.

3. **Nits can be seen, especially behind the ears, at the nape of the neck, and close to the hair shaft.**

4. **Often there are scratch marks and inflammatory papules as a result of the itching and scratching of the scalp.**

5. Head lice can be found in short and long hair and in coarse, curly hair.

TEST-TAKING HINT: Pediculosis capitis is common in classrooms. Because of the frequency, many schools require the nurse to see the louse walking on the scalp before exclusion from the classroom is permitted. Nits can be confused with dandruff, hair spray, and lint.

59. 1. Enuresis is bed-wetting, which can have an array of causes.

2. It is important to rule out sexual abuse before deciding on the attention deficit-hyperactivity disorder diagnosis. It is also important to have a health-care provider (HCP) do a complete physical examination and have both the teacher and the family complete behavioral checklists before making that diagnosis.

3. It is important to rule out a learning disability before deciding on the attention deficit-hyperactivity disorder diagnosis. It is also important to have a health-care provider (HCP) do a complete physical examination and have both the teacher and the family complete behavioral checklists before making that diagnosis.

4. **The most likely diagnosis is attention deficit-hyperactivity disorder because the child has the classic symptoms.**

TEST-TAKING HINT: Classic symptoms of attention deficit-hyperactivity disorder are impulsiveness (talking loudly), inattentiveness (difficulty organizing work), hyperactive-impulsive behavior (moodiness and being unable to finish assigned class work).

60. 1. **Extrapyramidal symptoms are motor neuron responses that go from the brain to the spinal cord and present as tics, jerkiness, incoordination, and loss of involuntary muscle control.**
2. The medication is given to control the inappropriate behaviors, such as aggressiveness. If the symptoms started with the medication, it would be important to report this to the provider.
3. The medication is given to control inappropriate behaviors, such as aggressiveness. If the symptoms started with the medication, it would be important to report this to the provider.
4. Thoughts of suicide would warrant further evaluation of the appropriate medication for treatment.

TEST-TAKING HINT: Pyramidal tracts control voluntary muscle movements, such as balance and walking. Extrapyramidal tracts are those that control involuntary motor movements, such as tics, twitches, and spasms.

61. **1, 5.**
1. **A Tanner stage II male (early puberty) shows signs of an enlarging penis and loosening of scrotal skin. Puberty occurs from age 9½ to 14 years for typical growing boys.**
2. Height spurts occur toward the end of mid-puberty.
3. Mid-puberty shows signs of breast enlargement (gynecomastia) due to elevated estrogen levels. This is temporary.
4. A deepening of the voice occurs with changes in the larynx toward the end of puberty.
5. **Enlarging scrotum and penis are characteristics of a Tanner II male.**

TEST-TAKING HINT: This is a Tanner stage II male.

62. **Anovulatory.**
Young women who have periods more frequently than every 21 days, after ruling out sexually transmitted diseases, are anovulatory. These young women have adequate estrogen levels but inadequate progesterone levels. Unopposed estrogen can place a young woman at risk for endometrial carcinoma.

TEST-TAKING HINT: The young woman is an athlete and has also lost weight.

63. 1. Using examples of short-term consequences, such as stained teeth, unpleasant odor, and stains on fingers, will emphasize the teens' most immediate needs of being accepted by their peers. These unpleasant effects may appear attractive.
2. Teens feel they are "invincible" and safe from harm.
3. **It is always best to focus on prevention of smoking and take a positive approach to how a teen might resist smoking. Peer support groups work well in redefining the teens' peer groups and give them tactics to use against smoking.**
4. Talking with parents is not always an option for a teen.

TEST-TAKING HINT: Teens are interested in becoming adults and are increasingly concerned about how their peer group sees them.

64. **3, 5.**
1. Skin testing is done by an allergist to help determine triggers for the asthma.
2. Taking PCO_2 levels would be helpful but would require the provider to order a blood gas.
3. A Biox level tells you what the oxygen concentration in the blood is, which aids in determining the treatment plan.
4. A metered dose inhaler is the device that is used to administer the medications.
5. **The Expert Panel recommends that peak flow monitoring be used in children with asthma to determine the severity of an exacerbation and to guide therapeutic decision making.**

TEST-TAKING HINT: The child has moderate asthma. The peak flowmeter is recommended for all children with moderate to severe asthma as a simple tool for offices and for patient home use.

65. **1, 3.**
1. **Leukotriene modifiers such as montelukast are given orally and are indicated for add-on to low-dose inhaled corticosteroids in moderate persistent asthma.**
2. The leukotriene modifiers should be given on a daily basis for effectiveness.
3. **The leukotriene modifiers are not to be used for acute asthma attacks.**
4. Although the parents should give up smoking for the sake of their child's asthma, it is not affected by the medication.

5. Chest physiotherapy is used for children who have cystic fibrosis. It can help with respiratory distress by loosening mucus in the lungs.

TEST-TAKING HINT: The child has moderate persistent asthma and is currently taking low-dose medications.

66. 1. **The ethical principle of double effect states that an action has good intentions and that a bad intention is permissible if the action itself is good or neutral, the good effect must not be produced by the bad effect, and there is a compelling reason to allow the bad effect to occur if the good effect is the primary reason for the action. The child may require doses of pain relievers higher than is considered safe in order to relieve the pain. If the child dies during this treatment, the overwhelming reason for the excess medication was to make the child comfortable and decrease the intense pain.**
2. Justice is the promotion of equity or fairness in every situation a nurse encounters, for example, fair allocation of resources, including appropriate staffing or mix of staff to all clients.
3. There is no principle of honesty. There is only acknowledgment of cultural differences in the dying process, honesty in dealing with the child and the family, and use of pain medication to relieve pain as indicated by the circumstances.
4. Beneficence is doing or active promotion of good, balancing the benefits and risks of harm, taking positive action to help others, a desire to do good.

TEST-TAKING HINT: The child is terminally ill and in great pain, and the nurse needs to treat the child's pain.

67. 1. The parents obviously want their son cared for in the best and safest manner possible.
2. The parents may not have other relatives who are able or willing to take care of the child.
3. **It is always best to ask the parents what plan of care has already been instituted.**
4. Many social service agencies have counselors who can assist parents with developing a specific plan and asking the right questions. Before offering this service it is important to ask if they already have a plan of care.

TEST-TAKING HINT: The parents are asking the nurse about a very personal decision. This is a very emotional issue and should be dealt with accordingly.

68. 1. All children with Down syndrome have mental retardation.
2. **Atlantoaxial instability is ligamentous laxity of the atlantoaxial joint. The symptoms of neck pain, torticollis, and loss of bowel and bladder control indicate that instability is already present. The purpose of the x-rays is to prevent symptoms by limiting activities if instability is present.**
3. Children with Down syndrome may have vision and hearing loss and should be screened before 2 years of age for both.
4. Children with Down syndrome attain puberty at the same age as do nondisabled children.

TEST-TAKING HINT: Children with Down syndrome have hypotonia, and the more active they become, the more they are at risk for displacement of the atlantoaxial joint.

69. 1. These are signs of increased intracranial pressure in an older child.
2. Confusion is not easily assessed in an infant.
3. These are signs of increased intracranial pressure in an older child.
4. **Previously undiagnosed, one of the first signs of hydrocephalus is a bulging fontanel, followed by irritability, poor feeding, and overall rapid head growth.**

TEST-TAKING HINT: The test taker should recognize that examination of fontanel and head circumference is a mainstay of the infant examination.

70. 1. No products that interfere with levels of consciousness are used so as not to confuse assessment.
2. The head of the crib is slightly elevated to help decrease intracranial pressure.
3. Infants with hydrocephalus are often irritable and do not sleep well.
4. **These may interfere with surgery and shunt placement.**

TEST-TAKING HINT: Answer 4 should be known by a nurse about any patient who is having surgery on the head.

71. 1. Dressings should be dry and free of drainage.
2. Once a shunt is determined to be functioning properly, head measurements are done at office visits.

3. Position the head on the side opposite the surgical site to prevent pressure on the shunt and valve. This provides better visibility to watch for signs of bleeding or infection.
4. Vital signs and neurological checks will be performed much more frequently, usually every 1 to 2 hours initially.

TEST-TAKING HINT: Knowing postoperative care, the test taker can eliminate answers 1 and 4.

72. **1, 2, 3, 5.**
    1. **Emesis and lethargy can be signs of increased intracranial pressure and may indicate an infectious process.**
    2. **A change in behavior can be a sign of increased intracranial pressure and can be a sign of shunt malfunction.**
    3. **Fever and irritability can be indications of a possible shunt infection.**
    4. Although diarrhea may be a sign of illness, it is usually not a shunt complication, nor is constipation.
    5. **Redness along the shunt system can be an indication of a possible infectious process.**

    TEST-TAKING HINT: The test taker should be able to identify signs of increased intracranial pressure and signs of infection.

73. 1. **The risk of shunt breakage or obstruction is extremely low.**
    2. There is no reason why athletics need be restricted. Recent studies have shown little evidence of shunt injury or malfunction with sport participation.
    3. The shunt is a sterile, closed system, without any external opening so there is no risk of infection from swimming.
    4. Even with the alert bracelet, close contacts should be aware to provide care if necessary.

    TEST-TAKING HINT: The test taker may assume a child with a shunt may be at higher risk of injury.

74. 1. Diapers are kept rolled down and out of the way during a lumbar puncture.
    2. **Airway, breathing, and circulation are always the priority during procedures.**
    3. Positioning the patient should facilitate the opening of the vertebral spaces, either by a lateral or sitting-type position.
    4. Conscious sedation is not utilized during a lumbar puncture.

    TEST-TAKING HINT: Cardiorespiratory status is always the priority in any procedure.

75. **1, 4, 5, 6, 2, 3.**
    1. **Always first priority to assess.**
    4. **Second aspect of ABC priority.**
    5. **Third aspect of ABC priority.**
    6. **Important after stabilization of the "ABC."**
    2. **Important but not first priority.**
    3. **Least important.**

    TEST-TAKING HINT: The test taker should always assess ABCs first.

76. **3, 4, 5.**
    1. Progressive but full recovery is possible, taking months to years.
    2. Neuromuscular progression is from feet to head.
    3. **Because of the progressive paralysis, immobility is a major concern.**
    4. **The respiratory tract muscles may become compromised with the progression.**
    5. **Adequate calorie intake is essential to prevent catabolism.**

    TEST-TAKING HINT: The test taker should be able to eliminate answer 1 because in nursing there are few absolutes. Just knowing that some sort of immobility is involved should lead the test taker to answers 3, 4, and 5.

77. 1. Multiple sclerosis appears initially as a neurological disorder.
    2. The offered signs and symptoms are not normal in any age-group.
    3. Myasthenia gravis is a neuromuscular disorder.
    4. **Butterfly rash, arthritic symptoms, Raynaud phenomenon (cold hands and feet), and headaches, when all are seen together, are indicative of systemic lupus erythematosus.**

    TEST-TAKING HINT: The test taker should know symptoms of all the involved diseases to determine which one it is.

78. **2, 4, 5, 6.**
    1. Low protein to keep BUN within normal range.
    2. **Low salt to help control blood pressure.**
    3. Worsens butterfly rash.
    4. **More susceptible to infections and a lowered immune response.**
    5. **Steroids are first-line treatment because of the anti-inflammatory effect.**
    6. **Antimalarials are used in mild SLE to control symptoms of arthritis, mouth ulcers, fever, and fatigue.**

TEST-TAKING HINT: Butterfly rash should be recognized as a sign of lupus erythematosus and that it will worsen with sun exposure.

79. **2, 5.**
    1. Required tetanus boosters are given at 5 years of age. If a "dirty" wound occurs before 10 years after the last dose, a booster is necessary.
    2. **Tetanus is a potentially fatal disease.**
    3. Puncture wounds are more susceptible to tetanus, especially in rural areas.
    4. This is a possible side effect of tetanus vaccine.
    5. **Because of the increase in incidence of pertussis in adolescents and adults, this is the vaccine of choice.**
    6. Td is no longer the vaccine of choice; DTaP is the vaccine used to help control the growing incidence of pertussis.

TEST-TAKING HINT: Pertussis outbreaks are occurring as immunity wanes, so there is a need to use diphtheria, pertussis, and tetanus for boosters.

80. **3, 4, 5, 6.**
    1. Pepto-Bismol contains bismuth subsalicylate, an aspirin component, and is contraindicated in children.
    2. Aspirin is contraindicated in children with viral symptoms because of the association with Reye syndrome.
    3. **Allow the body to rid itself of harmful agents. This is first-line advice.**
    4. **Pepto-Bismol contains bismuth subsalicylate, an aspirin component.**
    5. **This is first-line advice if there is no vomiting.**
    6. **Reye syndrome is associated with aspirin use and viral illness in children.**

TEST-TAKING HINT: Many people are unaware of the aspirin in Pepto-Bismol and the link to Reye syndrome.

81. 1. **If infection extends into the area of the cranial nerves, increased pressure may cause sensory deficits.**
    2. Although this is a possible complication, it is not the most common.
    3. Although there is often purpura and petechiae with meningitis, there is no intracranial bleeding.
    4. This condition is usually an injury incurred during the neonatal period.

TEST-TAKING HINT: The test taker should know about complications in children with bacterial meningitis. With meningitis there is an increase in intracranial pressure, which can put pressure on the cranial nerves.

82. 1. A delay in administering antibiotics can be fatal.
    2. Cerebrospinal fluid cultures may require up to 3 days to determine the causative agent.
    3. **Immediate antibiotic therapy is necessary to prevent death and avoid disabilities.**
    4. Antibiotic choice is based on the most likely causative agent for that particular age-group. If the culture indicates a resistant organism, the antibiotic can be changed.

TEST-TAKING HINT: The test taker may be tempted to choose answer 2 if the urgency of early treatment is not understood.

83. 1. Although these are the correct drugs, they are not administered simultaneously.
    2. **These continue to be the drugs of choice for in-hospital management of tonic-clonic activity. These are the recommended methods of administration; diazepam compromises intravenous tubing.**
    3. Phenobarbital is not the drug of choice for in-hospital management of tonic-clonic activity.
    4. Intravenous phenytoin is given by slow intravenous push. Dextrose causes phenytoin to precipitate.

TEST-TAKING HINT: The test taker needs to know emergency care of a child having tonic-clonic seizures.

84. 1. Trying to insert something into a seizing person's mouth can lead to injury.
    2. Anyone having a seizure should be rolled onto the side.
    3. **If a child has seizure activity at school, the parent should be called as soon as possible.**
    4. Growth spurts occur, and medications will need to be adjusted. Teachers should be made aware and notify a parent or guardian if they notice even mild seizure activity.

TEST-TAKING HINT: Answer 4 can be eliminated because the test taker should recognize the need for the nurse to know what to do during the child's seizure. Also, seizure activity lasting more than 5 minutes requires medical attention.

85. 1. **Tonic-clonic seizures consist of sustained, generalized stiffening of the muscles in symmetric, rhythmic contractions and relaxations of major muscle groups. Level of consciousness is impaired.**
2. Absence seizures are characterized by a blank stare and no muscle activity.
3. Atonic seizures are characterized by an abrupt loss of tone.
4. Akinetic seizure is also known as an atonic seizure.
5. Myoclonic seizures are characterized by sudden contractures of a muscle or muscle group.
6. Infantile spasms occur during the first year of life.

TEST-TAKING HINT: Answer 6 can be eliminated by the age of the child depicted.

86. 1. Infantile seizures occur during the first year of life.
2. Febrile seizures occur in young children, usually before 4 years.
3. **There is no change in the level of consciousness; motor symptoms are evident.**
4. No sensory involvement is depicted.
5. Atonic seizures are characterized by an abrupt loss of tone.
6. Absence seizures are characterized by a blank stare with no muscle activity.

TEST-TAKING HINT: Answers 1 and 2 can be eliminated by the age of the patient depicted.

87. 1. This statement indicates that the parents understand the potential severe consequences of receiving a second concussion while recovering from the first one. Football is a contact sport in which there is an increased risk of concussion. The child should not participate in contact sports until cleared by the physician.
2. **Short-term memory loss is a frequent side effect of concussions. Until effects of the concussion have subsided and the child is cleared by a physician, the child should not take school tests that often rely on short-term memory.**
3. Headaches can occur for up to 6 months after the initial impact. Headaches that continue to worsen, however, could be indicative of the development of other injuries.

4. This statement indicates that the parents understand the potential severe consequences of receiving a second concussion while recovering from the first one.

TEST-TAKING HINT: Because answers 1 and 4 have the same rationale, the choice is further limited to either answer 2 or 3.

88. 1, 2, 3, 6, 7.
1. **As the shunt malfunctions and cerebrospinal fluid builds up, the child will exhibit symptoms of increased intracranial pressure. Vomiting is one of the possible signs of increased intracranial pressure.**
2. **As the shunt malfunctions and cerebrospinal fluid builds up, the child will exhibit symptoms of increased intracranial pressure. Irritability and change in neurological status are two of the possible signs of increased intracranial pressure.**
3. **As the shunt malfunctions and cerebrospinal fluid builds up, the child will exhibit symptoms of increased intracranial pressure. Poor feeding is one of the possible signs of increased intracranial pressure.**
4. As the shunt malfunctions and cerebrospinal fluid builds up, the child will exhibit symptoms of increased intracranial pressure. Headache is very difficult to assess in an infant.
5. A sunken fontanel is a sign of dehydration. With increased intracranial pressure, the brain is edematous and expands in size. This would result in an enlarged rather than a sunken fontanel.
6. **As the shunt malfunctions and cerebrospinal fluid builds up, the child will exhibit symptoms of increased intracranial pressure. Seizure is one possible sign of increased intracranial pressure.**
7. **As the shunt malfunctions and cerebrospinal fluid builds up, the child will exhibit symptoms of increased intracranial pressure. A declining neurological status evidenced by the inability to wake a child up is one of the possible signs of increased intracranial pressure.**
8. A declining neurological status is a sign of increased intracranial pressure. Hyperactivity is not a sign of a declining neurological status.

TEST-TAKING HINT: The test taker needs to know signs of increased intracranial pressure in an infant.

89. **Allergies.**
Infants should be introduced to solid foods after 6 months of age. Iron-fortified infant cereals are recommended first, followed by the introduction of vegetables, then fruits. New foods should be introduced about every 3 to 5 days so the caregiver has the opportunity to identify any food allergies the baby may have.

TEST-TAKING HINT: The question requires knowledge of the nutritional needs of an infant as well as the safety concerns that involve children of this age.

90. **Vastus lateralis.**
The vastus lateralis muscle can be used for immunizations of children of all ages. It is a particularly good choice for infants because it is the most developed muscle for this age-group. This area is also appealing because it has few major nerves and blood vessels.

TEST-TAKING HINT: The test taker must have knowledge of intramuscular injection sites and acceptable volumes for children of varying ages.

91. **Rear-facing.**
An infant should always ride in a rear-facing car seat until 2 years of age.

TEST-TAKING HINT: The question requires knowledge of infant safety.

92. **Concrete operations.**
During the concrete operations stage of cognitive development, the school-age child is able to take into account another person's point of view. School-age children are also able to classify, sort, and organize facts in order to use them for problem-solving.

TEST-TAKING HINT: The question requires knowledge of Piaget's stages of cognitive development.

93. **Toilet-training.**
Freud believed that during the anal-urethral stage of psychosexual development, a child must achieve toilet-training. Freud believed that children may have long-lasting difficulties if they do not master toilet-training.

TEST-TAKING HINT: The question requires knowledge of Freud's stages of development.

94. **Partial or focal seizures.**
Seizures originating in both hemispheres are called generalized seizures.

TEST-TAKING HINT: The question requires knowledge of names of different seizure types.

95. **Nuchal rigidity.**
Nuchal rigidity is assessed when a child has a fever or appears septic.

TEST-TAKING HINT: The test taker needs to know how a health-care provider commonly assesses for meningitis.

96. **2, 4.**
1. Brain tumors are the most common solid tumor. Leukemia is the most common malignancy in the United States.
2. **Although an exact cause is unknown, an association has been linked to paints and radiation.**
3. The manifestations can vary, depending on where the tumor is located.
4. **Brain tumors in children usually occur below the cerebellum. Brain tumors in adults usually occur above the cerebellum.**
5. Symptoms of brain tumors can appear rapidly or slowly, depending on whether the tumor is fast- or slow-growing.

TEST-TAKING HINT: The test taker can eliminate answer 1 because brain tumors are not the most common malignancy in the United States.

97. **1, 2.**
1. **Cerebral palsy is the most common chronic disorder of childhood.**
2. **There is an increased risk of cerebral palsy in infants with hyperbilirubinemia.**
3. Cerebral palsy is a nonprogressive chronic disorder.
4. Approximately 75% of children with cerebral palsy experience learning disabilities.
5. There is no familial tendency seen in children with cerebral palsy.

TEST-TAKING HINT: The test taker needs to have a good knowledge of cerebral palsy.

98. **4, 5.**
1. Although it can be caused by a variety of organisms, encephalitis is usually a viral infection.
2. Encephalitis is an acute disease.
3. Encephalitis is most commonly seen after a herpes infection in the newborn population. It is often seen after a varicella infection in older children.

4. **Newborns diagnosed with encephalitis often have extensive neurological problems.**
5. **Encephalitis can be seen with meningitis.**

TEST-TAKING HINT: The test taker should be led to answers 4 and 5 by knowing that encephalitis is usually viral in origin.

99. 1. Support to grieving families varies with the needs of the family. General guidelines in support of grieving families are to deal openly with their feelings and accept the family's grief response. Do not avoid them and avoid judgmental or rationalizing statements. Focus on their feelings. Provide referral to self-help groups or professional help if appropriate.
    2. Support to grieving families varies with the needs of the family. General guidelines in support of grieving families are to deal openly with their feelings and accept the family's grief response. Do not avoid them and avoid judgmental or rationalizing statements. Focus on their feelings. Provide referral to self-help groups or professional help if appropriate.
    3. Support to grieving families varies with the needs of the family. General guidelines in support of grieving families are to deal openly with their feelings and accept the family's grief response. Do not avoid them and avoid judgmental or rationalizing statements. Focus on their feelings. Provide referral to self-help groups or professional help if appropriate.
    4. **Support to grieving families varies with the needs of the family. General guidelines in support of grieving families are to deal openly with their feelings and accept the family's grief response. Do not avoid them and avoid judgmental or rationalizing statements. Focus on their feelings. Provide referral to self-help groups or professional help if appropriate.**

TEST-TAKING HINT: The test taker should understand that answers 1, 2, and 3 are incorrect. General guidelines in support of grieving families are to deal openly with their feelings of grief, pain, guilt, anger, or loss. Stay with the family, either sitting quietly or talking, if they indicate a need to talk. Avoid offering rationalizations for the child's terminal illness.

Glossary of English Words Commonly Encountered on Nursing Examinations

Abnormality — defect, irregularity, anomaly, oddity

Absence — nonappearance, lack, nonattendance

Abundant — plentiful, rich, profuse

Accelerate — go faster, speed up, increase, hasten

Accumulate — build up, collect, gather

Accurate — precise, correct, exact

Achievement — accomplishment, success, reaching, attainment

Acknowledge — admit, recognize, accept, reply

Activate — start, turn on, stimulate

Adequate — sufficient, ample, plenty, enough

Angle — slant, approach, direction, point of view

Application — use, treatment, request, claim

Approximately — about, around, in the region of, more or less, roughly speaking

Arrange — position, place, organize, display

Associated — linked, related

Attention — notice, concentration, awareness, thought

Authority — power, right, influence, clout, expert

Avoid — keep away from, evade, let alone

Balanced — stable, neutral, steady, fair, impartial

Barrier — barricade, blockage, obstruction, obstacle

Best — most excellent, most important, greatest

Capable — able, competent, accomplished

Capacity — ability, capability, aptitude, role, power, size

Central — middle, mid, innermost, vital

Challenge — confront, dare, dispute, test, defy, face up to

Characteristic — trait, feature, attribute, quality, typical

Circular — round, spherical, globular

Collect — gather, assemble, amass, accumulate, bring together

Commitment — promise, vow, dedication, obligation, pledge, assurance

Commonly — usually, normally, frequently, generally, universally

Compare — contrast, evaluate, match up to, weigh or judge against

Compartment — section, part, cubicle, booth, stall

Complex — difficult, multifaceted, compound, multipart, intricate

Complexity — difficulty, intricacy, complication

Component — part, element, factor, section, constituent

Comprehensive — complete, inclusive, broad, thorough

Conceal — hide, cover up, obscure, mask, suppress, secrete

Conceptualize — to form an idea

Concern — worry, anxiety, fear, alarm, distress, unease, trepidation

Concisely — briefly, in a few words, succinctly

Conclude — make a judgment based on reason, finish

Confidence — self-assurance, certainty, poise, self-reliance

Congruent — matching, fitting, going together well

Consequence — result, effect, outcome, end result

Constituents — elements, component, parts that make up a whole

Contain — hold, enclose, surround, include, control, limit

Continual — repeated, constant, persistent, recurrent, frequent

Continuous — constant, incessant, nonstop, unremitting, permanent

Contribute — be a factor, add, give

Convene — assemble, call together, summon, organize, arrange

Convenience — expediency, handiness, ease

Coordinate — organize, direct, manage, bring together

Create — make, invent, establish, generate, produce, fashion, build, construct

Creative — imaginative, original, inspired, inventive, resourceful, productive, innovative

Critical — serious, grave, significant, dangerous, life threatening

Cue — signal, reminder, prompt, sign, indication

Curiosity — inquisitiveness, interest, nosiness, snooping

Damage — injure, harm, hurt, break, wound

Deduct — subtract, take away, remove, withhold

Deficient — lacking, wanting, underprovided, scarce, faulty

Defining — important, crucial, major, essential, significant, central

Defuse — resolve, calm, soothe, neutralize, rescue, mollify

Delay — hold up, wait, hinder, postpone, slow down, hesitate, linger

Demand — insist, claim, require, command, stipulate, ask

Describe — explain, tell, express, illustrate, depict, portray

Design — plan, invent, intend, aim, propose, devise

Desirable — wanted, pleasing, enviable, popular, sought after, attractive, advantageous

Detail — feature, aspect, element, factor, facet

Deteriorate — worsen, decline, weaken

Determine — decide, conclude, resolve, agree on

Dexterity — skillfulness, handiness, agility, deftness

Dignity — self-respect, self-esteem, decorum, formality, poise

Dimension — aspect, measurement

Diminish — reduce, lessen, weaken, detract, moderate

Discharge — release, dismiss, set free

Discontinue — stop, cease, halt, suspend, terminate, withdraw

Disorder — complaint, problem, confusion, chaos

Display — show, exhibit, demonstrate, present, put on view

Dispose — to get rid of, arrange, order, set out

Dissatisfaction — displeasure, discontent, unhappiness, disappointment

Distinguish — to separate and classify, recognize

Distract — divert, sidetrack, entertain

Distress — suffering, trouble, anguish, misery, agony, concern, sorrow

Distribute — deliver, spread out, hand out, issue, dispense

Disturbed — troubled, unstable, concerned, worried, distressed, anxious, uneasy

Diversional — serving to distract

Don — put on, dress oneself in

Dramatic — spectacular

Drape — cover, wrap, dress, swathe

Dysfunction — abnormal, impaired

Edge — perimeter, boundary, periphery, brink, border, rim

Effective — successful, useful, helpful, valuable

Efficient — not wasteful, effective, competent, resourceful, capable

Elasticity — stretch, spring, suppleness, flexibility

Eliminate — get rid of, eradicate, abolish, remove, purge

Embarrass — make uncomfortable, make self-conscious, humiliate, mortify

Emerge — appear, come, materialize, become known

Emphasize — call attention to, accentuate, stress, highlight

Ensure — make certain, guarantee

Environment — setting, surroundings, location, atmosphere, milieu, situation

Episode — event, incident, occurrence, experience

Essential — necessary, fundamental, vital, important, crucial, critical, indispensable

Etiology — assigned cause, origin

Exaggerate — overstate, inflate

Excel — to stand out, shine, surpass, outclass

Excessive — extreme, too much, unwarranted

Exertion — intense or prolonged physical effort

Exhibit — show signs of, reveal, display

Expand — get bigger, enlarge, spread out, increase, swell, inflate

Expect — wait for, anticipate, imagine

Expectation — hope, anticipation, belief, prospect, probability

Experience — knowledge, skill, occurrence, know-how

Expose — lay open, leave unprotected, allow to be seen, reveal, disclose, exhibit

External — outside, exterior, outer

Facilitate — make easy, make possible, help, assist

Factor — part, feature, reason, cause, think, issue

Focus — center, focal point, hub

Fragment — piece, portion, section, part, splinter, chip

Function — purpose, role, job, task

Furnish — supply, provide, give, deliver, equip

Further — additional, more, extra, added, supplementary

Generalize — to take a broad view, simplify, to make inferences from particulars

Generate — make, produce, create

Gentle — mild, calm, tender

Girth — circumference, bulk, weight

Highest — uppermost, maximum, peak, main

Hinder — hold back, delay, hamper, obstruct, impede

Humane — caring, kind, gentle, compassionate, benevolent, civilized

Ignore — pay no attention to, disregard, overlook, discount

Imbalance — unevenness, inequality, disparity

Immediate — insistent, urgent, direct

Impair — damage, harm, weaken

Implantation — to put in

Impotent — powerless, weak, incapable, ineffective, unable

Inadvertent — unintentional, chance, unplanned, accidental

Include — comprise, take in, contain

Indicate — point out, sign of, designate, specify, show

Ineffective — unproductive, unsuccessful, useless, vain, futile

Inevitable — predictable, to be expected, unavoidable, foreseeable

Influence — power, pressure, sway, manipulate, affect, effect

Initiate — start, begin, open, commence, instigate

Insert — put in, add, supplement, introduce

Inspect — look over, check, examine

Inspire — motivate, energize, encourage, enthuse

Institutionalize — to place in a facility for treatment

Integrate — put together, mix, add, combine, assimilate

Integrity — honesty

Interfere — get in the way, hinder, obstruct, impede, hamper

Interpret — explain the meaning of, to make understandable

Intervention — action, activity

Intolerance — bigotry, prejudice, narrow-mindedness

Involuntary — instinctive, reflex, unintentional, automatic, uncontrolled

Irreversible — permanent, irrevocable, irreparable, unalterable

Irritability — sensitivity to stimuli, fretful, quick excitability

Justify — explain in accordance with reason

Likely — probably, possible, expected

Liquefy — to change into or make more fluid

Logical — using reason

Longevity — long life

Lowest — inferior in rank

Maintain — continue, uphold, preserve, sustain, retain

Majority — the greater part of

Mention — talk about, refer to, state, cite, declare, point out

Minimal — least, smallest, nominal, negligible, token

Minimize — reduce, diminish, lessen, curtail, decrease to smallest possible

Mobilize — activate, organize, assemble, gather together, rally

Modify — change, adapt, adjust, revise, alter

Moist — slightly wet, damp

Multiple — many, numerous, several, various

Natural — normal, ordinary, unaffected

Negative — no, harmful, downbeat, pessimistic

Negotiate — bargain, talk, discuss, consult, cooperate, settle

Notice — become aware of, see, observe, discern, detect

Notify — inform, tell, alert, advise, warn, report

Nurture — care for, raise, rear, foster

Obsess — preoccupy, consume

Occupy — live in, inhabit, reside in, engage in

Occurrence — event, incident, happening

Odorous — scented, stinking, aromatic

Offensive — unpleasant, distasteful, nasty, disgusting

Opportunity — chance, prospect, break

Organize — put in order, arrange, sort out, categorize, classify

Origin — source, starting point, cause, beginning, derivation

Pace — speed

Parameter — limit, factor, limitation, issue

Participant — member, contributor, partaker, applicant

Perspective — viewpoint, view, perception

Position — place, location, point, spot, situation

Practice — do, carry out, perform, apply, follow

Precipitate — to cause to happen, to bring on, hasten, abrupt, sudden

Predetermine — fix or set beforehand

Predictable — expected, knowable

Preference — favorite, liking, first choice

Prepare — get ready, plan, make, train, arrange, organize

Prescribe — set down, stipulate, order, recommend, impose

Previous — earlier, prior, before, preceding

Primarily — first, above all, mainly, mostly, largely, principally, predominantly

Primary — first, main, basic, chief, most important, key, prime, major, crucial

Priority — main concern, giving first attention to, order of importance

Production — making, creation, construction, assembly

Profuse — a lot of, plentiful, copious, abundant, generous, prolific, bountiful

Prolong — extend, delay, put off, lengthen, draw out

Promote — encourage, support, endorse, sponsor

Proportion — ratio, amount, quantity, part of, percentage, section of

Provide — give, offer, supply, make available

Rationalize — explain, reason

Realistic — practical, sensible, reasonable

Receive — get, accept, take delivery of, obtain

Recognize — acknowledge, appreciate, identify, aware of

Recovery — healing, mending, improvement, recuperation, renewal

Reduce — decrease, lessen, ease, moderate, diminish

Reestablish — reinstate, restore, return, bring back

Regard — consider, look upon, relate to, respect

Regular — usual, normal, ordinary, standard, expected, conventional

Relative — comparative, family member

Relevance — importance of

Reluctant — unwilling, hesitant, disinclined, indisposed, adverse

Reminisce — to recall and review remembered experiences

Remove — take away, get rid of, eliminate, eradicate

Reposition — move, relocate, change position

Require — need, want, necessitate

Resist — oppose, defend against, keep from, refuse to go along with, defy

Resolution — decree, solution, decision, ruling, promise

Resolve — make up your mind, solve, determine, decide

Response — reply, answer, reaction, retort

Restore — reinstate, reestablish, bring back, return to, refurbish

Restrict — limit, confine, curb, control, contain, hold back, hamper

Retract — take back, draw in, withdraw, apologize

Reveal — make known, disclose, divulge, expose, tell, make public

Review — appraisal, reconsider, evaluation, assessment, examination, analysis

Ritual — custom, ceremony, formal procedure

Rotate — turn, go around, spin, swivel

Routine — usual, habit, custom, practice

Satisfaction — approval, fulfillment, pleasure, happiness

Satisfy — please, convince, fulfill, make happy, gratify

Secure — safe, protected, fixed firmly, sheltered, confident, obtain

Sequential — chronological, in order of occurrence

Significant — important, major, considerable, noteworthy, momentous

Slight — small, slim, minor, unimportant, insignificant, insult, snub

Source — basis, foundation, starting place, cause

Specific — exact, particular, detail, explicit, definite

Stable — steady, even, constant

Statistics — figures, data, information

Subtract — take away, deduct

Success — achievement, victory, accomplishment

Surround — enclose, encircle, contain

Suspect — think, believe, suppose, guess, deduce, infer, distrust, doubtful

Sustain — maintain, carry on, prolong, continue, nourish, suffer

Synonymous — same as, identical, equal, tantamount

Systemic — affecting the entire organism

Thorough — careful, detailed, methodical, systematic, meticulous, comprehensive, exhaustive

Tilt — tip, slant, slope, lean, angle, incline

Translucent — see-through, transparent, clear

Unique — one and only, sole, exclusive, distinctive

Universal — general, widespread, common, worldwide

Unoccupied — vacant, not busy, empty

Unrelated — unconnected, unlinked, distinct, dissimilar, irrelevant

Unresolved — unsettled, uncertain, unsolved, unclear, in doubt

Utilize — make use of, employ

Various — numerous, variety, range of, mixture of, assortment of

Verbalize — express, voice, speak, articulate

Verify — confirm, make sure, prove, attest to, validate, substantiate, corroborate, authenticate

Vigorous — forceful, strong, brisk, energetic

Volume — quantity, amount, size

Withdraw — remove, pull out, take out, extract

Index

Note: Page numbers followed by *f* refer to figures; page numbers followed by *t* refer to tables; page numbers followed by *b* refer to boxes; page numbers followed by *p* refer to procedures.

A